ACUPUNCTURE IN THE TREATMENT OF CHILDREN

Acupuncture in the Treatment of Children

Third Edition

Julian Scott and Teresa Barlow

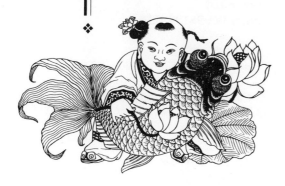

Eastland Press, Incorporated
P.O. Box 99749, Seattle, WA 98199 USA

Chinese Medicine Publications
22 Cromwell Road, Hove BN3 3EB England

Library of Congress Catalog Card Number: 98-74564
International Standard Book Number: 0-939616-30-0
Printed in the United States of America

2   4   6   8   10   9   7   5   3   1

Book design by Gary Niemeier

❖ Table of Contents

❖

❖ Foreword

Pediatrics has formed a specialized subject in Chinese medicine since the Song dynasty (960-1279). Chinese doctors recognized the differences between children and adults in diagnosis and treatment, and skillfully adapted their methods to the treatment of children. Their clinical experience is reported in many textbooks.

After 1949 the status of public health in China was horrific and China's new government had to deal with staggering social and economic problems. In particular, as always happens in times of crisis, children's health suffered immensely. The perinatal mortality rate was an astounding 200-300 per thousand, infanticide and child-selling were widespread, and there was an enormous legacy of infectious and parasitic diseases (smallpox, measles, diphtheria, scarlet fever, cholera, schistosomiasis, etc.)

China's new government dealt with these problems resolutely, and their achievements in the fields of public health and child welfare are too well known to be repeated here. Traditional Chinese medicine played an important role in the treatment and prevention of children's diseases. Many important textbooks on pediatrics were published after 1949, drawing on the experience of the old doctors and integrating it with present conditions.

None of these pediatric texts has ever been translated into English; indeed, some Western schools of acupuncture have gone so far as to say that children under seven should not be treated with acupuncture. This is a great waste of resources, since acupuncture is a safe and effective mode of treatment for many children's diseases.

Julian Scott has done an immensely valuable service for all of us who practice acupuncture in the West. Drawing from a variety of ancient and modern pediatric textbooks dating from the Ming dynasty to the present day, he has produced a very clear and useful textbook for the diagnosis and treatment of children with acupuncture. The experience of Chinese doctors is skillfully adapted to contemporary conditions in the West, and to the needs of Western children. Furthermore, Julian's own clinical experience adds to this traditional knowledge.

This book is a valuable contribution to the diffusion of traditional Chinese medicine in the West, and an important step in the process of adapting Chinese medicine to Western conditions, which is ultimately the crucial requirement for its survival and continued growth.

Giovanni Maciocia

❖

❖ Introduction

Introduction to the first edition

This book is intended for those who are already practicing acupuncture and have some familiarity with the theory and practice of traditional Chinese medicine. Many practitioners in the West advise against treating children, but in my (JPS) experience acupuncture is safe, effective, and gentle compared with most other available therapies.

I first used acupuncture on children when my own started on their childhood diseases, and since then I have had a special interest in the field. This interest led to the founding of a clinic for the treatment of children in Brighton in 1984. At the time of writing, the clinic is open only one day a week, so most of the patients come with chronic conditions. My experience in treating many acute disorders is correspondingly limited. Where my own experience is lacking, I have tried to substitute from Chinese doctors and Chinese texts; the book is thus something of a pastiche. In other circumstances I would have waited to build up a wealth of experience before writing a book, but present knowledge in the West about the treatment of children with acupuncture is scanty, and many children are going without treatment, or undergoing violent treatment unnecessarily. It is hoped that this book will encourage others to treat children and relieve this needless suffering.

Many people have helped me understand the treatment of children. I would especially like to thank Dr. Zhang Caiyun who taught me in Nanjing; Kate Diamantopolou for her support in the children's clinic; Paul Rausenberger who provided the impetus to carry out many of the translations; and Peter Deadman who has helped at all stages in the production.

Introduction to the second edition

A few years further on, and a little more experience, have given me the opportunity to fill out certain sections of the first edition. I have tried to explain in greater depth the differences between treating children and treating adults. For some of the illnesses described, I have found that the patterns given in the Chinese texts do not apply to Western children with different upbringing. I have rewritten these sections so that they will be more relevant. I am still lamentably short of experience with respect to acute febrile diseases, and these sections remain more or less unchanged.

Regarding style, the extra or miscellaneous (off-channel) points are identified first in *pinyin* followed by the widely used alphanumeric designation from *Acupuncture: A Comprehensive Text.*

At the end of the book I have included some case histories of patients from my practice, along with brief discussions. They are not a collection of my best cases, but have been chosen to show what is likely to happen when acupuncture works and when it does not.

Introduction to the third edition

In this third edition we explore a number of new topics, and review many of the old ones with fresh perspective.

We have tried to make the book more fun to read, avoiding (as best we could) those stilted expressions that seem to arise naturally in translations of Chinese medical texts. In its place we have substituted genuine English—the sort a patient can understand!

Next, we have described what actually happens in the Western clinic. How many treatments before you can expect results? What should you say when the patient complains? When must you insist on using needles, and when is moxa or massage enough?

We have also introduced patterns of disease that we see in the clinic, but which are not described in Chinese texts. One of these patterns, which we call hyperactive Spleen qi deficiency, arises from a combination of junk food, computer games, and lack of discipline—a combination that is not yet common in China. Throughout the book we have introduced new patterns of this sort, whenever we have experienced them. We have done our best to make it clear which information comes from China and which from our fertile imaginations.

Finally, this edition focuses more on our own experience at clinics in England and the United States. It is perhaps for this reason more than any other that we feel this book will be of benefit to all practitioners: it is based on the realities of the Western clinic. If we say that something works, it is because we have actually found it to work. It is an experience that we would like to share with others, so that you too may do your part in treating the countless children who need help.

Part One

Fundamentals

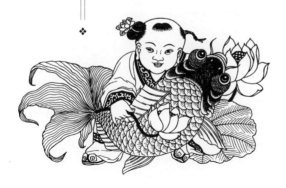

1 ❖ Differences Between Children and Adults

INTRODUCTION

Chinese medicine abounds in sayings or proverbs which sum up an important subject. In the English language, we have lost some of this richness of expression, although it used to be commonplace for people to say such things as "an apple a day keeps the doctor away" or "a stitch in time saves nine." Chinese medicine, however, has a saying or quotation for almost every situation. In this section we will summarize the medical differences between children and adults with these well-tried sayings, and then expand upon them to show what they mean in clinical practice. Most of the sayings are four or five characters long in Chinese, which is characteristic of the classical language used in traditional Chinese medicine. We have tried to preserve this flavor in translation.

小儿脾不足
xǐao ér pí bù zú

"Children's Spleen is often insufficient."

The Spleen governs the entire process of digestion, absorption of nutrients, and 'postnatal energy' (sometimes translated as 'acquired energy'). Before birth, children do not have to digest food they take all they need from their mothers. After birth, eating and absorbing food in order to grow is their main problem in life. This means that the Spleen has to work very hard. As a result, Spleen-related disorders are extremely common, so much so that one Chinese doctor has said, "Treatment of children is simple—all they suffer from is indigestion." In a similar vein, Dr. J. F. Shen has observed,"Children can only catch cold or have bad digestion."

Looking ahead to some of the problems described in later chapters, it can be said that one of the most common

3

digestive disturbances occurring in babies and toddlers is accumulation disorder *(jī)*, which is similar to the 'retention of food' disorder in adults. (The other most common pattern is Spleen qi deficiency.) This happens because a baby's digestive system is working so close to maximum capacity that it only needs a small extra stress to become overloaded.

小儿阴不足
xiǎo ér yīn bù zú

"Children's yin is often insufficient."

Children are extremely yang compared to adults—they are active, vigorous, always moving, and demanding attention. Because their yin is often insufficient, it is easy for them to come down with hot diseases (such as fevers) and convulsions. As a result, in China and other developing countries, yin deficiency is often seen in babies and children. It is rarely encountered among these age groups in the West, however, because febrile diseases are usually treated immediately with antibiotics. While it is true that such treatment may in turn give rise to other problems, it has the great advantage of avoiding the severe condition of yin deficiency, which is difficult to treat, especially with acupuncture. Perhaps for Western children another saying should be added: "children's yang is often insufficient." It seems to us that the hot patterns which were common in the West fifty years ago have now been replaced by cold patterns. Even illnesses such as otitis media are now frequently cold in origin.

脏腑娇弱
气易出道
zàng fǔ jiāo ruò,
qì yì chū dào

"Organs are fragile and soft, qi easily leaves its path."

This saying expresses the fact that because children are delicate, it is easy for external factors to disturb their qi. They can quickly become overheated in hot weather or catch a chill in cold weather. They are more susceptible to viruses than adults and are easily affected by changes in diet.

In babies we see another phenomenon during illness when the qi leaves its path: a wholesale breakdown in the production of qi. In Chinese this is described as a failure of the qi mechanism *(qì jī)*. It is seen especially in digestive disorders, which can cause a drastic reduction in a baby's energy and may give rise to any number of qi-deficient diseases.

发病容易
传变迅速
fā bìng róng yì,
chúan biàn xùn sù

"Children easily become ill, and their illnesses quickly become serious."

This saying follows from the previous one and expresses the fact that the rate at which illness progresses can be alarming. In febrile diseases the temperature can quickly shoot up; chest complaints can rapidly develop into pneumonia and threaten the child's life; and diarrhea can swiftly become severe and endanger life.

**脏腑清灵
易趋康复**
*zàng fǔ qīng líng,
yì qū kāng fú*

"Yin and yang organs are clear and spirited. They easily and quickly regain their health."

Although children's illnesses can quickly become serious, they can just as readily respond to all forms of treatment. Even when a disease appears to be hopeless, children can easily and rapidly recover.

We have talked so far in terms of physical disease, but this saying emphasizes the close link between health and the spirit. Thus, it is easy for children to be affected by the seven emotions. For example, they can suddenly fly into a rage and make themselves ill, or just as suddenly become overwhelmed by grief. They are, moreover, greatly influenced by the emotions of those around them, especially their parents. Any anxiety or irritation the parents feel is soon reflected in their children.

As we will see in the section on development, children under the age of seven have little awareness of their emotions, and even less control over them. It is this that makes children so susceptible to picking up the emotions of those around them. Many a mother has experienced this phenomenon, where her baby reflects her own emotional state, being happy when she is happy, and irritable when she is irritable.

肝常有余
gān cháng yǒu yú

"Liver often has illness."

This saying is usually understood to mean that it is easy for children to have convulsions. The term which we translate as 'illness' *(yú)* means surplus and refers to wind, as the Liver is the organ associated with that pathogenic influence. Even in the United Kingdom, up to five percent of children suffer from febrile convulsions at one time or another, despite the early use of modern medicines to reduce fever. In Chinese medicine convulsions are a manifestation of the stirring of Liver wind. Actually, many of the other Liver diseases that adults suffer from (e.g., stagnation of Liver qi or Liver invading the Stomach or Spleen) are rarely present in children. To read the Chinese books, one would get the impression that the only Liver disease children manifest is Liver wind, and that they never suffer from stagnation of Liver qi due to emotional constraint. This is not completely true in Western practice, where children are brought up differently, but it is generally true that children do not restrain their emotions nearly as much as adults.

By contrast, it is easy in children for food to become stagnant, leading to accumulation disorder or even childhood nutritional impairment. These disorders often have many symptoms similar to those of stagnant Liver qi, but are thought to be due to an entirely different cause, namely, the struggle to digest food.

It cannot be overstated that problems which look like Liver yang (with red face and tantrums, among other symptoms) are only rarely associated with a Liver pattern, but are usually related to accumulation disorder, which is to say, indigestion. Thus, in adults, stress and restrained emotions lead to anger and indigestion, while in children it is the indigestion that leads to anger and emotional outbursts. This has important implications when it comes to treatment, for accumulation disorder is a factor underlying a wide range of diseases from indigestion to asthma and eczema, to name but a few.

治母以治子
zhì mǔ yǐ zhì zǐ

"Treat the mother to treat the child."

During the first years of life a child receives energy from its parents (usually the mother) to supply any deficiency in time of illness. It is therefore normal for a mother to feel ill and exhausted when her child is ill. This is clearly seen in clinical practice, where it is not unknown for the mother to feel benefit from the treatment of her child even before her child does.

On the other hand, the energy that a mother supplies to her child will reflect the mother's imbalances: if the mother is ill, her baby will more easily become ill. When treating young children, one should therefore always consider the mother and child as a single unit, each dependent on the other.

Case History

A four-year-old child came to the clinic for treatment of asthma, always accompanied by his father. I determined that it would take about ten treatments, given once a week, to cure him. Treatment was going well until about the sixth or seventh visit, after which no progress was made. He was much better than when he first came, but still had a catarrhal cough. This 'steady state' continued for another ten treatments, when, by chance, the boy was brought by his mother. It was immediately clear that she had a severe lung problem (bronchiectasis in biomedicine; Liver invading the Lungs in Chinese medicine). She consented to treatment, and as her health improved, so did that of her son (see Case 7 in Chapter 47).

Childhood Development: Common Ages for Illnesses to Appear

There are certain common ages for illnesses to occur which are related to the stage of development of the child and to the particular problems the child is facing.

Six months

Underlying many problems at this age is the accumulation disorder, for it is around six months that the digestive system is under maximum stress. The baby is still growing very rapidly but has additional demands on its energy. More hours are spent awake, and there is more movement, with the child lifting itself up. With the commencement of weaning, the digestive system is adapting to new foods, and the child's first contact with infectious disease and immunization usually occurs at this time.

All of these stresses can easily overload the digestive system and lead to the development of accumulation disorder or Spleen qi deficiency. This, in turn, often leads to other disorders (e.g., asthma, eczema, diarrhea, or vomiting) and the practitioner will find that such illnesses will not respond to treatment until the digestion is cured.

Two years

At around two years children start to speak and become aware of their individuality as distinct entities. They begin to have desires of their own, other than the simple ones of eating and sleeping, and also begin to test their will against those around them. They start to want things for themselves. This phase is often described as the 'terrible twos'.

The diseases which accompany this transition are of the febrile type, which are an expression of the relationship between will power and Kidney yang. The more strong-willed and determined a child is, the more heat there is, and thus the more the child is prone to diseases of heat. It is not uncommon at this age for children to get a series of one- or two-day fevers throughout the year. These fevers should not be taken seriously. They can usually be distinguished from recurrent fevers associated with a lingering pathogenic factor by the extroverted character of the child and the absence of swollen glands in the neck.

Seven years

At around seven years children start to become aware of emotions as separate from themselves and begin trying to control these emotions. In fact, the years up to about the age of twelve are concerned with developing a constructive control over the emotions. These years are often the healthiest in a child's life, for it has left the childhood diseases behind and has not yet confronted those diseases associated with adulthood. The main problems that do occur in this period—like stress due to anxiety or over-work at school—are more characteristic of adults.

Puberty

The transition from childhood to adulthood is a difficult one in Western society. This is the best age for separation from the parents to begin, but in modern society this is often very difficult. The diseases that occur at this age are usually due to overwork at school or to emotional problems within or outside the family. It may be helpful for children to receive treatment once a month for about a year to help them through this transition. This is discussed at greater length in Chapter 43.

Differences Between Western and Oriental Children

One of my teachers said, "Your children are not taught to endure." Children are indeed the same the world over, but their upbringing varies in different countries. In the West there is very little in the way of discipline or boundaries. Children are not taught to endure pain, nor to sit still and keep quiet. This makes it much harder for the practitioner, whether acupuncturist or herbalist, for not only have the children not been taught to endure the small amount of pain from an acupuncture needle, but neither have their parents. This means that much time is spent persuading and cajoling the parents into having their children treated. It is very hard for many parents to see that the small amount of pain associated with a few treatments is insignificant compared to a lifetime of disease.

This is just one example of the many differences in the lives of Oriental and Western children. Other differences include a radically different diet, less exposure to television, lack of exercise, and a very different medical system. All of these will influence the development of disease. They explain why many of the disease patterns seen in China are not found in the West and vice versa. In this book we have tried to describe these different patterns and how to treat them.

❖

2 ❖ Causes of Disease in Children

INTRODUCTION

The question "What is the cause of disease?" has many answers, each of them correct and often complementary to the others. A doctor trained in Western biomedicine might look for an external cause such as a virus, while a homeopathic doctor might look for a hereditary miasma, and a Buddhist for a lesson not yet learned. A doctor of Chinese medicine would regard all of these as valid causes of disease and would consider it his or her task to decide which one was most important in a particular case.

In this section we will discuss some common causes of disease as they present in our children's clinic. It is thus based primarily on experience rather than on Chinese textbooks. In my experience treating both adults and children I have found that if a cause of a particular disorder can be identified, then the proper treatment can be provided and the prognosis determined with more certainty.

The treatment of asthma will serve as an example. One very common cause of asthma is the accumulated effect of recurrent lung infections, while another cause is the reflection in the child of strained relations between the parents. The treatment, prognosis, and advice to parents would be very different in the two cases. There is an appropriate saying in Chinese medicine, "Treat diseases of the Heart with Heart medicine." 'Diseases of the Heart' is usually taken to mean those illnesses associated with emotions such as unhappiness, and 'Heart medicine' is taken to mean warmth and love.

External Pathogenic Factors

Diseases associated with the six external pathogenic factors include many that would be classified as infectious, which, until the beginning of this century, were among the principal causes of illness and death in both children and adults. This situation has been radically changed in the developed world through better living standards, hygiene, and the invention of antibiotics. Nevertheless, the external pathogenic factors are still a very common cause of disease, even if they are now less feared. We will discuss them only briefly here because they are the same in adults as in children, the main difference being that children are more susceptible to them than are adults. Children also have more contact with infectious diseases in their play groups.

Wind

Wind is characterized by sudden onset and rapid progression of symptoms, and is often a primary cause of disease. It attacks the upper and outer parts of the body first and may then quickly penetrate to the interior. Since it attacks the exterior part of the body, it is met by the protective qi, resulting in symptoms which reflect disturbance in the circulation of protective qi, such as chills and fever. Wind disorders which remain at the exterior (or superficial) level are treated by the method of releasing or relieving the exterior, which usually involves causing the person to sweat. Wind readily combines with other pathogenic factors, especially cold, dampness, and heat.

Cold

Cold is a yin pathogenic factor and is contracting in nature. The contraction often causes severe, tight pain. For example, in influenza of the cold type there are often tight pains in the head, and in diarrhea of the cold type there may be contracting abdominal pains. Cold weather by itself is now a relatively uncommon cause of disease in children, but when it does occur, it may be treated by the method of expelling the cold. (The seven star needle, moxibustion, or cupping may be used for this purpose.) Cold commonly attacks in combination with wind, which drives it into the body. Wind-cold disorders of this type are treated by expelling the wind and warming the cold. One of the most common causes of cold in children is the consumption of ice-cold food and drinks, as well as cold energy foods and medicines.

Dryness

Dryness is a yang pathogenic factor that consumes yin. It most commonly affects the Lungs and is characterized by dryness of the skin, especially around the mouth, and by hard, dry coughs. It is most common during hot, dry summers and cold, dry winters, and amongst those who live in centrally-heated buildings. It is treated by moistening the Lungs.

Heat

Heat is a yang pathogenic factor characterized by fever and redness, and in children is more serious than cold. In children it is easy for any external pathogenic factor to transform into heat, and since their yin is insufficient, hot diseases can progress rapidly. Among other things, heat (without wind) can arise from exposure to heat in hot climates, remaining in the sun too long, accumulation disorder, and eating hot foods (see Appendix 2). When combined with wind as wind-heat, it can take a rapid course in children and requires prompt treatment. Heat disorders are usually treated by clearing the heat, for which acupuncture is especially effective.

Summerheat

Summerheat is a yang pathogenic factor characterized by sudden, extremely high fever with headache and frequently diarrhea. It is relatively uncommon in the temperate climate of Britain, but ironically can occur in winter when children go into overheated buildings. The most common manifestation is sunstroke, which rarely proceeds to the diarrhea stage, but which is dangerous if it does.

Dampness

Dampness is a yin pathogenic factor characterized by heaviness and by watery or sticky discharges. Children who live in seaside towns and damp houses are particularly susceptible. Dampness is usually treated by draining the dampness and tonifying the Spleen.

Lingering pathogenic factors

When an illness is left untreated, is checked by inappropriate treatment which prevents it from running its natural course, or is only partially treated, it may leave behind some trace of the original disease. For example, acute tonsillitis that is untreated, or treated with antibiotics, can lead to chronic tonsillitis where the tonsils are permanently swollen. These conditions are regarded in Chinese medicine as ones in which the pathogenic factor lingers *(yú)* or is not completely cleared from the body. In every clinic in which we have worked, this is the most common single cause of chronic disease.

For those trained in Western medicine this is a difficult concept to understand. The original disease has been cured, and yet it leaves behind an imbalance which is like a remnant or echo of the original disease. This stumbling block can be removed, however, if one forgets the idea of 'germs' causing disease and thinks instead of pathogenic factors. It is then easy to imagine an attenuated or weakened version of the pathogenic factor still lingering or hiding in the body.

This phenomenon also occurs in adults, and is behind such conditions as post-viral syndrome. When adults describe the sensations they feel, they say things like "I have not completely got rid of the disease," or "I still feel that there is some of the disease left."

Adults find it easier to throw out the pathogenic factor completely, as they can remember what it feels like to be healthy and know what measures are required to return to health. Babies and young children, however, have short memories and often cannot remember what it is like to be healthy; they do not know what they are aiming for.

This pattern is now so common that we have provided a more detailed description of the symptoms and treatments in Chapter 3.

Immunizations

Like lingering pathogenic factors, immunizations are such a common cause of disease in children that we have provided a fuller discussion of this subject in Chapter 19. The key to understanding their long-term effects resides within the pattern of lingering pathogenic factors.

Emotional Factors

As mentioned in the previous chapter, there is little discussion of children's emotions in traditional Chinese medical textbooks. Obviously, this is not because children do not have emotions, but because they usually do not restrain their emotions. This means that it is very rare to see in them the pattern of restraint of Liver qi. Indeed, if a child under seven years does restrain its emotions, it is generally not the child's problem, but a problem of the parents in not listening to the child's demands. However, if a child is living in a highly-charged emotional environment, for example, if the marriage is on the point of breaking up, these strong emotions will be reflected in the child. This is commonly seen in children with asthma and tonsillitis. Jealousy toward a sibling is also a common cause of problems (see Case 17 in Chapter 47). Another factor, which is rarely talked about and very difficult to detect, is sexual relations between one of the parents and the child. (A recent survey in the United Kingdom estimated that one child in five had been subjected to incest.) This can give rise to severe emotional disturbances on the mental level, and insomnia and urogenital disorders on the physical level.

Food

The main problem that children face in coming into the world is eating and digesting enough food to support growth. The primary ways through which food can cause illness are listed below. They almost always lead to accumulation disorder or Spleen qi deficiency, since it requires only a small disturbance to overload a child's delicate digestive system, which is working close to maximum capacity.

Too little food

It is uncommon in the developed world for a child not to have enough food, but this can be a cause of illness when the mother has insufficient breast milk or where the child shows little interest in food. It can also be a problem in older children when they are growing rapidly.

Too much food

One of the most common causes of diarrhea and digestive disturbances is overfeeding. It is a natural instinct for mothers to give their children as much food as they demand, but this instinct must at times be curbed.

Irregular feeding

There is a saying in Chinese medicine, "Irregular feeding injures the Spleen." Some babies and children are fed on demand with virtually no interval between feedings. Whenever a child shows the least agitation or discontent, he or she is offered the breast. Many mothers in the West find it very difficult to say no to their children, even if it means damaging their health. As a general rule, there should be an interval of at least two hours between feedings. If a child is constantly snacking (whether solid food or breast milk) this is likely to weaken the qi of the Stomach as well as the Spleen.

Unsuitable milk

Unsuitable milk means milk that the child has difficulty digesting. It includes cow's milk, prepared dried milk, and even the mother's own milk. The mother's milk can cause abdominal pain if she feeds the baby when she is very anxious or distressed. These emotions can cause the milk to be acidic or bitter. Similarly, if the mother has a history of gallbladder trouble, her milk may be indigestible and bitter. Cow's milk and prepared dried milk are sometimes too rich for newborn babies, and can cause colic or excessive phlegm. If this is suspected, goat's milk or soy milk should be tried.

Early weaning

The age when solid foods should be introduced into the diet varies enormously and may be as early as two months in a rapidly growing child, or as late as six months in a child with poor digestion. Unfortunately, there is commercial pressure from baby food manufacturers to give a varied diet from as early as two weeks. A child with a strong digestion can cope with this, but a weaker child may have difficulty.

Weaned on unsuitable foods

It is wrongly assumed by the mother that food which is good for her will also be good for the baby. This is not always the case. Common pitfalls include:

Whole foods—A baby's digestion is very delicate, and it is often difficult for it to digest rough whole foods such as brown rice or whole wheat bread. This can lead to the pattern of accumulation disorder. If possible, babies should be weaned first on more digestible foods, and only later given rougher foods. For parents determined to give their baby whole foods, millet is the best grain to start with.

Hot or cold energy foods—Some foods, such as bananas or yogurt, are regarded as having cold 'energy', while others, such as red meat and spices, are regarded as being hot (see Appendix 2). If the child is naturally of a cold disposition, cold foods may cause digestive distress; conversely, if the child is naturally hot, foods that are heating may cause further heat.

Physically cold foods—Many parents do not realize the damaging effect of eating food straight from the refrigerator, or continuously drinking ice-cold water. As a consequence, many children develop a cold and deficient Spleen from an early age.

Fruit juice—There is a growing trend to give children fruit juice rather than water when they are thirsty. There is no doubt that children love this (and it does keep them quiet), but it can lead to symptoms such as a sore mouth, poor digestion, poor appetite, diarrhea, and insomnia.

Food allergies

If a child is allergic to a food, even a small amount will cause some trouble. Common food allergies and their associated symptoms include the following:

- cow's milk: catarrh, abdominal pain, insomnia, eczema, violent behavior
- bananas: catarrh, abdominal pain
- gluten: in mild cases catarrh, irritability, depression; in severe cases diarrhea, malnutrition
- food additives: hyperactivity, irritability, restlessness
- citric acid: hyperactivity
- refined sugar: catarrh, lack of energy, listlessness

- peanuts and peanut butter: skin rash, sudden swelling of the tongue, anaphylactic shock
- tomatoes: asthma
- shellfish (crabs, mussels, etc.): irritability, insomnia, hyperactivity, vomiting, skin rash*

Food allergies are sometimes difficult to detect. Among the uncommon allergies we have seen are the following:

- chicken: eczema
- honey: asthma, diarrhea

Allergies seem to be on the rise. There are many possible reasons for this. One is the general degradation in the quality of food, with entirely new strains being genetically engineered for their high yield, with little thought to their digestibility. Another reason is the general weakening of the digestive system from the irregular and unsuitable foods listed above, and from the overuse of antibiotics.

Other Factors

Overstrain

This is not an easy cause to discover, because it is usually due to the parents' expectations of the child. Common situations where this occurs are the following:

- children who want to be top of the class. This is more common among girls than boys, whose ambitions are more likely to be leader of the pack on the playground, and may appear after about the age of seven.
- children of successful parents who want them to have many opportunities and take them from one activity to another in their spare time
- going to bed too late, often with excessive reading
- too much television, leading to an overstimulated mind and underexercised body
- the eldest child of a large family who has to take on much of the housekeeping work

Poor upbringing

The task of a parent is complicated, more so now than at any previous time. Families are scattered and have difficulty passing on the traditional ways of upbringing, while educationalists offer conflicting advice. Common ways in which poor upbringing can cause illness include the following:

- not enough fresh air and physical exercise, leading to tiredness and lack of stamina. As the urban environment

*Shellfish are thought to contain poisons which affect the nervous system and should be avoided by children and nursing mothers.

becomes more dangerous, parents are often unwilling to let their children walk to school or play outdoors. As a consequence, their bodies and muscles may become weak and soft.

- not enough sleep, leading to agitation and problems of yin deficiency
- overstimulation (especially television), leading to problems of yin deficiency. Television is especially pernicious because the stimulation of the programs is aggravated by the electromagnetic stress of being exposed to a rapidly changing, high-voltage electric field.
- insufficient discipline, leading to insecurity and restraint of Liver qi. Under the age of about seven, most children are happiest in environments where the boundaries and rules are clearly drawn. It was explained to me by one doctor that if a child is restricted or disciplined too much, it may readily suffer from uprising of Liver qi or even Liver yang. On the other hand, if the child is not given clear boundaries, as is often the case in the West, then the child has to make its own boundaries at an early age, and this can lead to restraint of Liver qi.
- overprotection, leading to asthma and problems of yang deficiency

Toxins

In Chinese medicine the term 'toxin' *(dú)* encompasses two causes of disease that we would regard as being rather separate, namely, toxins from poisonous plants and metals, and diseases such as measles, hepatitis, and encephalitis. Some toxins, such as lead and pesticides, should never have been introduced into the body in the first place and will inevitably cause serious damage. However, there is another class of toxin which naturally accumulates in the body during pregnancy. These toxins, although potentially harmful to the child, can be expelled during childhood rashes, such as measles and chicken pox. Although these diseases are potentially dangerous, for most children they are very beneficial. It is true that the external nature of childhood infectious diseases has been recognized in Chinese medicine in recent times, and prescriptions frequently include herbs that 'expel pathogenic wind', but one of the most important parts of the medicine has always been to expel or release toxins. (We return to this subject in later chapters.) Other common toxins and their effects include the following:

- contaminated foods: food poisoning
- food additives: hyperactivity, lethargy
- tobacco smoke: tonsillitis
- cavity wall insulation: asthma, catarrhal conditions, tonsillitis
- paint and gasoline fumes: headaches, sore throat

Heredity and birth

Many diseases run in families and can be passed on from generation to generation. The most common ones we have seen are asthma and eczema. While these are easy to recognize, there are others which are less acute and harder to discern. For example, many children have symptoms of chronic damp-heat with intermittent green discharge for which there is no apparent cause in their lives. This can often be traced to some similar problem in one of the parents. Similarly, a hereditary disposition to pulmonary tuberculosis is often found in children, with the characteristic white face, red lips, and temper tantrums. When a problem is traced to hereditary disposition or a disorder that occurred in pregnancy, it can still be treated with acupuncture, but the treatment will be more difficult and may take longer.

Problems associated with gestation and birth are listed below.

Womb diseases—If the mother contracts any disease during or shortly before pregnancy, some part of the disease may be passed on to the child in the form of a lingering pathogenic factor.

Womb heat—If the mother consumes too much hot or spicy foods, if the weather is uncomfortably hot, or if the mother herself has a hot disposition, this can be passed on to the child in the form of womb heat. Common symptoms include tantrums, insomnia, and vomiting (hot type).

Womb toxin—If the mother consumes unsuitable foods or stimulants, this too may affect the child. For example, overconsumption of oranges or shellfish can lead to hyperactivity (see Chapter 31).

Shock in utero—If the mother receives a shock (emotional or physical) during pregnancy, especially in the last few months, this can be passed on to the child. (For characteristic signs and symptoms, see Chapters 4 and 27.)

Premature birth—Neither the Lungs nor the digestive tract of a premature baby are fully formed. As a result, it is very common for these babies to suffer from deficient qi.

Birth trauma—Especially violent or difficult births can give rise to shock, although this is not always the case. The most common effect of a difficult birth is qi deficiency in the child. This seems to be aggravated by the use of analgesics by the mother, which gives rise to qi deficiency and internal cold. Many cases of insomnia due to qi deficiency or cold can be traced to the use of analgesics. In severe cases, there may even be brain damage and epilepsy.

There are also problems associated with the period just after birth.

Overanxiety—If the mother is overanxious or highly strung, this can be passed on to the child. For example, if a shock occurs to the mother during or shortly after birth, the child can also show the symptoms of shock. In this case it is the mother who needs treatment.

Lack of love from parents—Some children are unwanted, and their parents are unable to show them any love. Apart from behavioral disorders, this may show as lack of qi or retarded growth.

Planned babies—With the practice of contraception it is possible to plan a family. Some parents take advantage of this, to the extent of planning even the month when the baby is to be born. Children who are conceived in this way are sometimes born with a weak constitution. It seems as though the babies are not really ready to be born, but are dragged into the world prematurely by the will power of their parents.

In addition to these functional diseases, there is a wide range of congenital abnormalities. In the past, such children frequently did not survive, but thanks to improved obstetrics and prenatal care, many now live. There is relatively little written about these children in the Chinese literature, but very often, what appear to be 'miracle' cures can be achieved with acupuncture. Thus, for example, holes in the heart can be repaired, pancreatic deficiency can be made good, or hydrocephalic children can be made normal, all by means of acupuncture. While it is too early to suggest a prognosis for all the many congenital abnormalities, it is always worth trying acupuncture before more invasive therapies are undertaken.

❖

3 ❖ Excess and Deficiency

TWO BASIC TYPES OF CHILD

In this chapter we will be looking at a fundamental concept: children can be described as basically strong in nature, or more delicate and weak. In Chinese medicine, this concept is expressed by using the terms excess *(shí)* and deficiency *(xū)*. We are accustomed to using these terms in connection with pathological states, as in a disease of excess or deficiency. However, they can also be used to describe the overall state of the person. You might say that it describes the personality to some extent. Excess children and adults tend to be strong and full of life and energy, and deficient, weak children and adults tend to be more fragile and quiet. Both types, however, may go through life never getting ill, and both may live to ripe old ages. The excess type will be shouting right up to the end, and the more deficient type will be quietly reading a book until they reach a hundred years.

This is a simple idea, and it is so simple that it is often overlooked. However, we are spending time discussing it because when a child becomes ill, the sort of illness that it gets is very often based on its type. And, most importantly for us, this will indicate the type of treatment that this particular child will need, that is, either to disperse or to tonify. For example, a child that is strong or *shí* in nature—full of life and energy, loving food, and very active—will, when it becomes sick, tend to have patterns of excess, such as wind-heat with high fever. Here one must disperse to cure the child. On the other hand, a more fragile or *xū* child will tend more toward patterns of deficiency, such as chronic diarrhea, where the cure requires tonification.

Of course, one differentiates between excess and deficiency in the treatment of adults as well, but with children it is much more important, for sometimes it is the only differentiation you can make when they are ill. It is, therefore, vital that you be able to recognize which type of child you are treating. Is this child strong and full of energy most of the time, or is it more of a fragile and delicate type? Obviously, the disease itself will influence your treatment. However, as you proceed through the case history, you should form a picture of either a strong or delicate child, and this is invaluable in making a diagnosis.

So let us now look at how to recognize these two types of child. Once again, let us stress these are not descriptions of sick children; they simply describe the personality or type of child that has come into the world.

Description of the Two Types

The descriptions that follow represent, as you might say, the "ideal." Obviously, not all excess-type children look exactly as described here; some are only slightly excessive in nature. The same applies to the deficient-type child: not all are as deficient as the profile; some are only slightly deficient.

Excess-type profile

- strong, sturdy
- alert
- eyes open and inquisitive
- good appetite, eat everything
- lots of energy
- often has red cheeks
- may make a nuisance of itself
- difficult to ignore
- strong reactions to pain
- when child does get ill, it tends to be severe

The excess type is basically a strong child with a good constitution. Consequently, these children appear strong and sturdy, the bone structure is good, and they feel solid and robust. They have a healthy interest in life and are basically glad that they have been born, and want plenty of everything that is going on. They appear alert and their eyes are open, ready to take in everything that is going on around. You feel when looking at the eyes that there is someone in there—a force to be reckoned with. Their appetite is good, and they have an enthusiasm for food.

These children often have red cheeks, which is traditionally a sign of good health, although we will see in a later chapter that very red cheeks are a sign of imbalance. They make a nuisance of themselves and are difficult to ignore. The reactions they provoke also tend to be strong. When the excess-type baby smiles at you, it is as if the sun has come out: you feel bathed in the child's cheerfulness. Likewise, when the child screams, the pain seems to go straight to your heart. You can't just ignore the screams; you have to go and do something about them.

If they are in pain, it tends to be rather strong, and they get strong reactions to everything. For example, if they get a fever, it is often quite high.

At an older age, these children are mischievous and inquisitive, and are always up to something!

Deficient-type profile
- quiet, even floppy, frail
- eyes dull
- pale
- need lots of sleep
- physical energy is low; often prefer to read or watch television
- tend toward artistic pursuits
- easy to be with
- poor appetite or choosy about food
- easily startled
- sensitive
- quick to cry
- may become ill easily, as the qi is deficient
- when they do get ill, it tends to be more deficient illnesses

The key feature of this type of child is that neither their energy nor their constitution is very strong. In addition, it appears as if these children do not really enjoy being in the material world, and so will often spend their time in a fantasy world or lose themselves in books. They often prefer to be by themselves and not want to interact as much with others. The manifestations vary from child to child; you may not notice anything particularly wrong about these children, but you do not really feel a huge amount of energy surrounding them. This is especially true when you look at their eyes, where you will often notice a dull quality, or, at any rate, a lack of vitality. In more extreme cases, there may even be an air of unhappiness about them—this is not a good sign, as children should not be that unhappy.

On the physical level you may find these children to be rather 'floppy'. In babies this means just floppiness, while in older children it means that they cannot, or just do not want to, sit up straight. They tend to sleep a lot, partly because their energy is not so strong, and partly as another way of escaping. Their lack of enthusiasm extends even to food, and they have poor appetites. (In older deficient-type children, the appetite may be greater, but they have no interest except in very basic foods, or will crave junk food.) This is actually a very important symptom.

When they experience pain, it tends to be rather dull, as they do not have the energy to experience strong sensation.

In contrast to the excess-type child, these children have a rather weak cry and are easier to ignore. The weak cry means not only weak in decibels—not very loud—but also weak in emotional content. The cry may even be a bit tiresome, and unlikely to cut right to the center of your heart.

Excess and Deficient Types in Illness

It is clear from these descriptions that strong, excess-type children have more qi with which to fight illness; thus, they tend to become ill less often than those children who are more fragile with deficient energy. The deficient-type children have fewer resources to fight off illness, and thus become ill more frequently. This is, of course, backed up by experience in the clinic, especially in Western clinics, where most of our patients are of the deficient type.

The sort of illnesses that appear vary from type to type as well. Fragile children tend to have more deficient-type illnesses, such as chronic loose stools (diarrhea) or chronic, weak-sounding coughs, whereas the strong type tend to have a stronger reaction to illness, such as a very high fever, a cough that is loud and severe, and pain that is violent.

Why is this Basic Differentiation so Important?

We find that by making this distinction it is easier to come to a clear diagnosis in the case of illness, and, more importantly, easier to determine the correct needle technique. This is because of the nature of healing in children. Simply put, for healing to occur, the child must have enough energy. When a deficient-type child becomes ill, one must first tonify. If, however, the child is more excessive in nature, then one can disperse or move the energy straight away. It is such a fundamental distinction, and so important in the treatment of children, that again and again one finds oneself asking the question, "Is this child basically excessive or deficient?"

It is also important in those very complex situations

when you are confronted with a really difficult case or a problem which is not covered in the books. By making this simple distinction, you have a foothold from which to start treatment: in the case of deficiency, tonify the qi, and in the case of excess, disperse or move the qi. Very simple, but extremely effective.

Reassess Every Time

We have discussed in this chapter how the basic energy often affects how a child becomes ill. What must also be realized is that when a child does become ill, it does not react to the disease in the same way as adults. Children are generally much more dynamic and more energetic than adults, but they are also that much more delicate, and their energy can easily be thrown out of balance. They may be fine at four in the afternoon, but by six they may be very ill with a raging fever. They respond very rapidly to illness, becoming ill very quickly. Often in a matter of hours, an illness in a young baby can become very serious, even life-threatening, if not treated properly. Thus, a child that you have determined to be a strong type after, say, a bad case of measles or an asthma attack, may actually now be more weak and deficient. In adults, this change from excess to deficiency is usually gradual and takes a long time, but with children it can happen over a short period of weeks or even days.

A child's response to treatment can likewise be rapid, changing from day to day as you treat it. In just one treatment, a deficient child may become one with ample energy.

Therefore, every time that a child comes to the clinic, even if the child has been seen many times before, it is important to make this differentiation afresh: is this child basically strong with an excess of energy, or is it more weak with a deficiency of energy? It is also a fundamental distinction when it comes to needle technique. If the child has a lot of energy, you can disperse the qi using a reducing technique, but if the child is deficient in qi, then you must tonify the qi, for then dispersing can be a serious mistake.

Uncertainty in Diagnosis

Very often in the clinic it is obvious whether a child is excessive or deficient. As you go through the case history, the symptoms match the appearance. However, there will be times when you are not quite so sure. It will happen that the child has some signs of excess and some signs of deficiency. When it comes to treatment, you may be uncertain whether to disperse or tonify. The Chinese texts have little to say about this beyond "half disperse, half tonify" or similar advice. But this advice applies to adults. When treating children there is another way of approaching the problem, and that is to be clear in your mind what you are trying to do.

This is what is meant by "principle of treatment" in Chinese textbooks. So often this principle of treatment appears to be just like a platitude. For example, after saying that the pattern is due to an external pathogenic factor, the principle of treatment may well be to "expel the pathogenic factor." It seems so obvious that it does not seem worth saying.

When treating children, however, this step often has a really useful function. For example, in the next section we describe a pattern called accumulation disorder, where the child is filled with lots of partly digested food. When treating a child like this, the principle of treatment is to expel the partly digested food—obvious enough. When you are treating a child who is part excessive and part deficient, the question you can ask yourself is, "Does the child have enough energy to expel the food, or do I need to build up the child's energy to help get rid of the food?" Put another way, "Should I disperse or tonify?" What will the child feel like after expelling all this food? Will it feel a sense of relief or will it feel exhausted? By going through a mental exercise of this kind, you can arrive at an appropriate treatment.

COMMON PATTERNS OF ILLNESS

Before we consider specific pediatric diseases, we need to look at five common patterns of illness in children. These patterns have very different presentations from the corresponding adult patterns, and are very often seen in the clinic.

Previously, we looked at two basic types of children who were not ill: the strong (excess) and the weak (deficient) types. The strong children are quite likely to grow into strong adults. The weak ones may have to take more care of their health in later life, but there is no basic reason why they should not live equally useful, productive, or long lives as their strong-natured counterparts. Yet what we have noticed in the clinic is that when these two basic types of children do become ill, they tend to manifest illness in specific ways, as befits their type.

The five common patterns of illness in children are:

- accumulation disorder: a condition of excess, usually seen in the excess-type child
- Spleen qi deficiency: a condition of deficiency, usually seen in the deficient-type child
- hyperactive Spleen qi deficiency: a condition of deficiency which, however, appears to be excessive
- hyperactive Kidney qi deficiency: a condition of deficiency which, however, appears to be excessive
- lingering pathogenic factor: a truly mixed pattern of excess and deficiency

The last pattern, lingering pathogenic factor, is different from the others. Here we are looking at the aftereffects of infectious disease, which can be much more devastating in children than in adults. Because of this difference, this pattern is discussed separately at the end of this chapter.

Etiology and Pathogenesis of the Basic Patterns

One of the basic premises of Chinese medicine is that all illnesses have a cause, and that this cause can nearly always be found in the life of the patient. For example, the cause of Liver qi stagnation in adults is usually the result of suppression of emotions, while Kidney yang deficiency is associated with overwork, excessive sex, or poor nourishment.

To find the cause of a problem in the lives of children, one has to look at their lives, which are very different from those of adults. Children do not have to worry about money, pay the mortgage, or repress their emotions; and they rarely suffer from overwork. But there are two huge problems which children face, especially those under the age of three: protecting themselves from pathogenic factors, and eating enough. The first problem will be discussed at length in the chapters on respiratory disease. It is the second problem that we will be discussing here, that is, how differences manifest in the digestive system.

To appreciate the magnitude of the problem facing the digestive system of a newborn baby, one need only consider the enormous weight gain during the first six months of life. In Britain, there is a rule of thumb that babies should double their weight in the first six months, and treble their birth weight by the end of their first year. It does not take much imagination to visualize the amount of food that a baby must consume, and the resulting strain put on the digestive system as it works flat out to accommodate the food. This helps explain why the very young often look like miniature sumo wrestlers!

Obviously, the digestive system is very important to a baby: it must eat a vast amount to survive, but because the digestive tract is working so hard, it can easily be thrown off balance. As the child grows, the system gradually becomes stronger, but only slowly.

The reason why this problem is so much more serious for babies and young children is because of the way they react to disturbances. There is a saying in Chinese medicine that in children, "the organs are fragile and soft, and the qi easily leaves it path." And another, that "children become ill easily, and their illnesses quickly become serious."

So if the digestion is upset, which happens quite easily in the very young, all sorts of problems can arise. Put another way, when one thing goes wrong, then everything goes wrong. The organs of the very young are like delicately tuned instruments that can go wrong with just the slightest disturbance. And when something goes wrong with the qi-generating mechanism in babies or young children, then the whole system stops working, and the production of qi almost stops. This can be devastating.

―――

The digestive system of a baby is delicate and yet has to work flat out in order to digest enough food. Thus, it is easily overworked and upset.

―――

When a digestive disturbance occurs in a baby or young child it will manifest as one of two basic patterns, depending on the type of the child. Because the digestive system is so fundamental to the health of a baby or young child, these patterns can cause many symptoms. The patterns are very commonly seen in the clinic and underlie diseases as diverse as asthma, eczema, vomiting, diarrhea, influenza, and whooping cough. Let us now look at each pattern in more detail.

ACCUMULATION DISORDER

Introduction

There are two obvious dysfunctions of the digestive tract: either the food moves through too fast and causes diarrhea, or it moves through too slowly and causes blockage. Intestinal blockage from accumulation is very common among babies and children. It corresponds roughly to the retention of food disorder *(shǐ zhì)* seen in adults. It is very common in Western children and is regarded as a major factor in a wide range of disorders including constipation, abdominal pain, intestinal parasites, vomiting, diarrhea, cough, and asthma. In fact, when treating young children, this disorder is so common that one should routinely check to see if it is present.

As mentioned earlier, accumulation disorder occurs with such frequency because a baby's digestion is working so close to its maximum capacity—a healthy baby should take enough food to double its weight in the first six months—that it only takes a small reduction in the child's level of qi to disrupt the qi mechanism. This extra stress may be due to many causes including emotional distress in the parents, infections, immunizations, and teething.

Accumulation disorder is a condition of excess, and is commonly found in the excess-type child. The importance of this cannot be overstated, for it implies that a dispersing or reducing needle technique is indicated to treat the disorder. If you try to treat a *deficient* child as if it is suffering from accumulation disorder (see Spleen qi deficiency, below), then at best your treatment will not work; more likely, however, you will make the child worse. In diagnosing this disorder, the key question is whether the child has enough qi to expel the accumulated food. If it does have enough energy, then treat it as a disorder of excess; if not, treat it as one of deficiency.

This pattern may have a sudden onset, accompanied by great discomfort. It is often brought on by overeating or external stress, but may also be a lingering condition, which becomes more or less severe as the child's energy fluctuates. Those children who are more susceptible often have very red cheeks. In England it is thought that very red cheeks (also called "high color") are a sign of good health; these children are therefore often not regarded as being ill.

Etiology & Pathogenesis

Etiology

Accumulation disorder is caused by food and milk blocking the digestion, which in turn disrupts the function of the Stomach and Spleen. This can occur as a result of irregular or voracious feeding; demand feeding; eating unripe, uncooked, or undercooked food; eating food that is too rich, too sweet, or too difficult to digest, such as brown bread or brown rice; eating unsuitable food at weaning; or eating when overexcited.

Both the types of food that are eaten and the regularity of meals are extremely important to a baby or young child.

Overfeeding. This is the most common cause of the disorder. Parents want to see their children eat well. There is a widespread belief that a child who eats a lot must be a healthy child. Also many parents make a subconscious link between love and food: "I give my child lots of food, therefore I give it lots of love."

Regularity of meals. A baby or young child needs time between each feeding or meal in order to assimilate the food. We find in the clinic that babies who are fed on demand and children that continually snack are much more prone to digestive disturbances. There is a saying in traditional Chinese medicine that the "Spleen likes regularity." Another way of putting it is that the Stomach needs to empty completely before being refilled, and that just takes time.

Type of foods. It may seem hard to believe, but we believe that 'whole' foods are unsuitable for many children under four years of age. We find that children have difficulty in digesting foods such as brown rice, brown bread, fruit, and salads, and many also find wheat bread to be indigestible. These foods are unsuitable for a child because they are simply too difficult to digest and assimilate, putting a strain on an already fragile digestive system.

We also find that children thrive on simple foods, and those that are easily digested. Appreciation of rich and exotic foods can come later in life when the energy of the Spleen is not so taxed.

Weaning too early. Children who show a great enthusiasm for food and a great interest in a wide range of foods are often weaned at an early age before their digestion can cope with the food. This can cause accumulation disorder. They may go on eating the food even though it is not being digested properly.

Stress. Events may put temporary stress on the child, either physically, such as by moving from house to house or by giving the child an immunization, or emotionally, such as a frightening accident or the death of someone close. The stress puts an added strain on the qi, and if the child continues to eat large amounts of food, this can lead to accumulation disorder in a short space of time.

======

At times of stress, the child should eat less food in order to avoid overloading its digestive system.

======

Immunization. This subject is discussed in detail in Chapter 19, but here it is worth pointing out that immunizations can lead to accumulation disorder. This happens simply because the child's qi is temporarily reduced while it copes with the immunization. If the child continues eating as much food as before, the digestion will be unable to cope with all the food; it thereupon accumulates in the Stomach and is not digested properly.

Pathogenesis

The common factor in all of these causes is that they put extra stress on the qi, especially that of the Spleen. A baby's digestive system is working very close to its maximum capacity, and it only needs a small extra stress to cause a problem. It is like a conveyor belt in a factory: if there is a "hiccup" in the production, then all the material piles up in one huge mess because it is incapable of processing the excess. The undigested food then decays and transforms into heat. It accumulates in the Intestines, and invades the Spleen and Stomach. The transportive and transformative functions become impaired, the digestion becomes unregulated, and blockage occurs. The food is then either not expelled (constipation) or expelled as green, smelly stools. The stools may become irregular, with diarrhea alternating with constipation.

Eventually the stagnating food leads to heat in the digestive system. The heat may then spread through the body where it gives rise to the following symptoms:

• red cheeks (from heat rising up through the Stomach, Large Intestine, and Small Intestine channels)
• irritability
• insomnia

The fluids can also stagnate and dry up, leading to phlegm. This gives rise to other symptoms:

• green nasal discharge
• other signs of phlegm, slippery pulse
• possibly cough

When there is stagnation over a period of time, this taxes the Liver's function of governing the free flow of qi, and the child becomes very irritable. One may also observe green around the mouth because a branch of the Liver channel encircles the mouth.

Signs & Symptoms

Babies

• vomits curdled milk
• interior of the mouth has a milky appearance
• abdomen swollen and feels like a drum

- no appetite
- stools smell sour or of apples
- stools often alternating between constipation and diarrhea
- baby smells of apples
- restless and irritable
- intermittent abdominal pain and crying
- both cheeks bright red
- often a pale, yellowish-green around the mouth
- often has nasal discharge

Tongue body: thin, red
Tongue coating: thick, white
Finger vein: purple, broad (see Chapter 4)

Treatment principle: reduce the accumulation due to milk and remove the obstruction

Toddlers (under four years)

- stools are green and sour-smelling (mild case), or rotten and stinking (severe case)
- facial color is greenish-yellow, possibly red cheeks
- feels stuffed up inside
- often has green nasal discharge
- restless, cries out loud, irritable
- vomits sour and rotten food
- abdominal pain that worsens with pressure, occurs with eating, and is relieved by passing stool
- in serious cases, there is low grade fever and burning in the palms of the hands
- possibly sweating in the evening and at night

Tongue coating: thick, greasy
Pulse: wiry, slippery
Finger vein: dull purple

Comments about the symptoms

- As we already mentioned, red cheeks are traditionally a sign of a healthy child. In our experience, an overall pink color to the face is healthy, but when the cheeks become much redder than the rest of the face it is a sign of accumulation disorder, and thus of an imbalance. (This is a big difference from adults, where red cheeks are usually a sign of yin deficiency.)
- The abdomen is very large and bloated as a result of the excess accumulated food, and the fermentation of the food, resulting in the production of gas.
- The stools smell foul because the food is not properly digested and goes bad inside the child. In mild cases, the stools (and even the whole baby) may smell of apples or of cider because the food ferments slightly inside the

child. In severe cases, the stools smell absolutely repulsive and acrid.

- 'Restless and irritable' is a term that appears so frequently in the literature that one sometimes forgets to visualize it. In a child this means thoroughly bad-tempered, impossible to be with, contrary, and refusing to do anything it is asked to do.

Priority of symptoms

In diagnosing accumulation disorder, some symptoms have more significance than others. For example, a child's bad temper may arise from many things: a strong will, upset in the family, overtired.

The bad temper and green color around the mouth are Liver symptoms. In fact, the behavior of a child with this pattern might bring to mind an adult pattern, stagnation of Liver qi. There is, however, a huge difference between them. In adults, it is the *restraint* of anger that gives rise to stagnation of Liver qi; the accumulation of food is a possible consequence. In children, on the other hand, it is the accumulation of food that gives rise to the stagnation of Liver qi, which in turn generates anger. In adults, it is enough to regulate the Liver, but in children, this simply does not work; the stagnant food must be cleared. Thus, for example, a point such as Liv-3 *(tai chong)* is helpful in treating stagnation of Liver qi in adults but is of no help in treating accumulation disorder in children.

Treatment

Treatment principle

Reduce the food stagnation and remove the obstruction

Main point

si feng (M-UE-9)

Method

All the textbooks say that this point should be treated with the triangular needle to withdraw a few drops of yellow fluid. In practice, it is sufficient to needle it with a broad gauge (28 or 30) filiform needle; moreover, it is unnecessary to squeeze out any fluid. Treatment may be given as often as every other day, on one hand each time. However, in practice, it is rare for this point to be used more than twice a week. It should be used no more than once every four days, and then on alternating hands. This is because of its length of action. Needling this point causes dispersement, and is especially suitable for treating the excessive pattern.

Other points

S-36 *(zu san li)*
S-25 *(tian shu)*   } Clears blockage by promoting the
CV-6 *(qi hai)*   } movement of qi

CV-12 *(zhong wan)*
B-25 *(da chang shu)*   } Clears blockage by promoting the
TB-6 *(zhi gou)*   movement of qi

Method   All with dispersing or moving technique

According to symptoms   P-6 *(nei guan)*   For vomiting
S-44 *(nei ting)*   For great heat

After each treatment, the patient may be irritable for twenty-four hours, followed by a discharge of foul-smelling stools. It is important to warn parents about this!

Usually *si feng* (M-UE-9) is sufficient. If the patient is quite violent, add Liv-2 *(xing jian)*. A mild purgative may be given to assist the treatment, but is rarely necessary.

Prognosis

For an acute attack, one to three treatments should be sufficient to clear the main symptoms; a total of six treatments is quite common. To prevent recurrence, it is essential that some dietary changes are made: less food, more suitable foods, and regular meals. For some children, regular treatment about once a month may be needed for up to a year.

Note

Accumulation disorder includes the condition which we would call constipation, but is more commonly characterized by irregularity, with days when no stools are passed followed by days with diarrhea.

SPLEEN QI DEFICIENCY

Introduction

This is perhaps now the most common chronic disorder in children who live in developed countries. They do not have sufficient qi to enable their digestive system to function properly. This means that they have poor appetites, loose stools, or constipation. It follows that they do not have much energy and are often floppy and pale faced.

Like accumulation disorder, this condition may appear in the clinic in many different guises, and may underlie many diseases. There are a variety of causes including heredity, recurrent acute attacks of accumulation disorder, and the transformation of other disorders. Other causes seen in the West are anesthetics given in childbirth, immunizations where there is no feverish reaction in the child, and the effects of being an unwanted child. This type of problem is almost continuous, and the child goes on for a long time without energy. It may present in the clinic as the basis of a serious disease, such as asthma. Sometimes, however, we see it before a serious disease manifests itself, when it should nonetheless be treated because it can easily lead to other problems.

Etiology & Pathogenesis

This condition is caused by any factor that injures the qi of the child.

Weak constitution and exhaustion. Some children are simply born with weak constitutions. They easily become tired.

Accumulation disorder. Long-term presence of the accumulation disorder can injure the digestive system and deplete the qi.

Illness. Recurrent infections, repeated illness, or a strong external pathogenic attack can deplete the qi of a baby or child, giving rise to Spleen qi deficiency. This is especially true if the child is treated with antibiotics.

Immunizations. The effect of immunizations is similar to that of a very strong external pathogenic attack, and can weaken the qi system.

Anesthetics. Anesthetics given during childbirth deplete the qi of the baby. They dull the senses of the mother, and have a dispersing effect on the qi of the baby. Similarly, a long and exhausting childbirth can deplete the baby's qi.

Unsuitable or irregular food. In China, insufficient food is a cause for Spleen qi deficiency. In the West, it is food with poor nutritional content. Also, continuous feeding—such as demand feeding of babies, or frequent snacking or 'grazing'—can weaken the qi of the Stomach.

Weak qi of the mother. Weakness of the mother's qi, often with anemia, is becoming increasingly common as more and more mothers work during pregnancy, often at very hard or stressful jobs. Fewer mothers now are aware of the need to rest during pregnancy.

Lack of qi development in older children. Children are spending less and less time playing out of class, and more and more time watching television and playing computer games. This means that they develop their mental faculties at a young age, but at the expense of developing their qi.

If the qi of the child is upset or weakened, the Spleen is then unable to function properly, leading to irregular or loose stools, or to constipation. There is simply not enough strength in the Spleen and the Intestines to properly transport and digest the food. In addition to disturbed digestion, the appetite is very poor. Furthermore, there is not enough qi to fight off external pathogenic factors. The child will thus suffer recurrent illnesses of all sorts, which will further weaken the qi. Long-term weakness of the Spleen will lead to phlegm and dampness, which in turn opens the way for many other diseases.

Signs & Symptoms

- pale or faded yellow face
- skin tone and limbs flabby, body lacks strength
- eyes dull
- lips pale, lower lip possibly protruding
- irregular stools, perhaps constipated for days at a time, or frequent loose stools
- stools do not usually smell bad, but are slippery and oily, or contain particles of undigested milk
- prefers to sleep during the day, but remain awake at night, often waking every two hours
- often lots of phlegm or dampness
- prone to coughs, colds, or other illnesses
- poor appetite or picky about food
- weak cry that is irritating or easy to ignore
- possibly vomiting

Tongue body: pale
Tongue coating: white, thick, greasy
Pulse: fine and weak, or fine and slippery
Finger vein: thin, blue, or not visible

Comments about the symptoms

- Many of the symptoms listed above are of the deficient type. The others relate to digestion.
- The stools do not usually smell bad, as there is complete absence of heat. It is like keeping food in a refrigerator—it does not go bad or rotten.
- The protruding lower lip is really a symptom of a malnutrition disorder *(gān),* but sometimes appears in Spleen qi deficiency as well.
- Sleeping a lot is characteristic of deficient types. As we will see in a later chapter, if the qi and blood are weak, the child wakes up many times at night.
- Being prone to coughs and colds is in fact a sign of weak protective qi, and thus of weak Lung qi. However, one often finds that if the Spleen qi is weak, then the overall qi is weak, including the Lung qi.

Treatment

Treatment principle

Strengthen the Spleen, augment the qi, and assist in clearing the waste.

Points

The most important thing here is to tonify the Spleen qi with points such as:

S-36 *(zu san li)*	Tonifies qi
CV-12 *(zhong wan)*	Strengthens the Spleen

Method

The needle technique is important. Care should be taken to tonify when the condition is one of deficiency. Indirect moxibustion can also be applied at CV-12 *(zhong wan)*.

Results of Treatment and Prognosis

The results obtained from treating Spleen qi deficiency are far less dramatic than when treating accumulation disorder. Usually the results are gradual, with the qi slowly becoming stronger. If the child was only slightly deficient in energy, then only three to five treatments may be necessary, possibly less if it is a very young baby. But very often the Spleen qi deficiency is quite severe, having persisted for a few months or even years. In these cases, ten, twenty, thirty, or even more treatments may be needed, depending on the strength of the child. In these cases, you must try to encourage the child to rest and to avoid constant stimulation: lots of television (which depletes the qi), late nights, and parties. If the child continually overdoes such things, your treatment will at best be much slower, and at worst totally ineffectual, and the child will continue to be ill.

It is important to be clear about the cause of the Spleen deficiency, since it must be removed. Sometimes this is very difficult. For example, if the child is at school and is being pushed too hard by ambitious parents, it may be difficult to convince them that this is not a good thing. With other distractions, such as computer games and television, it is very hard to explain to the child why it should play fewer games or watch less television. Stopping the child from doing so, and coping with the ensuing tantrums, can prove to be too much for some parents.

THE ENERGETIC LINK BETWEEN PARENTS AND CHILD

As mentioned earlier in the chapter, to explain the common patterns of hyperactive Spleen qi deficiency and hyperactive Kidney qi deficiency, we must first look at the relationship between parents and child.[1]

During the first year or two of life the relationship between mother and child is very strong. In these formative years the child cannot be regarded autonomously, but always as a couple, that is, as mother-child. If a child has a problem, the mother is intimately bound up in that problem. During this time, mother and child share energy as though they are still linked by an invisible umbilical cord. It is this energy flow that enables the child to thrive. Understanding this flow is the key to understanding some illnesses, and some unusual patterns in a child's behavior.

Just as this energy connection enables the child to thrive normally, when the child has an illness, there is an extra flow to help the child. For example, when the child is struggling against a disease such as measles, or going through a difficult transition such as teething, it needs more energy. It cannot produce the energy by itself, and being so small, there are no reserves. So it calls on its parents for the extra energy. This is freely given through the tender care and nursing from the parents, and it enables the child to overcome the illness quickly.

What mothers and fathers seem to do is to take some of the suffering of their children onto themselves. Parents actually feel the pain and suffering of their child. At the same time, they actively give out healing energy to the child. They give, without any thought of holding back, as much energy as the child needs to get through the illness. Thus, during a child's illness, the important parent in the relationship is likely to feel the illness as well, and will also feel quite unnaturally exhausted from giving her or his own energy to the child to help it through the illness.

This common link between parents and their children leads to a situation we often see in the clinic where the child is ill and weak and the important parent is tired or exhausted. However, we also see another situation which arises if a child does not have proper care or support from the parents during an illness. Perhaps the child is sent back to school too soon, or the parents are too busy to give much of their energy so the child has to fight the illness on its own. Here, the child is seen to be ill and weak while the

---

1. We refer to the mother throughout this section. This is not to say that the father is unimportant, since he is just as energetically linked to the child. However, the mother does seem to have a special connection. Nevertheless, occasionally we do find that it is not the mother who is critical to the development of the pattern; rather, it is the parent that makes the strongest connection to the child in the first year of life, which could be the father.

Case History

An example of the close bond between mother and child can be seen in the flow of breast milk. One of the mothers who came to our clinic was very materialistic and did not believe in psychic energies or anything that could not be measured. One evening, she left her two-month-old baby at home with a baby sitter and went out to the pub for the first time since the birth of her first child. She was half way through her drink when suddenly her milk started to flow and she felt a great need to get back to her child. When she got home five minutes later, she was very shocked to find that her baby had woken up hungry five minutes before, just when her milk started to flow.

important parent is in good or even radiant health. It is helpful to distinguish these two situations to see how each can best be helped with acupuncture, as this will aid in understanding the final two patterns we will discuss. Again, the two situations are:

• child is ill and weak, parent is exhausted
• child is ill and weak, parent is in radiant health

We will now look at these two situations and how acupuncture can help in each case.

Child is Ill and Weak, Parent is Exhausted

This is a very common pattern. It will occur when the child is ill for some reason or other, and the mother is pouring all of her available energy into the child. You will notice that the mother has great anxiety about her child.

Alternatively, it may come about because the mother herself is exhausted, perhaps anemic. For example, if this is her second or third child, it is very possible that she would not have had time to recover her energy after the latest birth. If the birth was difficult and the child was born with qi deficiency, then both mother and child would start off in a deficient condition. If the baby does not sleep well, then the mother will have broken nights as well, but has to look after the other children during the day. Thus, she has no chance to recover. Since she is tired, the baby has no one to supply the missing qi, so the infant never recovers from a difficult start.

The following is a typical symptom picture:

Child
• pale face
• poor appetite or choosy about food
• possibly loose stools

- listless
- easily tires
- sleeps a lot during the day
- disturbed sleep at night

Mother

- tired
- gray face
- dispirited and very worried
- hair lacks luster

Treatment

Treatment principle

Tonify the qi of the child

Points

S-36 *(zu san li)*	Tonifies qi
CV-12 *(zhong wan)*	Strengthens the Spleen

Method

These points are treated with the tonifying method. Additionally, indirect moxibustion can be applied at CV-12 *(zhong wan)*.

If there is severe Spleen qi deficiency, with the child exhausted, dispirited, and especially dribbling from the mouth (with the mouth hanging open most of the time), you should add:

B-20 *(pi shu)*

Method

Use the tonifying method if you can. These children do not like being needled on the back, and make rather a fuss and wriggle around. In these circumstances, it is quite difficult to be sure that you are really tonifying. However, even when the treatment progresses in this manner, it does seem to be effective.

Results of treatment

Usually there is steady progress. If the mother is exhausted when she first comes in, you may find that it is the mother who starts to feel some improvement. She may feel better before the child does, and before there is any change in symptoms. Conversely, if the mother is in radiant health, you may notice the opposite sequence, as described below.

Child is Ill and Weak, Parent is in Radiant Health

This is an unnatural state of affairs. Normally, if a child is deficient it will claim some energy from the mother and she will start to feel tired. In this case, however, for some reason the mother is withholding energy—perhaps the child is unwanted, is of the "wrong" sex, or interferes with the mother's career. Normally in this situation, the child would make a fuss and start to claim energy from the mother. But when the child becomes exhausted, or if the situation has been going on for a long time, the child loses spirit and so cannot make enough contact with its mother to be able to claim any qi.

The treatment given is the same as above, but the effects of treatment in this situation are quite surprising. Simply by tonifying the qi of the child, one can make enormous changes in the family dynamics. If the treatment is successful, the first thing to happen is that the contact between mother and child is restored, and the child is able to tap into the energy of the mother. Very quickly the child becomes well, but correspondingly the mother becomes exhausted, as she pours her energy into the child who needs it. It does sound a bit unfair to the mother, but be reassured, this state of affairs is temporary. As the child gets well, its energy demands on the mother will diminish, and the mother's energy returns.

There is another possibility, which is that the child really does need more energy from the mother than she is able to give in her present circumstances. For example, a mother might be putting all her energy into a stressful career or managing a large family, and simply does not have any spare time for the child. What happens then is that she will usually reassess her circumstances and reduce her energy expenditure in other quarters so that she can nurture her child. Put quite simply, the mother realizes that she loves her child more than she thought, and is prepared to make changes because of that love.

After this little detour, we will now return to a discussion of the next two common patterns.

HYPERACTIVE SPLEEN QI DEFICIENCY

The third basic pattern of illness in children is that of hyperactive Spleen qi deficiency. It is really an extension of the Spleen qi deficiency pattern, but with some significant differences. There is also an associated pattern—hyperactive Kidney deficiency—which we will talk about later, as it is the fourth basic pattern and is itself a further development of hyperactive Spleen qi deficiency. You will not find either of these patterns mentioned in the Chinese textbooks, probably because these types of children do not exist in China. This should give you some idea as to how these patterns arise: they are the result of the Western way of raising children.

The paradox of this pattern is that from the symptoms, the child would appear to be completely deficient, that is, it has a poor appetite and thin arms and legs, and is often ill. Yet from its behavior, it would seem as though the child had plenty of energy. What is in fact happening is that the child has learned how to tap into the energy of the parents and other adults in its environment. The child does not generate its own energy—it cannot generate much energy with such weak Spleen qi—but manages to live off the surplus energy of the adults around it.

Signs & Symptoms

- pale face
- possible nasal discharge
- often small for age
- thin arms and legs
- appetite small or very picky about foods
- often either constipated or has loose, watery stools

Behavior

- alternately bold and coy
- resists going to sleep, maybe not sleepy until 10 or 11 P.M.
- enjoys being the center of attention
- manipulative—able to find the weakest spot in adults!

As can be seen, the symptoms are clearly those of Spleen qi deficiency, while the behavior is not. The behavior is somewhat manipulative and is aimed (albeit subconsciously) at getting the adults around it to give off some energy.

This pattern is becoming more and more common, and arises from many reasons. One is that parents now find it difficult to draw boundaries. A "yes" is a "yes," but a "no" is a "maybe." The child instinctively knows this and exploits it mercilessly to provide energy.

Another reason is overstimulation from all sorts of external causes—food, television, school, and out-of-school activities. Sometimes the stimulation comes from taking such medications as Ventolin.

Although these children are often laughing or giggling, it seems to us that they are not really happy, but would be happier with clear boundaries. When parents can really develop clear routines and boundaries for their children, it is often found that their health improves a lot.

Treatment

Treatment principle | Tonify the Spleen

Points | S-36 *(zu san li)*   Tonifies qi
CV-12 *(zhong wan)*   Strengthens the Spleen

Method | These points are treated with the tonifying method. Additionally, indirect moxibustion can be applied at CV-12 *(zhong wan)*.

Even though the behavior is hyperactive, the result of tonification is to calm the child down. Another result is that the parents will start to feel better as the child is less of a drain on their energy. However, there are problems with the treatment.

• It can be difficult to actually treat these children. The parents are often somewhat indecisive, either by nature or because they have become totally exhausted by their child. So when the time comes for treatment, the child often starts to behave badly. Even though the child does not fear treatment at all, it sees an opportunity for grabbing more energy. The child starts to complain and to pretend to be fearful of the needles. The parents are then thrown into a quandary: should they or should they not have their child treated? They may even ask their child if it wants to have acupuncture treatment. The child responds with a wonderful performance, with floods of crocodile tears. This performance can make treating these children very difficult. Not only can it make the present treatment difficult, but sometimes the children manipulate themselves out of further treatment.

• The results of treatment are not so predictable. Since a proper cure depends on establishing clear boundaries for the child, this requires to a certain extent that the parents learn from the new situation. Usually they can, and it is just exhaustion which has prevented them from being firm, but sometimes discipline is so far removed from their own idea of upbringing that they find it impossible to impose it.

Problems Facing Parents

Finding a proper routine for the child, establishing clear boundaries, and imposing discipline are all very difficult now. Advice, and the old rules of behavior which grandparents are accustomed to, may not be appropriate. Simple rules and harsh discipline were suitable for a time when life was simpler and harder than it is now. When the weather was cold, it was necessary to wrap up well, for if you got cold, it was almost impossible to get warm again. Now there is no difficulty in getting warm, and so some parents have gone quite to the opposite extreme and allow their children to go swimming in winter even if they have a respiratory infection.

Likewise, in the past if a child got overtired, it could easily get seriously ill, so parents made quite sure that their children went to bed on time. Now there is not the same health risk when children become overtired, so there is not the same urgent necessity to get them into bed. And when a child cannot get to sleep, it will get sympathy, but there will not be the same pressure to get it back into bed. The child senses this instinctively, and so plays up in order to receive the energy that goes with the sympathy. If the parent allows this to happen too often, it soon becomes a habit, one which is difficult to break.

This little example from sleep patterns is repeated in other areas of life, the child sucks more and more energy from the parents, and the hyperactive Spleen qi deficient pattern is born.

HYPERACTIVE KIDNEY QI DEFICIENCY

This pattern is very similar to the previous one, with the same causes and energy flows. The difference is that the deficiency has become a bit deeper, and the child is more exhausted. It is a very common pattern.

Signs & Symptoms

Typical symptoms will include those listed for hyperactive Spleen qi deficiency, plus:

- face is bright white
- dark pools around eyes
- thin
- nervous, tearful
- hypersensitive
- insomnia: takes an hour or more to go to sleep, even when tired
- terrified of needles and even of moxibustion!

Treatment

There are even bigger problems facing the practitioner here than with previous patterns, since the child really is afraid of needles (as is often the case with Kidney deficiency). That, combined with an ability to manipulate parents, means that needles can rarely be used. The only option is to use moxibustion or to massage the points.

Points

CV-12 *(zhong wan)*
B-23 *(shen shu)*

Occasionally, when a child is not too nervous, moxibustion on salt can also be performed at CV-8 *(shen que).*

Prognosis

Surprisingly, with treatment, these children do progress. There is, of course, the same problem over establishing boundaries, but in our experience, most of the children ` get better.

Other Causes of Hyperactivity

It is worth mentioning other factors which aggravate hyperactivity and should therefore be avoided:

• sugar in the diet
• artificial colorings and flavorings
• overstimulation
• watching television

Usually the mother is aware of these factors. However, she is so worn down by the continual drain from her children that she just does not have the strength and determination to keep them away from things that she knows are harmful.

Note

The type of hyperactivity discussed here is just one of many patterns. This subject is discussed at greater length in Chapter 31.

LINGERING PATHOGENIC FACTORS

Introduction

In this section we look at the sequela of infectious diseases in children, or in Chinese medical terms, invasion by pathogenic factors. We will see that children are affected in much the same way as adults, but often much more strongly: an infection which might keep an adult in bed with a fever for a few days can cause lasting damage to a child. Indeed, it often happens that children are permanently thrown out of balance.

Here we will study the normal process of invasion by a pathogenic factor and then introduce the concept of lingering pathogenic factor, a pathogenic factor which has not quite been expelled. (It has some similarities to the biomedical idea of post-viral syndrome.) We will see that there are three possible patterns left behind after an illness:

1. Spleen qi deficiency
2. Retention of phlegm
3. Retention of very thick phlegm[2]

Pathogenesis of an Invasion

During the invasion

To understand the aftereffects of an infectious disease, it is helpful to look at the normal process that occurs during invasion of a pathogenic factor. It is thought that a pathogenic factor enters through the skin, the superficial layer, where it is met by the protective qi, which resides in this superficial layer, and goes no further. The effect of this invasion is to obstruct the normal flow of qi in the skin, giving rise to two further symptoms: shivering (with aversion to drafts) and phlegm.

- The shivering and aversion to drafts results from the skin not working well. The protective qi has been temporarily vanquished from its place in the skin, so it is no longer available to protect against drafts and wind.
- Phlegm arises because the pathogenic factor sits in the skin and superficial layer, causing stagnation of fluids. The stagnant fluids quickly transform into phlegm. (An alternative explanation is that the pathogenic factor enters the Lung channel and causes a functional disturbance, impairing the Lung's function of causing the fluids to descend and disperse through the body.)
- The next stage in the illness, which occurs spontaneously in a healthy child, but may need the assistance of medicine or treatment in a weaker child, is for the protective qi to fight back and expel the pathogenic factor. Symptoms associated with this stage are fever and sweating. Fever arises because of the heat generated in the struggle between the protective qi and the pathogenic factor, and the sweating is a sign of the pathogenic factor being expelled.

These processes and symptoms—shivering, phlegm, fever, and sweating—are characteristic of the invasion of almost all pathogenic factors.

---

2. We use this term interchangeably with lingering pathogenic factor.

Immediately after the invasion

The processes just described also explain the characteristic patterns that are seen after such an invasion: a *combination* of qi deficiency and phlegm. In the qi-deficient pattern, weakness is the predominant symptom, such that although there may be lots of phlegm, the child is simply too weak to cough it up. The qi deficiency occurs because so much qi is used in expelling the pathogenic factor. There is a saying in Chinese medicine, "Any long illness injures the qi."

In the phlegm pattern, there may be tiredness, but the dominant symptom is the huge amount of phlegm. The child obviously has got some qi and is trying to cough the phlegm up, but there is so much of it that the child does not have a chance to get rid of it all. In the phlegmy soup left behind in the child you may also see some heat, and, very rarely, yin deficiency.

Summary of Stages

First stage

- shivering
- phlegm

Second stage

- fever
- sweating

Recovery

- qi deficiency
- phlegm
- possibly heat
- possibly yin deficiency

Signs & Symptoms

Lung and Spleen qi deficiency

- tiredness
- lethargy
- no interest in life
- no interest in food
- runny nose
- cough (weak)
- child is shy
- possibly loose stools

Pulse

- weak

Retention of phlegm

- very snotty nose
- cough with lots of gurgling noise
- mouth breathing
- wants things, but is dissatisfied
- wants to eat, but is choosy
- stools may be glistening (because of phlegm)
- glands enlarged

Pulse

- full, slippery

In adults, these patterns are usually present for only a few weeks after an illness, while in children they may persist for months or years in the absence of treatment.

In healthy children, the two conditions mentioned above will right themselves: the qi will gradually recover, the phlegm will slowly resolve, and, given time, the child will regain perfect health. However, in some children this does not happen. If, for example, the child is weakened by being sent back to school too soon, or because the disease was treated with antibiotics, the child never recovers completely, that is, it never really gets rid of the pathogenic factor. Many months (even years) later, the imbalance caused by the original disease is still present.

What is then left behind is the thick phlegm pattern. To explain this phenomenon, the Chinese have devised the concept of lingering pathogenic factor. The idea is that the original pathogenic factor has been overcome but not completely expelled. Still lurking in the body is a very much weakened or dormant pathogenic factor. It is weakened to the point that it rarely causes any specific trouble, except that it has a strong effect in blocking the flow of qi and fluids, and can alter the character of the child.

The symptoms of this pattern include:

• didn't completely recover from an illness
• qi is a bit weak, but not drastically so
• some phlegm, but not huge amount
• mild symptoms (such as sore throat, tickling cough, or earache) which worsen when the child is tired. These symptoms are often an *echo* of the original illness.
• swollen glands
• child's character is subtly altered
• sudden collapse of energy for no apparent reason, which lasts for a few hours
• intermittent abdominal pain

Qi is a bit weak. This is because the qi has not fully recovered after the illness. Moreover, the pathogenic factor sits in the channels and interferes with the production of qi.

Some phlegm, but not a huge amount. The phlegm which was present after the illness has largely, but not completely, been cleared from the body. What is left behind is generally very thick phlegm, which is especially difficult to clear.

Mild symptoms which worsen when tired. The original pathogenic factor has not been completely cleared. Additionally, the site where the pathogenic factor resides is weakened by the invasion. So, for example, after tonsillitis, the tonsils will be swollen because the pathogenic factor is still there, and the qi in the tonsils is weakened because the pathogenic factor obstructs the flow of qi.

A lingering pathogenic factor can persist through one's entire life. Once the imbalance occurs, it can take root. There are opportunities for expelling it, especially at the seven- and fourteen-year transition periods, but very often, in the absence of treatment, the imbalance remains, year after year. As the child grows from toddler to adulthood, the symptoms may wane and disappear because the general strength of the child increases. We may say that the symptoms are then submerged. For appropriate treatments at the seven- and fourteen-year transitions, see Chapter 43.

But it often happens that the symptoms reappear later in life when the qi is weakened, for example, at a time of great stress and exhaustion, or in old age. The lingering pathogenic factor can be likened to rocks on the sea bed. When the tide of energy is low, the rocks appear. As the energy increases, the tide comes in and submerges the rocks. But should the energy wane, as happens in old age, the rocks will reappear as the tide goes out.

One of my teachers, Dr. J. F. Shen, uses the analogy of a burglar. He likens the invasion of a pathogenic factor to a burglar coming into a house. The proper way to expel such an intruder is to open the doors and windows and chase him out. (The medical analogy being the expulsion of a pathogenic factor by sweating or diaphoresis.) But if the expulsion goes wrong, the burglar is stunned before being expelled. For the time being he causes no trouble, but he may wake at any moment and start trouble all over again.

Case History

I was asked to treat a child with asthma and eczema. Both conditions were quite variable, being worse at certain times than at others. The girl was ten-years old and a very good swimmer, so much so that she was undergoing intensive training. She was already on the county team and hoped to make it onto the national team. She had to do this in a few years, for the best age for women swimmers is between the ages of twelve and fourteen.

There were, of course, many factors contributing to the asthma and eczema, including reaction to the chlorine in the swimming pools, but the one feature which stood out was that all her symptoms were worse when she got tired. It did not matter if the tiredness was caused by swimming too much, by having a row with her parents, or by simply staying out too late at night. Regardless of why the tiredness occurred, her asthma and eczema got worse. In other words, *as the tide of her energy went out, the rocks of the illness started to appear!*

Swollen glands. This occurs because the pathogenic factor also lurks in the channels, where it obstructs the circulation of fluids and thereby gives rise to phlegm. The phlegm which accumulates in this way is generally very thick and sticky. A measure of its stickiness can be gained by actually feeling the glands. If they are soft and spongy, the phlegm is relatively soft. If they are hard and slippery (like pearls or oiled ball-bearings), then the phlegm in the system is very tough and viscous. (*Note:* the glands also swell during an active stage of invasion by a pathogenic factor.)

Subtle character change. This is perhaps the most insidious change. It happens because the whole balance of energy between the organs and channels is changed. This then causes a reaction in the emotional pattern of the child. Even when the child's energy is good, it is still "colored." It is as though the child's inner light, instead of being pure, is seen through stained glass. If this subtle change in character lasts through the fourteen-year transition period, it can entirely color the way the person relates to other people and to the world. Part of the cause of many broken marriages and tempestuous relationships is a lingering pathogenic factor.

Sudden collapse of energy. This occurs because, from time to time, the energy of the body is diverted toward fighting the lingering pathogenic factor.

Case History

Quite early on in my practice of treating children, a one-year-old girl was brought to me for treatment of eczema. She looked adorable, had great big brown eyes, smiled and gurgled, and never complained. The only problem was rather unsightly eczema on her arms and legs, which caused her to wake up and scratch at night.

I do not remember exactly what treatment I gave her, but I do remember the response very well. It was not particularly dramatic, but after several treatments when the eczema was much improved, the mother came to me and said, "What have you done to my lovely baby? When I brought her to you, she had a beautiful temper—cheerful and happy all the time. Now you have turned her into a monster. She is really demanding and I don't have a moment's peace!" She was only half serious (fortunately), but I was somewhat unnerved at the time. In retrospect, I can see what a really important change had taken place. If this child had not been treated, she would have developed the habit of being "nice" to people and concealing her true feelings. This might have continued through her entire life.

Intermittent abdominal pain. This occurs because the glands (or channels) in the abdomen are congested with phlegm, which interferes with the circulation of qi in the abdomen.

Other Symptoms Associated with Thick Phlegm

Superimposed on this pattern of thick phlegm may be either hot or cold symptoms (flavors in the soup). It is very common for a pathogenic factor to have a hot or cold aspect; thus, the common invasions are either wind-heat or wind-cold. In babies and children, such an invasion can give rise to a long-term change in the balance between heat and cold in the body. After an invasion of wind-heat, there are often heat symptoms left behind, while after an invasion of wind-cold, it is cold symptoms that often remain. This is especially true if antibiotics are used in treating the illness. In addition, heat symptoms are especially prominent if the pathogenic factor penetrates deeper and transforms into phlegm-heat invading the Lungs (bronchitis) or heat invading the Heart (meningitis).

Heat

- irritability, short temper
- insecurity, clinging to mother
- restlessness, even to the point of hyperactivity
- insomnia (hot type): difficulty in falling asleep, light sleeper
- red face; if heat affects the Lungs, then white face with red lips
- difficulty concentrating
- crossed eyes

Cold

- grumpy, whining
- colicky pains
- wakes up at night sweating from tummy pains
- pale face
- nasal discharge
- poor appetite
- loose stools
- vacant eyes

A symptom that one often sees is a rather vacant look in the child's eyes, showing a lack of spirit. They are not quite "with it." Whenever you see this sign, you should suspect a lingering pathogenic factor.

Examples of lingering pathogenic factors

Typically, these are diseases that recur again and again at regular intervals, maybe as often as every month. Examples include:

- chronic tonsillitis
- chronic otitis media
- chronic 'tickly' cough, which worsens when tired
- chronic cystitis

Why Does a Lingering Pathogenic Factor Take Hold?

The basic cause is clearly the invasion of a pathogenic factor and the difficulty in expelling it. But we may ask, Why are children more frequently affected in this way than are adults? There are, in fact, two main components: internal factors and external factors.

Internal factors

A child finds it difficult to recover completely because time seems to last much longer for a child. A fever may last the same time (a few days) in an adult and in a child, but for the child, a few days seem like a much longer time. Relative to its age, the days are ten to twenty times longer! For this reason, the child may well find it difficult to remember back to a time when all was well. For them, the illness has gone on for so long that it has obliterated from their memory the feeling of being really happy and well, and at ease with the world.

External factors

These are more straightforward. The child may have difficulty in recovering qi for a number of reasons:

- the child may have a weak constitution
- the mother and other adults around the child may be exhausted, and have no spare qi to give the child
- adults who care for the child may simply not have enough time in their busy lives to care fully for the child during convalescence
- the child was sent back to school too soon

There are also several reasons why a child may develop chronic phlegm:

- the child is given a diet containing a lot of phlegm-producing foods, for example, cow's milk, cheese, bananas
- the child lives in a very damp place
- the parents and adults around the child feel very gloomy and depressed

Recurring Attacks

Another effect of a lingering pathogenic factor is *local* weakening of qi. For example, after tonsillitis, the pathogenic factor may sit in the tonsils where it gives rise to local weakness of qi. This means that if another pathogenic factor should invade the Lung system, it will find that there is weakness in the throat and tonsils, and it will quickly go there. The arrival of this new external pathogenic factor has the effect of waking up the dormant pathogenic factor, and the original tonsillitis flares up once again. Likewise, children who have a lingering pathogenic factor in the Lungs after a respiratory infection may come down with another Lung problem, then another, and another.

This problem of repeated attacks is especially common in children who are treated with antibiotics. The antibiotics may stun the pathogenic factor but not completely expel it. This is not to say that antibiotics should never be used, but that they are limited in their effect. They are very helpful in clearing heat, but they are of no use in clearing phlegm or in restoring an imbalance. Thus, the treatment of illness with antibiotics very often gives rise to a lingering pathogenic factor.

Summary

The main patterns seen after an invasion of a pathogenic factor are qi deficiency or phlegm. After a period of time, these patterns will often resolve themselves in healthy children. However, some children are left with a pattern of thick phlegm, which we call a lingering pathogenic factor. Additionally, the pathogenic factor may leave behind aspects of either heat or cold.

Treatment

The treatments listed here are intended to serve only as guides, and apply mainly to lingering pathogenic factors affecting the Lungs. As we saw earlier, a lingering pathogenic factor can affect any part of the body—tonsils, ears, Lungs, and even the Intestines and Bladder. In the case of the Intestines and Bladder, treatment would be quite different from that shown below.

LUNG AND SPLEEN QI DEFICIENCY

Treatment principle	Tonify the Lungs and Spleen

Main points	L-9 *(tai yuan)*	Earth point of the Lung channel; tonifies Lung qi
	S-36 *(zu san li)*	Tonifies Stomach and Spleen qi

Method — The tonifying, or reinforcing, method is used; treatment is given once or twice a week.

Secondary points	L-5 *(chi ze)*	Water point of the Lung channel; can be used to tonify the Lungs
	B-13 *(fei shu)*	Removes phlegm

Treatment principle — Clear the phlegm

Points — L-7 *(lie que)*
S-40 *(feng long)*

Method — Even or dispersing method is used; treat once or twice a week.

Thick phlegm — Here the phlegm is so thick that it is often not apparent.

Points — Points are used which soften the phlegm, three of which are often used together:

bai lao (M-HN-30)
B-18 *(gan shu)*
B-20 *(pi shu)*

Bai lao (M-HN-30) is an extra (miscellaneous) point located on the neck, one unit on either side of the midline, and two units above GV-14 *(da zhui)*. It is used to treat swollen glands, and has a very marked effect on moving and softening phlegm which has congealed into hard lumps in the glands. After using this point, you often see an increase in the amount of phlegm that is coughed up.

The back *shū* points of the Liver and Spleen, B-18 *(gan shu)* and B-20 *(pi shu)*, respectively, are generally used for tonifying their associated organs. However, when needled with an even technique or a moving technique, they have the effect of softening very thick phlegm.

Priorities in Treatment

First, treat the qi deficient or phlegm pattern; only later on should you treat the thick phlegm, which is to say, the lingering pathogenic factor. There is no point in treating the lingering pathogenic factor if the child is weak—it simply does not have the strength to throw out the lingering pathogenic factor. Also, there is no point in treating the lingering pathogenic factor if there is lots of phlegm. The effect of such treatment will just be to increase the amount of phlegm.

Effects of Treatment

Lung and Spleen qi deficiency

Treatment will have a gradual effect. Slowly, over a period of about ten to fifteen treatments, the child will get better. Very often the pattern changes, from deficiency to phlegm, and sometimes to the thick phlegm pattern.

Phlegm

The first effect of treatment is that some of the phlegm will be cleared. Commonly, the child coughs a lot. Sometimes the stools become loose and glistening, almost diarrhea-like, as the phlegm is passed out through the stools.

As with the deficiency pattern, it may take ten to fifteen treatments to resolve, although if the condition is of recent origin, it may take much less. In addition, this pattern may well evolve into the thick phlegm pattern.

Thick phlegm (lingering pathogenic factor)

The primary aim of treatment is to soften the phlegm. This means that if the treatment is successful, the hard phlegm which was so viscous that it could not be coughed up, now becomes softer, and there will be more signs of phlegm. In some cases, so much phlegm will be liberated that a quite severe, but productive, cough results. If this should happen the treatment must be changed, for the pattern has reverted back to phlegm. The thick phlegm pattern generally takes longer to cure, which is to say, from twenty to thirty treatments.

You will see that, during the course of treatment, it is common for a child who first came with one pattern to return the next time with a different pattern. It is important to take note of what is actually going on and to change your treatment each time, if necessary.

Behavioral changes

There is another common effect that one sees when treating lingering pathogenic factors, namely, bad behavior and emotional disturbances. During the course of treatment, often after about four or five treatments, the child becomes bad tempered and shows stubbornness and irritability. This can be disturbing to the parents, who may feel that you have made their child worse than it was before treatment started.

In fact, this behavior is a sign that the treatment is really beginning to work. What is happening is that the child is starting to get in touch with its emotions, and for the first time in perhaps many years has enough energy to do something with them, to express them, to say what he or she feels, and to do something about changing the child's place in the family.

At first the child tends to overreact, being much more stubborn than it needs to be, or using much more violent methods than are necessary. However, you can reassure parents that this behavior will eventually settle down over a period of a few months.

Case History

Curing a child with a lingering pathogenic factor is sometimes very easy and sometimes very difficult. It is easy when the child has a straightforward pattern and is basically a straightforward child living in a happy family atmosphere. But the patients that we saw in our London clinic did not always belong to this category. Most of the children had inadequate diets (because of the poor quality of the nonorganic foods), suffered from the effects of atmospheric pollution, and lived in families where every member was stressed out. This made the cure much more difficult. A good example of this was a boy I treated who was suffering from chronic tonsillitis.

The pattern was for this child to suffer an attack of acute tonsillitis. There would be mild fever, great pain in the throat, and enormously swollen tonsils that contained pustules; meanwhile, he felt thoroughly dreadful. These attacks would come every month or two, and each time were treated with antibiotics. He came to me when he was eleven years old, by which time he had taken countless courses of antibiotics.

In view of the chronic nature of the problem, I predicted a period of six or more months to cure him. Little did I know! It took many more than six months. As it turned out, he had circumstances in his life which compounded his illness: he was in a state of almost permanent rage.

It was clear that his bosom was filled with anger and bitterness, and from the very first treatment, he used to describe dreadful ways in which he would like to murder the various members of his class at school. For example, he described in vivid detail the pleasure he would get from seeing one person's arms dissolve in acid!

At first I thought this was due to the obviously stressed state of his parents. But as time went on, it became clear that there was another cause, just as important: he was one of only six boys in his class, in a group of over seventy girls. For some reason, the girls had turned against the boys (as a group) and took great pleasure in taunting them. It was a reenactment of Thurber's *War of the Sexes*! In addition to this, he had more than an hour and a half of travel each way to school at the beginning and end of the day.

So, at school his rage boiled up but was not allowed to be expressed any further than the throat. At home, his parents were so tense that they were the ones that needed comforting by him! Small wonder that the heat and phlegm collected in the throat and gave rise to tonsillitis.

The parents were in fact very pleased with the treatment. The tonsils did not go down at first, but since the first treatment, he never had one attack of acute tonsillitis again.

His treatment continued, once every two to three weeks, for over two years. During this time his anger subsided quite a bit, but was still always there, smoldering beneath the surface. Sometimes it would flare up after a bad incident at school or a violent program on television. At the end of this, he at last moved to a new school, where he was much happier. Treatment continued for a few more sessions, during which the tonsils started to go down. He is now happy, and the tonsils have shrunk to a normal size.

A comment about the treatment: although the treatment did not make any difference to his symptom of swollen (but not inflamed) tonsils while he was going to a school he hated, it nevertheless had a very supportive role at this time. It enabled him to bounce up as soon as the external stress was taken away. Without the continued treatment, it is likely that the pattern of repeated attacks of acute tonsillitis would have recurred, so that when he reached the all-important transitions at puberty, his health would have taken a turn for the worse, rather than for the better.

Advice

There are two areas where advice can be helpful in getting over a lingering pathogenic factor, and these relate to the two main components, phlegm and qi deficiency.

Overcoming phlegm

The main advice is to avoid phlegm-producing foods, in particular:

- cow's milk
- cow's cheese
- sugar (including in biscuits and cakes)
- bananas
- more than one orange a week
- peanuts, including peanut butter

Parents sometimes resist this advice, saying that they have tried doing this already, but that it did not make any difference. Even though this may be the case, it is really worth trying again during the course of treatment. You can explain that simply giving up these foods may not be enough to cure a case of really thick phlegm or qi deficiency, but it will certainly help in the cure when receiving some treatment.

Overcoming qi deficiency

The main advice is to make sure that the child does not become too exhausted. This may mean keeping the child out of school, reducing its workload at school, or its activities after school, until the condition is resolved. In very young children, it may mean spending more time with the child. *But be careful:* this advice may be unwelcome when both parents work!

Effects of Antibiotics

In an ideal world, infectious diseases in children—invasion by pathogenic factors—would be treated by a natural medicine. In practice, they are usually treated with antibiotics, which are an imperfect medicine. Granted, in some situations antibiotics are a wonder drug. There is no doubt that millions of people have been saved from an early death by the timely use of antibiotics. But these wonderful results should not blind us to their imperfections. All antibiotics of course have well-documented side effects, such as liver damage, and some people are allergic to this or that antibiotic. Likewise, there are longer-term effects which seem to be implicated in the use of antibiotics, such as diabetes.

But there are some effects which are so common that they seem to go unreported. These are (in terms of Chinese medicine) the weakening of qi and increasing of dampness. The wonderful aspect of antibiotics (again in terms of Chinese medicine) is that they expel pathogenic heat. However, in doing so, they inevitably weaken the qi of the body. This effect is quite variable: some people react very strongly, feeling very tired and depressed when taking antibiotics, while others are hardly affected at all.

The other effect of antibiotics is to create dampness, since all antibiotics are products of fungi or molds. Consequently, they have to be grown in extremely damp conditions. Clinically, the accumulation of dampness manifests as diarrhea.

Symptoms

Symptoms of qi injury include:

- tired
- lethargic
- depressed
- grumpy
- choosy about food
- pale or green-gray face
- lots of catarrh

Symptoms of accumulation of dampness include:

- poor appetite
- loose stools or diarrhea
- runny nose

Symptoms of reaction

If a child has a tendency to cold disorders, or if some cold is left behind from another illness, the cooling and dispersing effect of antibiotics may aggravate the associated symptoms. In particular, one commonly sees:

- abdominal pain
- cold-type insomnia

APPENDIX

Accumulation Disorder (Excess Type)

For the sake of completeness, we mention here a pattern which is sometimes precipitated by an invasion of a pathogenic factor: accumulation disorder. As explained earlier, babies and toddlers need to consume a lot of food, and it is easy for accumulation disorder to arise. Common causes include rough food, unsuitable food, and irregular feeding. Accumulation disorder will occur whenever the amount of food consumed exceeds the capacity of the Spleen to transform it. In simple terms, if you eat too much food, you get tummy problems!

What sometimes happens during an infectious disease, especially if it is relatively mild, is that the child goes on eating just as much as it did before. But during the disease, much of the child's qi is being diverted to strengthening the protective qi to fight off the pathogenic factor. Consequently, there is much less qi available for digesting food. If the child then continues eating as much as before, accumulation disorder will arise.

Advice for parents

Reduce the food intake during infectious diseases to avoid accumulation disorder.

❖

4 ❖ Diagnosis

Woman:	"Could you cure this disease?"
Doctor:	"What is impossible for me? You have an ailment of the heart, and I have medicine of the heart. Turn your face to the light and let me have a good look."

When she had turned her face to the doctor, he gave it but a casual look, since he was a high official, and she a woman unrelated to him, so that it was against the rules of propriety that he should allow her to come too close to him.

—*from* Dee Goong An, *an 18th century Chinese detective novel*

INTRODUCTION

The diagnosis of children follows the same pattern as the diagnosis of adults: look, hear, ask, and feel. Of these, looking at the face and asking questions of the parents are the most important. Hearing is relatively less important, for the child's speech patterns are often changed when in an unfamiliar clinic. Feeling is also less important because of the difficulty in taking the pulse.

The following section on diagnostic features is based on *Pediatrics in Traditional Chinese Medicine (Zhong yi er ke xue)* by the Shanghai College of Traditional Chinese Medicine, with additions from our own experience in treating Western children. It is important when treating children with acupuncture to be familiar with the basics of Western (biomedical) diagnostics. This subject is not within the scope of this book, but I strongly recommend that the reader spend some time with basic pediatric texts in Western medicine.

Diagnosis of children is at once more difficult and easier than diagnosis of adults. It is more difficult because there are fewer signs and symptoms, and because children often have trouble describing their symptoms accurately. For example, I asked a child if he ever had a tummy ache. "Yes," he replied, "quite often!" A little later I asked him where he felt the tummy ache. "Oh, usually in my feet!" It is also more difficult because the mother is usually worried and is anxious for the child to be cured quickly. On the other hand, diagnosis of children is easier because their illnesses are usually simple.

LOOKING

When treating children, the looking phase of diagnosis is the most important of the four diagnoses, for two reasons. As will be made clear in the section on treatment, the most important single factor is determining whether the baby or child is strong or weak, that is, excessive or deficient. This is more important for children than for adults, where often the most important factor is the affected organ, rather than the overall level of qi. Diagnosing precisely what is wrong can often be done by asking the mother, but the level of qi is best determined by looking. This can usually be done in a few seconds, but they are the most important seconds of the diagnosis.

The second reason for carefully observing the child is to determine the success (or otherwise) of treatment. After the first few treatments, the parent may initially notice no change in the child; but if the treatments are having an effect, you will easily be able to tell this by simply looking, for the child will look healthier, its energy will be better, its eyes brighter, and the colors on the face less vivid.

Practical Aspects

There is an art to looking diagnosis, which begins at the moment you set eyes on the parent and child. At this stage you have to be very gentle, looking mainly at the parent. Look at the child only out of the corner of your eye, or just fleetingly. Children are very sensitive to being looked at, and if you give them a long hard stare, they will feel shy and may even burst into tears. This is a bad start!

As you look at the parent and child you should be doing two things. First, you should be absorbing the general feel. Just be there with the parent and child and try to get an idea of what it is like to be the parent and what it is like to be the child. Is the child loved by its parent? Is the child lonely, afraid, angry? And so on. Just let your intuition come into play.

At the same time as you are doing this, try and get the logical part of your mind to work—first of all, on the basic question of deficiency versus excess. Then, if you are happy with that answer, refine it further, and try to decide roughly what pattern the child has. One of the keys to diagnosis is knowing what you are looking for, and in this book we have made a list of the patterns that are common to children (see Appendix 1). As time goes on and you gain experience in handling and treating children, you can often identify the basic pattern before the parent and child have sat down.

In order to reach this stage of proficiency, here is a piece of advice: *believe what you see.* When treating adults, it can be difficult to figure out what the pattern is. Only by putting together the results of all four diagnostic methods can you decide with any degree of certainty. But with children it is different. Since they are so young, they have not had time to collect a whole heap of problems. Therefore, it is common for a child's appearance to be an accurate representation of what is really going on.

As the tables below illustrate, the interpretation of information gathered from looking at children can be slightly different from that of adults. This is to be expected owing to the differences in their physiologies. Rashes, however, are interpreted exactly the same.

Face and spirit (shén)

Looking at the face is the single most important part of diagnosis. This should begin with a general look at the whole face to take in the overall condition of the child, with a special look at the eyes, which show the child's spirit, and thus its will to get better. Broadly speaking, one will see either:

- an active child with a strong spirit, bright eyes, and a quick response; any disease such a child has will be mild
- a tired and sleepy child with a withered spirit, expressionless eyes, and little or no response to people or stimuli; this denotes a serious disease
- a characteristic glazed quality to the eyes that denotes the presence of a lingering pathogenic factor; this will gradually clear as the child's health improves

Facial color—In children these characteristics can change very rapidly, and are among the truest reflections of health. They are better than the tongue, which often does not change very much and can sometimes be difficult to get a look at; and are also better than the pulse, which is both difficult to determine and can change with the child's thoughts and feelings. Some aspects of facial color are related to race.

Body movement

Under this heading it is customary to include growth and development, motion, posture, and activity. Omitted from the table are the growth and development patterns as viewed by Western medicine, since this information can be found in many other books. There are also many other aspects of motion, posture, and activity which may quickly lead to a diagnosis, but are very difficult to describe.

The orifices

Looking at the orifices is a very important aspect of the examination. This includes not only the tongue, but also the oral cavity, ears, nose, eyes, and the two 'yin orifices' (the areas around the urethra and anus).

Finger vein or capillary

This is one diagnostic feature which is quite different in adults and children. It refers to the capillary that appears on the dorsal surface of the hand, somewhere in the region between LI-4 *(he gu)* and LI-3 *(san jian)*. In adults and healthy children there is no capillary there, but in some children the capillary is present and looks like a vein. At the end of the Ming dynasty, great importance was attached to this form of diagnosis, and about ten pages of the *Great Compendium of Acupuncture and Moxibustion (Zhen jiu da cheng)* are devoted to this subject alone. At present, this form of diagnosis is considered unreliable, except for the following features:

Three regions or 'gates'. If the vein described above spreads past the 'wind gate', the disease is mild. If it spreads past the 'qi gate', the disease is severe. And if it spreads past the 'life gate', the disease is life-threatening (see Fig. 4.1).

In my experience, the presence of a vein is an indication of a pathogenic factor—either violent, as with acute disease, or mild, as with a lingering pathogenic factor. However, the vein is not always there when it should be, and its absence should not be taken to mean the absence of a pathogenic factor.

HOW TO FIND IT

When you first look for the capillary it may not be visible, or is only faintly so. It can be made more visible by gently stroking along the line of the Large Intestine channel. This is usually done upwardly, toward the chest, in the direction of flow of the channel.

WHEN CAN IT BE OBSERVED?

It is commonly seen up to the age of three. Beyond that

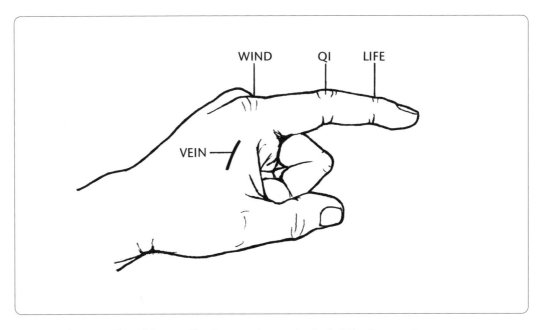

WIND   QI   LIFE

VEIN —

Fig. 4.1   *The three regions or 'gates' of the finger vein*

age, the capillary is rarely seen. If you do see it in older children (say, in a seven- or eight-year old), it has relatively greater significance.

DIFFERENT SHAPES

Length. The longer it is, the more active the pathogenic factor. If it goes past the knuckle joint, it is quite serious. If it goes right into the finger, it is really very serious and indicates a life-threatening condition.

Width. The broader it is, the stronger the pathogenic factor.

Color. The blacker it is, the hotter or more stagnant the pathogenic factor. By contrast, the redder it is, the colder the pathogenic factor. (This is opposite of what you might expect.) Finally, the fainter it is, the weaker the pathogenic factor (right).

Excretions

Although mentioned under the looking phase of diagnosis, this information is more commonly

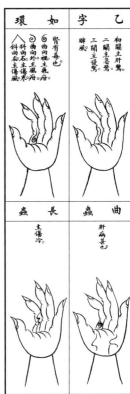

gathered by asking. Do not forget to ask about this, even though some patients may find it slightly embarrassing. As we will see below, this information is sometimes extremely important.

In the following tables are listed the diagnostic features mentioned in *Pediatrics in Traditional Chinese Medicine*. Many of these are the same for children as for adults. Those features which are either different in children, or especially significant in them, are indicated with a check mark (√).

TABLE 4.1

FACIAL COLOR

Red Face

Pink-red and shiny with glistening skin	A healthy child
Deep red	Heat. In practice, this is not very common and usually relates to heat from excess in febrile disease.
√Deep red with white forehead	Internal heat with Lung deficiency
√Deep red with green or yellow around the mouth	Usually accumulation disorder, but may be Liver yang rising
√Cheeks red most of the time	Accumulation disorder. In adults, red cheeks (often translated as 'malar flush') are an indication of yin deficiency. In Western children, however, this is rarely the case, but is an indication of accumulation disorder with the undigested food transforming into heat.
Cheeks red only in the afternoon	Damp-heat or internal heat from yin deficiency
Both cheeks bright red with remainder of face bright white, limbs cold, and rigid with cold sweats	Empty yang rising. This is seen in severe Lung disease such as pneumonia and tuberculosis. In the clinic, a less acute form of this pattern can be observed, often with only mild, recurrent symptoms. This is found in families with a history of pulmonary tuberculosis and in children who have been immunized against tuberculosis. In traditional Chinese medicine it is associated with the pattern of Lung yin deficiency and is often accompanied by symptoms of chronic sore throat, tonsillitis, and enuresis.
√One cheek red	Teething

Pale Face

Pale	Mostly cold or deficiency
White and puffy	Yang deficiency, dampness (extremely common)
White face and cold limbs	Collapse of yang

Yellow Face

Dark yellow	Usually dampness
Bright yellow	Internal damp-heat rising up, that is, yang dampness (jaundice)
Dull yellow	Damp-cold obstruction, that is, yin dampness (jaundice)
Dull yellow-grey	Long-term Spleen deficiency
√Dull yellow with white powdery patches on the cheeks, just lateral to the mouth	Intestinal parasites or thick phlegm

Qīng

In Chinese the color *qīng* (   ), usually translated as green or blue-green, can range from the greenish color of a person about to be sick, to the bluish color that is seen on the cheeks of some men who must shave frequently. The color is always dull. Below I have tried to distinguish shades of *qīng* in accordance with Western color classifications.

Qīng-bluish	Cold
Qīng-grey	Pain. Very occasionally this color is seen in children who have had a very bad shock. When there is blue-grey above the lips only, it denotes pain from indigestion.
Qīng-cyanotic	Blood stasis
Qīng-clear blue (slightly bluer than a vein)	Shock
Qīng-purplish-dull, shaking, no spirit	Convulsions
√Qīng-blue to grey with parts of the face white, furrowed brow, shouting	Internal cold, abdominal pain
Qīng-cyanotic with blue lips, panting, shortness of breath	Stagnant qi and blood, with obstruction of the Lung qi (pneumonia)

TABLE 4.2

BODY MOVEMENT/APPEARANCE

Big head, thin neck, big belly, thin chest and limbs	Childhood nutritional impairment
Hair dry and thin, easily falls out	Insufficient blood
√Excessive sleeping, motionless, and expressionless	Long-term disease which has led to weakness. Sometimes seen when the mother has been given too much anesthetic during childbirth.
Cannot move neck, shaking limbs, arched neck and back	Convulsions
Restless, touching, belly, shouting	Acute abdominal pain (may be an emergency)
√Clinging to mother	In itself it means fright or fear, although most commonly it arises from heat in the system affecting the Heart. May also be due to shock or insecurity from some factor such as discord between parents.
√Violent behavior	Interior heat from excess (common in boys). This includes hyperactive children as well as the more benign 'terrible twos'.
Beautiful or handsome, calm at interview but panic stricken with needle treatment, violent temper	Water does not control fire (often hereditary tuberculosis factor)
√Poor growth	Congenital weakness, unwanted child. If a child is unwanted by its parents, as sometimes happens to children of successful professionals, the parents may withdraw the supply of energy that children need to thrive, and consequently growth may stop. May also be due to lingering pathogenic factor from immunization (see Chapter 19).

TABLE 4.3

THE ORIFICES

Mouth

Inflammation	Heart and Spleen have accumulated heat; floating heat from deficiency

Spots	Mouth ulcer, or Koplik's spot, which is an indication of measles
Tonsils	Inspect for tonsillitis, diphtheria
Throat	When red may indicate wind-heat or yin deficiency
√*Dribbling at the mouth*	Dampness. If there is really excessive dribbling, dampness has combined with greater Spleen deficiency. B-20 *(pi shu)* is often needled.
√*Mouth hangs open*	Extreme qi deficiency, often associated with mental disturbance
√*Lips deep red, with white face*	Internal heat; usually indicates lingering pathogenic factor
Lips pale	Cold from deficiency
√*Lower lip protruding*	Constipation; childhood nutritional impairment; extreme stage of accumulation disorder
Gums red and swollen	Stomach heat
Breathing from the mouth	Nasal cavities blocked by thick phlegm

Tongue

Traditionally, one can use the normal rules of tongue diagnosis in children.

Tongue body	Clinically, the tongue body of Western children is several shades redder than for the same condition in adults. Thus, a red tongue is normal; what would be a normal color for an adult indicates cold in a child; and a hot disorder in a child is indicated by a red color rarely seen in adults. The most reliable feature is a red tip to the tongue, which always denotes either mental irritation or wind-heat.
Tongue coating	The coating of the tongue is an unreliable indicator in children. Often there is just a normal thin, white coating on the tongue, even though the child is suffering from phlegm, dampness, or retention of food. In contrast, some babies may have a greasy tongue coating most of the time, even when in good health.
√*Features and cracks on the tongue*	If there is any feature—such as a crack—on the tongue, it is usually of significance. For example, even the faintest crack at the end of the tongue can indicate Heart deficiency.

Ears

√*Purulent and foul discharge*	Damp-heat either in the Liver and Gallbladder channels, or as a lingering pathogenic factor

Dark brown discharge	Liver childhood nutritional impairment or accumulation disorder with phlegm which invades the Liver and Gallbladder channels
√*A low and small ear*	Poor constitution
√*Tip of ear below the level of the eyes*	Constitution is very weak. In earlier times this signified that the child would likely die before its first birthday. With higher living standards and hygiene, the child will now normally survive. However, the child will be frail, and when it contracts an illness, it is a long and difficult process to cure. Sometimes, as the child grows stronger, the position of the ear may rise, reflecting the stronger constitution.

Nose

Watery discharge	Wind-cold, dampness
√*Thick white discharge*	Phlegm
√*Thick yellow discharge*	Wind-heat, heat in Intestines
√*Thick green discharge*	Phlegm with stagnation affecting the Liver
√*Thick green-blue discharge*	Lung childhood nutritional impairment, that is, extreme accumulation disorder with Lung deficiency
Alar flaring	Lung heat
Nose dry and irritated	Lung heat, wind-heat
Crusts below nose	Chronic catarrh
Lingering boil on cheek	A sign of tuberculosis in the family (the tuberculous miasm of homeopathy). Often accompanies Lung weakness, or indicates stagnation of Liver qi.

Eyes

Inflammation	Internal heat, wind-heat
√*Blue sclera*	Liver heat
Yellow sclera	Dampness
√*Black spots in sclera*	Intestinal parasites
√*Whites of eyes show while sleeping*	Spleen yang deficiency
√*Red and dry skin in between eyebrows*	Localized internal heat, which may lead to convulsions
Puffy bags below the eyes	Kidney and Spleen deficiency, dampness collects; usually congenital (e.g., premature birth) or nephritis

√*Sunken eyes*	Body fluids exhausted, dehydration; in chronic disease, extreme Kidney weakness
Dark (black) circles around the eyes	Kidney deficiency: with red cheeks, yin deficiency; with white cheeks, yang deficiency
Brown around the eyes	Usually steroid poisoning
√*Blue below the eyes*	Shock (distinguish carefully between blue of shock and black of exhaustion)
√*Blue between the eyes*	Shock, possibly before birth
√*Green between the eyes*	Dampness (often difficult to distinguish from blue; refer to other symptoms)
Watery eyes	Accumulation of dampness internally, or attack of external wind-dampness, that is, a cold in the head
Gluey discharge from eyes	Internal phlegm rising up to the eyes, or external attack of damp-heat
Photophobia with watery eyes	Measles, womb heat
Dry eyes	Liver yin deficiency, Liver childhood nutritional impairment
Pale eyelids on inside	Blood deficiency

Two Yin (Anus and Urethral Orifice)

Yellow skin in genital area	Dampness or damp-heat
√*Recurrent diaper rash, in spite of careful hygiene*	Damp-heat in the Liver channel, often from accumulation disorder
Sore and irritated anus	Heat in the Intestines
√*Anal itching, worse at night*	Pinworms

TABLE 4.4

	FINGER VEIN
Superficial	Exterior disease
Deep	Interior disease
Dark red or purple	Heat
Black	Heat congestion, food congestion
Pale red	Cold
Broad	Excess
Narrow	Deficiency

TABLE 4.5

EXCRETIONS

Stools

Yellow and soft, not dry or oily	Normal for babies
√*Green*	Wind-cold or injury to the Spleen from overfeeding, accumulation disorder
√*Thin, watery, flecked with white*	Further injury to the Spleen from overfeeding
√*White masses in stool*	Stagnation in the Stomach
Watery and yellow with bad smell	Damp-heat obstruction
√*Stools like soy sauce in babies, with occasional crying*	Intestinal prolapse
√*Irregular stools, maybe missing a day, then loose and bad-smelling*	Accumulation disorder
Stools dry and in pieces	Heat from excess or yin deficiency
Itching anus	Intestinal parasites, usually thread worms (pinworms)
Undigested food in stools	Spleen qi deficiency. The Spleen yang is insufficient to digest the food. In mild cases, only raisins and raw carrots come through. In severe cases, other foods come through as well. This symptom also occurs when the diet is totally inappropriate.
Shiny stools	Phlegm in the digestive system

Urine

Dark or yellow, painful	Damp-heat
Turbid as though containing milk	Spleen yang deficiency, unregulated diet
Red	Probably blood in urine
Dark yellow	Damp-heat pouring down (jaundice)

TABLE 4.6

RASHES

Red	Heat
Raised	Dampness
Oozes watery fluid	Dampness
Itching	Wind, stagnation of blood and qi
Purple	Heat in blood, or Spleen not controlling the blood
	Note: rashes with a clearly defined edge are more difficult to cure than those with an indistinct edge.

TABLE 4.7

HEARING AND SMELLING

Voice

Strong voice	Excess
Weak voice	Deficiency
Shouting	Pain
√*Voice too low in pitch by school age*	Kidney deficiency. (The Lung qi controls the strength of the voice, and the Kidney essence controls the timbre.)
Hoarse voice	Wind-heat (may also sound low in pitch)
Gurgling noises	Phlegm
Loss of voice	Externally contracted sore throat or yin deficiency

Speech

Incessant talking, but intelligible	Heat affects the Heart
Incoherent babbling (delirium)	Pathogenic heat at the yang brightness organ stage or at the nutritive level
√*Poor grammar, forgets words, late development*	Possible brain damage. However, if other signs and symptoms are present, this indicates phlegm clouding the Heart, in which case it is curable.

Breathing

Gurgling	Phlegm in the bronchi
√*Sniffling, snoring*	Phlegm in the nose
√*Mouth breathing*	Nasal cavities blocked by phlegm; swollen adenoids due to lingering pathogenic factor

Smells

√*Breath smells like bad eggs*	Stomach heat
√*Burping sour gas or smells like bad eggs*	Too much rich food, injury from food, accumulation disorder
√*Smell of bad apples (sour)*	Too much rich food, accumulation disorder, injury from food
√*Stools have foul smell*	Heat due to accumulation or damp-heat
Urine has foul smell	Damp-heat pouring down
Urine is without smell and is copious	Spleen and Kidneys cold from deficiency

---

TABLE 4.8

ASKING

The asking phase of diagnosis is almost the same for children as it is for adults, but this information is usually obtained from the parents. Below, I have generally listed only the major headings as a reminder of what to ask.

1. Hot or Cold

2. Perspiration

3. Head Area

Sweating of the head area only after feeding	Heat in the Stomach, or Heart qi deficiency
Sweating of the head at night	May not be pathological
Pain	
Dizziness	
Consciousness	

Learning ability	If a child grows rapidly, its learning ability may be temporarily retarded, and if it grows slowly, its learning ability may be advanced. The deficits are usually made up later.

4. Food and Drink

√*Poor appetite*	Spleen qi deficiency
√*Choosy about food*	Spleen qi deficiency
√*Irregular appetite*	Phlegm, lingering pathogenic factor, glandular congestion
Abdominal distention after meals	Spleen qi deficiency, accumulation disorder
Good appetite but irregular stools	Stomach strong, Spleen weak
Vomits a little after feeding	Water in Stomach, Stomach yang deficiency; or mother's milk is too watery
√*Vomits a lot of partly digested food*	Accumulation disorder, Spleen cold from deficiency
√*Vomits water*	Phlegm accumulation
Vomit is foul-smelling	Accumulation of heat in the Spleen and Stomach
Dry heaves	Yin deficiency with depletion of fluids

5. Chest and Abdomen

Stifling sensation, pain, distention

6. Hearing

Poor hearing often denotes phlegm

7. Family Illnesses
8. Sleep

Not enough sleep	Leads to qi deficiency and then to Kidney deficiency
Too much sleep	Spleen yang deficiency, dampness
Grinds teeth in sleep	Stagnation in the Intestines, intestinal worms
Insomnia	See Chapter 27
Dreams of fighting things	Accumulation disorder, Spleen cold from deficiency, or reaction to a violent television program or movie
Vivid dreams	Heart heat, yin deficiency

9. Pregnancy, Birth, and Postnatal

Prenatal	Health of mother, shock, rashes, infectious diseases, anemia
Birth	Unusual features, trauma, anesthetics, caesarian, long labor
Postnatal	Jaundice, appetite, breast feeding, breathing, immunizations, childhood diseases

10. Family circumstances

Living conditions, brothers and sisters, family stress, family conditions (e.g., one-parent family)

TABLE 4.9

TOUCHING (PALPATION)

In adults this means primarily taking the pulse. In children, however, this is not possible before about the age of three, and even at this age, the practitioner's finger is likely to cover all three positions at the same time. Moreover, with very young children, there is a thick layer of subcutaneous fat which makes pulse-taking difficult. By three, however, the pulse is worth taking; one can determine the speed and whether it is superficial or deep, strong or weak, and sometimes slippery or not. Each of these characteristics has the same significance as in adults, except that at three years of age the normal pulse rate is about 100 to 120, at five years it is 80 to 90, and even up to puberty a slightly rapid pulse is normal. Beyond about the age of five, normal pulse diagnosis is possible, provided that the child can keep still. The positions and qualities have the same significance as in adults.

Of more importance in children is feeling the lymph glands, back, abdomen, and limbs.

Examining the Lymph Glands

As you will see on the next page, swollen lymph glands are a sign of a pathogenic factor: either an active pathogenic factor, as in wind-heat, or a passive lingering pathogenic factor. What is not so clear is that examination of the lymph glands in the neck should be part of your routine examination of children. It should certainly be done at the first appointment, and thereafter periodically during the course of treatment to see how they are getting on.

Here, we will show how to examine these glands. It is not difficult, but should always be done. There are three sets of glands (which is a slightly misleading word, as we actually feel the lymph nodes) in the neck that we commonly examine:

1. submaxillary, which are midway between the angle and the tip of the mandible
2. cervical chains
3. tonsillar, which are located at the angle of the mandible.

How to palpate the glands (Fig. 4.2)

Use the pads of your fingers. Move the skin over the underlying tissue in each area, rather than moving your fingers over the skin. The child should be relaxed, with the neck flexed slightly forward, and if necessary slightly toward the side. You can usually examine both sides at once.

Feeling the Back and Abdomen

In older children, have the child stand in front of you, facing sideways. Place one hand on the chest and one opposite, on the back. Quickly run your hands down the whole of the torso and notice the shape and energy of the abdomen and the back, especially the lower back. Feel the back for strength and hollows (Fig. 4.3).

Feeling the Limbs

Gently palpate the arms and legs for tone quality, and to feel the size of the bones. It will tell you a lot about the level of qi and accumulation of dampness, among other things.

Lymph Glands (Nodes)

Examine especially in the neck and groin. These should be examined routinely in all babies and children.

Swollen when there is a fever

External pathogenic factor

Swollen but not painful

Glandular congestion, lingering pathogenic factor

Swollen and painful

Phlegm toxin

Swollen and painful below jaw

Parotitis

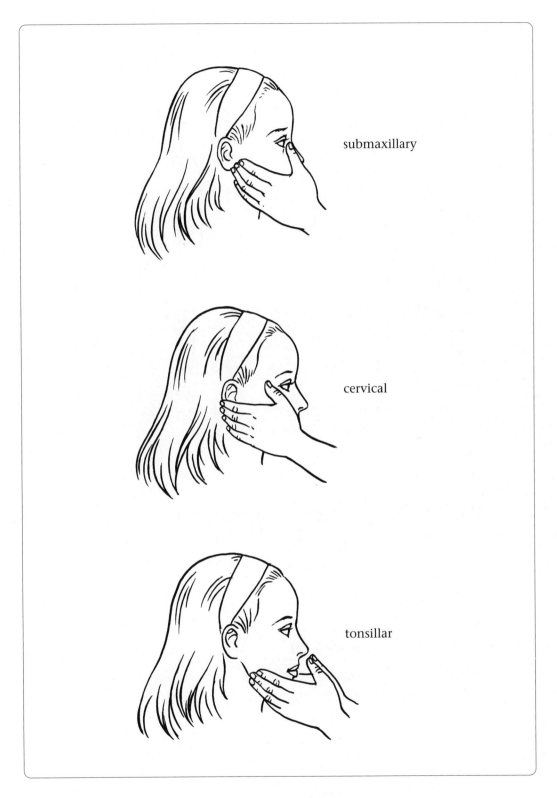

Fig. 4.2   *Feeling the lymph glands (nodes)*

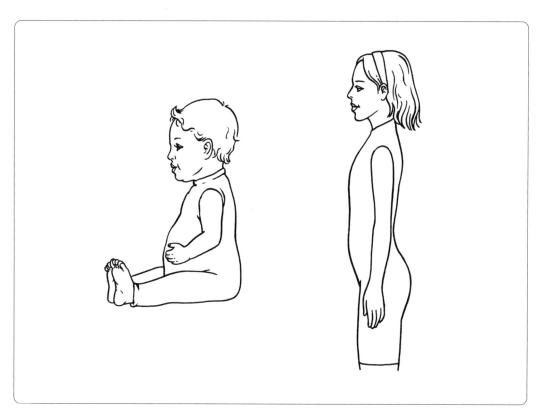

Fig. 4.3   *Feeling the back*

Skin

Cold with sweating	Insufficient yang qi
Hot without sweating	Fever in patterns of superficial excess
Palms and soles hot	Yin deficiency, heat from excess at the yang brightness stage
Skin shows pitting when pressed	Edema

Head Area

Palpate the head area carefully to inspect the fontanel for closure. Closure should be complete by eighteen months to two years.

Chest and Abdomen

Concave chest	Rickets. Abdomen should be soft and tender and not painful on palpation.

Abdominal pain, relieved by palpation	Deficiency or cold
Abdominal pain, aggravated by palpation	Excess, worms

Back

Areas of cold or tenderness	Externally contracted disease (cupping helpful)
Lower back hollow with tight but weak muscles	Kidney deficiency
Lower abdomen tight but not distended	This is often seen in children who suffer from enuresis, and is a key sign of Kidney and Bladder weakness. As the child gets stronger, this tightness is replaced by a more flexible quality.
Back curved in	A child should be able to stand up straight without effort. A curved back means, at the very least, that the child's qi is weak. Usually the curvature is in the lumbar region, where it indicates Kidney qi weakness.

Arms and Legs

Inspect the arms and legs for function and reflexes, and for swollen joints. Feel the tone of the muscles, which is an indication of the overall level of qi. Feel the squashy feeling associated with dampness, and for the characteristic 'dead' feeling of limbs affected by brain or nerve damage.

TABLE 4.10

THE FIVE TYPES OF CHILDHOOD NUTRITIONAL IMPAIRMENT

This table lists the commonly observed types of childhood nutritional impairment *(gān)* that affect the five yin organs. This list has been developed over the centuries and is reproduced here more or less as it appears in the *Great Compendium of Acupuncture and Moxibustion (Zhen jiu da cheng)*. The same list can be found in modern textbooks on children's diseases, often accompanied by a note that knowledge of these patterns can be useful in situations where it is difficult to arrive at a clear diagnosis.

Liver

Main illness	Wind
Facial color	Qīng
Pulse and stools	Wiry; green
General symptoms	Fingernails blue-green Eyes diseased and watery Shakes head and rubs eyes Discharge of thick, dark fluid from ears Large blue veins on abdomen
Other symptoms	*Excess:* eyes diseased and painful, shouts, acute attack of rigid neck and back, twitching with violence *Deficiency:* grinds teeth, much sighing *Heat:* sclera of eyes blue, gasping for breath, foul breath

Heart

Main illness	Convulsions, heat
Facial color	Red
Pulse and stools	Rapid; dry
General symptoms	Fever and agitation Snaps teeth and moves tongue Sweating, thirst Sores in mouth, foul breath Body thin
Other symptoms	*Excess:* fever, thirst, weeping, likes lying face upward, convulsions *Deficiency:* lying down, palpitations *Heat:* high fever, Heart and chest hot, thirst, prefers cold drinks, eyelids tremble, eyes red, shuts eyes and sleeps, delirious

Spleen

Main illness	Tiredness
Facial color	Yellow
Pulse and stools	Slow; rotten, glutinous diarrhea
General symptoms	Emaciated, flesh wasted Stomach and abdomen hard and full; head appears too large, and neck too thin

Other symptoms	*Excess:* tired, cannot think, body hot, thirst with desire to drink, diarrhea with yellow color
	Deficiency: vomiting, diarrhea with white color, sleeps with eyes showing
	Heat: sclera of eyes yellow, urine red

Lung

Main illness	Asthma
Facial color	White
Pulse	Floating
General symptoms	Coughing Breath smells fishy Withered hair, white hair Blue-green discharge from nose Sores in nostrils Vomiting
Other symptoms	*Excess:* gurgling and difficulty in breathing, cough, chest full and oppressed, thirst with no desire to drink, copious nasal discharge
	Deficiency: choking, difficult to breathe in and easy to breathe out, asthma with shallow breathing, skin and hair dry and withered

Kidney

Main illness	Cold from deficiency
Facial color	Black (ashen)
Pulse and stools	Deep; diarrhea
General symptoms	Feet cold and discolored Incomplete closing of fontanel
Other symptoms	*Heat:* acute asthma, breathing not calm, nose dry or epistaxis, hand rubs eyebrows, eyes, nose, and face
	Deficiency: urine clear

❖

5 ❖ Using Acupuncture in the Treatment of Children

INTRODUCTION

For a variety of reasons that are often ill-founded, acupuncture is not widely used in the Western world in the treatment of children. Some believe that it is too much of an intrusion into the baby's body or that it is too painful or traumatic. In fact, acupuncture is a gentle method of treating babies and children, and can be used from the moment they are born. It is not, perhaps, as gentle as homeopathy; but compared to Western medicine, which, even before treatment is considered, may involve the insertion of large needles for diagnostic blood tests, the near-painless insertion of very fine needles in acupuncture is indeed a gentle technique.

Even in China, acupuncture is used only rarely on children. There are two reasons for this: first, there is the choice of Chinese herbs, which the long-suffering children are trained to drink from an early age. Second, the needles available in China are much coarser than the ultrafine Japanese needles available in the West. With thick needles it is easy to cause pain and difficult to tonify, but with thin ones, it is much easier to tonify and pain-free needling is possible.

It is true that acupuncture must be used with caution on babies and children, for the needles have a relatively stronger effect than on adults. However, anyone who has seen acupuncture in practice knows that the alarm that a minority of children experience is worth the speed of cure.

It is also important to bear in mind that although children cry when they experience pain, they do not fear it as many adults do. A child's life is full of pain, for in the very early years all unpleasant sensations are experienced as pain—whether it be hunger, wet diapers, indigestion, falling over, or loneliness. Thus, much as younger children may dislike acupuncture, for many the trauma is no worse than having their face roughly washed.

Acupuncture can be used at any age for a wide range of diseases. The youngest patient seen in our Brighton clinic was less than one week old. The discussion of disorders in this book represents only an introduction to the most commonly seen pediatric diseases; just because a problem is not mentioned here does not mean that it is one for which acupuncture is ineffective. For example, we have treated a number of rare congenital disorders, some of them with great success. A brief survey of illnesses treated with acupuncture is provided in Chapter 6.

The basis of this book is traditional Chinese medicine as it has evolved over centuries of time. Chinese medicine was not born from the brain of one person, nor did it come into the world fully formed. It has developed over thousands of years during which new ideas were constantly raised and tested in clinical practice. Ideas found to be worthless were rejected, and those that were useful were absorbed. Thus, many different ideas are incorporated in the body of traditional Chinese medicine, some of which appear to be mutually incompatible. Although this poses a stumbling block for the Western-trained mind, it can be avoided if one remembers that each idea is only a rule of thumb that is useful in a particular situation.

One of the constant features of traditional Chinese medicine has been the immediate interaction between diagnosis and treatment. Indeed, the Chinese phrase which is loosely translated as diagnosis is more accurately rendered as 'differentiation of patterns and determination of treatment', since the two are regarded as one and the same act. The conclusion to be drawn from this is obvious: when using acupuncture (or any of the other Chinese medical techniques), always use the traditional method of diagnosis. For those trained in Western medicine there is a temptation to use Western diagnosis as the basis for prescribing acupuncture treatment, but this will not bring particularly good or reliable results. This is not to say that Western diagnostic techniques are useless to the practitioner of acupuncture—quite the contrary. These tests serve to enrich one's understanding of Chinese medicine. But in the practice of acupuncture, they should never be allowed to replace the differentiation of patterns.

Preparation for Treatment

When treating children it is worth spending a little more time in preparing oneself than one would in treating adults. Indeed, if you are treating children and adults in the same day, it is a good idea to pause for a few minutes before treating the child. Preparation should consist of exercises to clear away bad thoughts and emotions, and to bring about a sense of calm (e.g., qi gong, meditation, taking a cup of tea and the like). If this is done, you will find that the children cry much less and are easier to handle during treatment. Babies and children are very sensitive to emotional states. If the practitioner is anxious or pressed for time, they will feel this and become restless and uncertain themselves.

Those of you who want to treat children but have none of your own would benefit from some special preparation. It is important to learn how to relate to children and how they think and perceive the world. For this reason it is useful to spend some time observing and playing with children at kindergarten or in play groups.

Practical Considerations

It can be a great joy to treat children, for they are so spontaneous and full of enthusiasm for life. In our experience, it is helpful to treat children and adults at different times. This is helpful both to the practitioner, who needs to approach children with a lighter manner and more spontaneity than adults, as well as to those patients who are old and infirm and need to be protected from hyperactive children.

Technical Considerations

Acupuncture can be nearly painless, but for this to be so it is essential that one develop a good needle technique. My (JPS) teacher in China, Dr. Zhang Caiyun, used to say that many people fear acupuncture because of the pain it causes, but that this fear is unnecessary. However, it is essential that one practice needle insertion to reduce pain. We encourage practitioners to needle themselves regularly to understand how much pain they are causing their patients.

How to avoid pain · It is an axiom of Chinese medicine that pain is caused by obstruction of qi. The key to reducing pain is to ensure that your own qi is flowing well, especially in your arms and fingers. In the accompanying illustrations we show some pictures of hands with the qi flowing reasonably well. You will notice that the fingers are very flexible, and that the joints of the fingers and wrist are never straight or bent back. They are always curved, in the same way that the joints are kept curved when practicing *tai ji*. This point cannot be emphasized too much: if the fingers are bent back, it means either a deficiency or lack of qi. In both cases, the child will feel much more pain.

Quick insertion | The skin is full of nerve endings that experience pain. A slow insertion through the surface layer is much more painful than a rapid insertion.

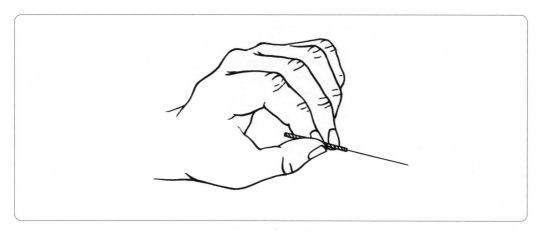

Fig. 5.1   *Joints are all bent and flexible*

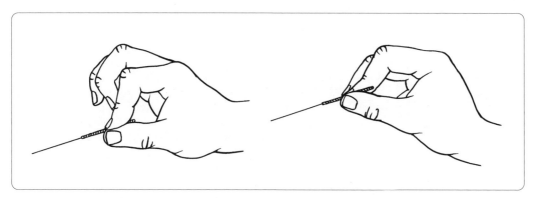

Fig. 5.2   *How not to hold the needle: the joint of the index finger is bent back, because the qi is stagnant. This will cause unnecessary pain.*

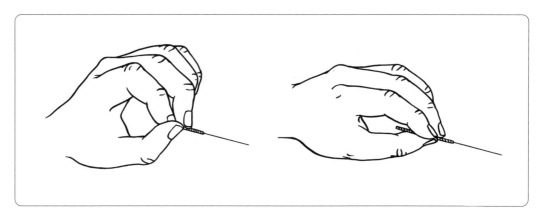

Fig. 5.3 *How the fingers extend during insertion. They should remain bent in a graceful curve at all times.*

The sequence below shows the insertion of needles in S-40 *(feng long)*. After the insertion, the practitioner lets go of the needle for a few seconds. This is because the child often wriggles at this stage. After the wriggling has settled down, the practitioner can grasp the needle again to perform the required qi manipulation.

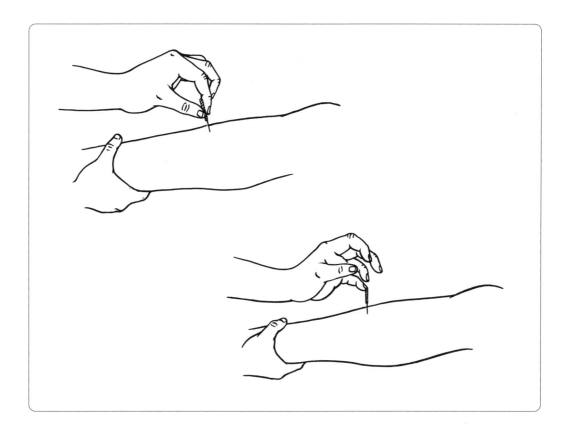

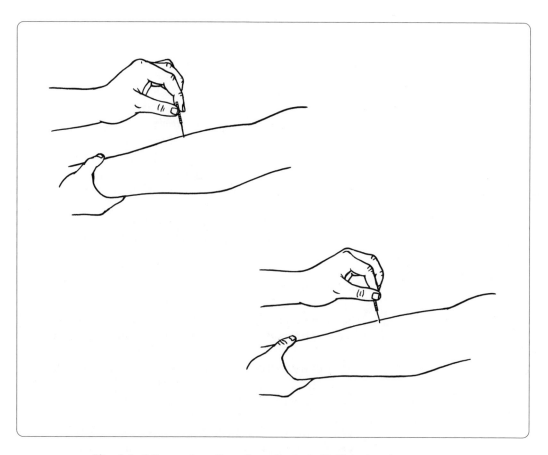

Fig. 5.4~5.7   *Insertion of needles in S-40 (feng long)*

Choice of needles

From birth to about five years of age, use 0.5-1 inch long 32 gauge (0.30mm diameter) Chinese needles with a very short handle. If finely-tapered Japanese needles are available, 34 gauge may be used instead. The short handle is preferred for babies, because although it is more difficult to manipulate and direct the qi, there is less risk of the needle catching on clothing (see below).

For children five to twelve years of age, use 1-inch long 32 gauge needles. These needles may seem rather thick, but a baby's skin is often quite tough and some force is needed to pierce the outer layer quickly. Thinner needles can easily bend and cause more pain.

Insertion

Insertion should be done quickly and forcefully. This is the most difficult part, for the needle should penetrate 0.5-1mm below the superficial layer of skin very rapidly. If the needle penetrates too slowly through the layer rich in nerves, or too deeply at high speed, a lot of pain will be experienced by the patient.

Babies' skin has a different texture from that of adults. It is more fine-grained, and there is a thicker and less firm subcutaneous layer of fat. This can make it very difficult to insert the needle, for the fine grain resists penetration, while the subcutaneous layer provides less support. It is helpful to grasp the skin firmly so that it does not move on insertion, and to use very finely-tapered and well-shaped needles.

When treating adults, the different stages of needling merge together into one fluid movement. When treating babies, each stage should be more discrete and separated. It is often helpful to pause briefly between stages. For example, in babies, especially when treating points on the legs, the practitioner should let go of the needle immediately after insertion. This will allow the baby time to kick and thrash its legs for a short while to relieve any discomfort it experiences from needle insertion. This is a situation where a short handled needle is most necessary. Babies and children often cry at this stage of the treatment. This crying is more often due to anger than to pain.

Further penetration

After penetrating the skin, the needle should be inserted to the required depth. These depths are the same (i.e., the same number of proportional units) as for adults.

Obtaining needle sensation (de qi)

When the needle has reached the required depth, the qi should be summoned in the normal way. It can be difficult to ascertain whether the qi has arrived. With experience, it can be felt as a heavy sensation in the hand used to manipulate the needle, and as a tingling feeling in the hand which is holding the baby's limb. It can also be ascertained by listening to the cry of the baby, which will change its note when the qi arrives. It must be explained to the mother that this cry is not one of pain, but of surprise at the unfamiliar sensation.

Tonification and dispersion

The most important differentiation to make when treating children is between deficiency and excess. The principles of treatment are simple: tonify in cases of deficiency, and disperse in cases of excess. It can be said that when treating children the choice of points is less important than whether to tonify or disperse. In clinical practice, it is sometimes difficult to maintain the objectivity required to make this very basic distinction, especially after hearing of the sufferings of a mother and child. One way to overcome this is to take a clear look at the child and ask yourself if there is enough qi available for the treatment you are about to give. Thus, in the case of accumulation disorder, you would ask whether there is enough strength to expel the accumulated food; or, in the case of asthma, whether there is enough strength to disperse the accumulated phlegm. If the answer is yes, then disperse; if the answer is no, then tonify.

To summarize, the choice of tonification or dispersion is relatively more important when treating children than adults. This is because the qi of a child is very strong in proportion to its small physical body, so that small manipulations of qi will have a relatively large effect on the body.

Retaining needles

After needle manipulation (if any), the needles are immediately withdrawn. There is generally no needle retention. As children get older, some retention may be considered for deficiency, but it is usually unnecessary under the age of ten.

Choice of points

It is said by some acupuncturists that the channels are not fully formed in children. To a certain extent this is true, and it is also true that differences in function among the points have not developed. The significance of this for the practitioner is that the choice of points is not so critical.

Number of points

Great care should be exercised with respect to the number of points chosen. For young babies, two points treated bilaterally (i.e., four insertions) is usually enough. Even for older children, there is rarely any need for more than six insertions per treatment. (The exception to this rule is in the treatment of paralysis following polio or hemiplegia.)

Frequency of treatment

In China, treatment is given every day or every other day, and there is no doubt that this brings the quickest results. However, this is not always practical for Western patients. Many of the treatments described in this book will be satisfactory for chronic diseases if given as infrequently as once a week—although the cure will certainly take longer. For acute disorders, treatment must be given frequently, maybe every two hours for problems like acute convulsions and febrile diseases.

Moxibustion

Direct moxibustion can be used on children as soon as they are old enough to tell you that they feel a burning sensation, provided they can hold still (usually about seven years). Under this age, indirect moxibustion should be used, with the right hand holding the moxibustion stick and the fingers of the left hand around the point to ascertain the degree of heating (Fig. 5.8). Moxibustion with ginger or garlic partitioning can also be used on babies, for there is less danger of burning the skin.

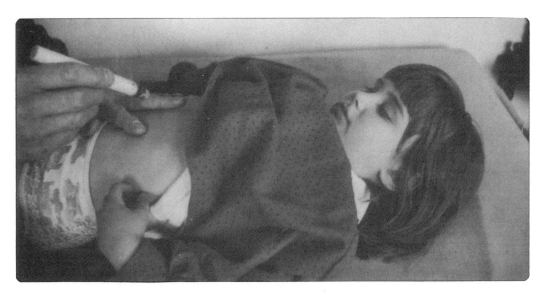

Fig. 5.8   *The practitioner's left hand monitors the heat during moxibustion*

*'Without heat'
moxibustion*

This technique is an extension of acupuncture, but might
better be called point irritation therapy. The principle is to
place a medicinal herb which is slightly irritating to the
skin on a point associated with the disease under treatment. The method is not widely used, but is convenient
for treating children and babies when needling is inappropriate. For example, it can be used for tonsillitis, where a
paste of crushed garlic is applied at LI-4 *(he gu)* for one to
two hours. It can also be used effectively for teething problems, where a powder of Fructus Evodiae Rutaecarpae *(wu
zhu yu)* moistened with vinegar is applied at the same
point and left on overnight. The herbs should be covered
with a waterproof plaster.

Massage of points

It is often asked whether one can massage the points
instead of doing acupuncture, and the answer is certainly
yes. For mild conditions, massage of the points is extremely effective. For most of the conditions described in this
book, however, massage is actually more painful than
acupuncture. Frequently, the points are spontaneously
tender, and for massage to be effective, at least two
minutes should be spent on each point, for a total of ten
to fifteen minutes per treatment. For many Western children, holding still for this length of time is more of a
penance than an acupuncture treatment.

*An important miscellan-
eous point for children*

The same miscellaneous or extra points (those outside the
channels) that are used for adults may be used for treating
children. There are a few miscellaneous points, however,

which are especially indicated for children. The location and usage of these points are described in the appropriate chapters. The exception is *si feng* (M-UE-9), which is so commonly used that we will describe it here.

Si Feng (M-UE-9)

Location: on the palmar surface, in the transverse creases of the proximal interphalangeal joints of the index, middle, ring, and little fingers (Fig. 5.9).

Indications: childhood nutritional impairment, accumulation disorder, pertussis, food allergies. This point has a strong dispersing action and should not be used where the child is extremely deficient .

Method: the Chinese textbooks recommend piercing with a triangular needle and withdrawing a few drops of clear yellow fluid. In practice, needling with a broad-gauge needle (32 or 30) is usually adequate for treating this point; and in practice the fluid comes out red! See Fig. 5.10 on how to hold the hand.

Note: pricking all four fingers on one hand constitutes a treatment.

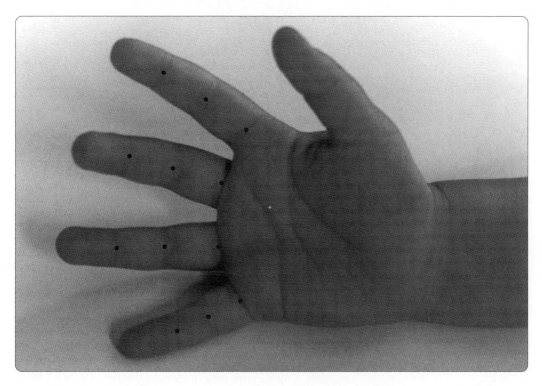

Fig. 5.9   *Location of the si feng points (M-UE-9)*

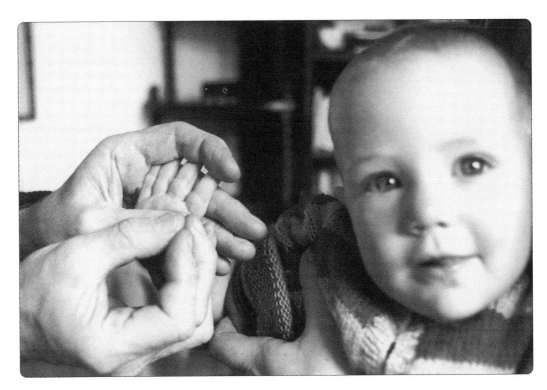

Fig. 5.10   *Method of holding the hand while needling si feng point (M-UE-9)*

Frequency of treatment: these points are powerful and their action continues for four to six days. However, for acute or serious disorders, treatment can be given every day.

Problems in Treating Children

The parents

Most children, although they do not relish acupuncture treatment, do not fear it either since they don't fear pain. Instead, it is usually the parents who are often very nervous and fearful for their children. As we have said before, it is important that the practitioner needle him- or herself to know the amount of pain that is being inflicted on the patient. For the same reason, in some cases it may be helpful to needle the parent.

The child

A minority of children have a great fear of needles. For these children the practitioner must decide if the treatment is worse than the illness or the alternative therapy, such as surgery. As a general rule, at least one needle should be inserted so that there is a basis for making a decision. Often, after one treatment, many children find that the needles are not so terrible after all.

The wriggling baby

Some babies, especially boys, are loath to be held or constrained in any way whatever. For such babies, being held still for needle insertion is far more trying than the needles themselves. These babies respond especially well to acupuncture, but some skill is needed to get the needle inserted.

Ask the parent to hold the child's arms, so that it does not push your hands away and cannot take the needle out once inserted. Locate the point quickly, keep your eye on the point, and wait until the baby is still for a fraction of a second, then quickly insert the needle and let go. The baby will resume its wriggling and writhing with the needle still in place, and you should wait until this settles before manipulating the qi, usually a dispersing technique if the baby has enough energy to wriggle that violently!

❖

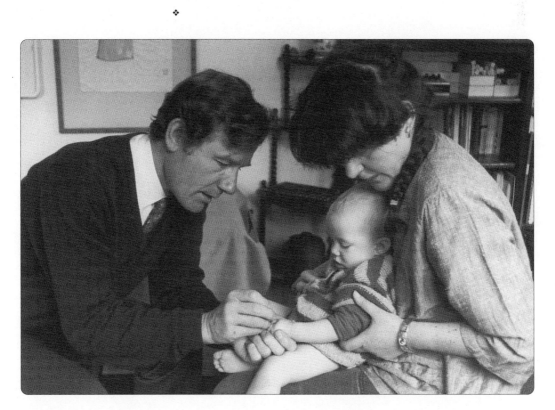

Fig. 5.11   *The baby is held on the mother's lap during treatment*

Part Two

The Treatment of Disease

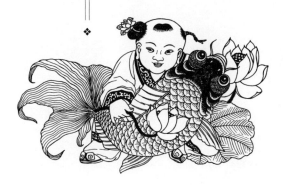

6 ❖ Outline of Common Patterns in Children

Pattern	Distinctive Symptoms
Digestive System	

<table>
<tr><td colspan="2">Digestive System</td></tr>
</table>

	Pattern	Distinctive Symptoms
	Digestive System	
Constipation	Excess	Active, pain is strong
	Cold	Pale face, not especially weak
	Deficient	Weak, shy
Diarrhea (acute)	External pathogenic factor	Sudden onset, often infectious
	Spleen and Stomach qi deficiency	Also pathogenic factor, frequent stools, bad odor
	Spleen and Kidney yang deficiency	Very weak, looks drained, serious illness
Diarrhea (chronic)	Injury from food	Possibly chronic, green stools
	Spleen and Stomach qi deficiency	Intermittent, chronic, undigested food in stools
Abdominal pain	Attack of cold	Sudden, often infectious, sensitive to food
	Blockage	Green stools or constipation
	Organ deficiency	Looks weak
	Worms	Patch on cheek, possibly cough
	Blood stasis	After injury or surgery

95

	Pattern	Distinctive Symptoms
Abdominal pain, cont.	Lingering pathogenic factor	Recurrent, dull pain, often exhausted for one to two hours
Vomiting	Obstruction of food	Often recurrent
	Cold from excess or deficiency	With abdominal pain; maybe an epidemic
	Stomach water	Vomits a little after each feeding
	Stomach phlegm	Signs of phlegm
	Heat	Red face
	Yin deficiency	Usually exhausted, glittering eyes
	Nervous	When excited

Respiratory System

	Pattern	Distinctive Symptoms
Influenza	Wind-cold	Cold signs
	Wind-heat • with phlegm • with accumulation • with fright	Heat signs • cough, nasal discharge • digestion disturbed • clingy
Cough (acute)	Wind-cold	Tickle in the throat
	Wind-heat	Sore, painful throat
	Wind-dampness	Copious nasal discharge
	Phlegm-heat	Acute bronchitis with painful chest
Cough (chronic)	Phlegm-dampness	Thick-sounding cough
	Lingering pathogenic factor	Hard cough
	Lung and Spleen qi deficiency	Weak, watery cough
Asthma (acute)	Spasm	Straightforward attack, whole chest seizes up, muscles in spasm
	Phlegm	Lots of phlegm, gurgling sounds
	Hot	Red face, feverish

	Pattern	Distinctive Symptoms
Asthma (chronic below age three)	Phlegm • Lungs only • accumulation disorder	Lots of phlegm apparent • stools and digestion normal • stools irregular
	Lung and Spleen qi deficiency • plain • hyperactive	 • poor appetite and lethargy • poor appetite with hyperactivity
	Lingering pathogenic factor • cold • hot	Swollen glands with no visible phlegm • cold signs • heat signs
Asthma (chronic above age five)	Lung qi deficiency	White face, frequent infections
	Spleen qi deficiency	Poor appetite
	Lingering pathogenic factor	Hard glands, no other major symptoms
	Kidney yang deficiency	Hunched shoulders
	Liver qi retarded	Worse with irritation
Tonsillitis (acute)	Wind-heat	Mild fever
	Lung and Stomach heat	Yang ming fever
Tonsillitis (chronic)	Lingering pathogenic factor	Swollen glands, recurrent infections
	Spleen qi deficiency	Exhaustion, recurrent infections
	Yin deficiency	Exhausted, overstimulated
Conjunctivitis	Wind-heat	Headache, fever
	Liver and Gallbladder fire	Red face, wiry pulse
Otitis media (acute)	External pathogenic factor	Sudden onset, floating pulse
	Liver and Gallbladder heat	Sudden onset, wiry pulse

	Pattern	Distinctive Symptoms
Otitis media (chronic)	Lingering pathogenic factor (excess)	Recurrent, glands swollen
	Spleen qi deficiency	Lethargic, phlegmatic
	Liver and Kidney yin deficiency	Excitable, hyperactive
Hay fever	Liver yang rising	Frequently flies into a rage
	Lingering pathogenic factor	Swollen glands, gray face
	Lung and Spleen qi deficiency	Droopy, probably has poor appetite

Miscellaneous Disorders

	Pattern	Distinctive Symptoms
Insomnia	Cold	Indigestion, so wakes up screaming
	Heat	Restless, afraid of the dark
	Fright	Bad dreams, blue between the eyes
	Deficiency	Wakes every two hours
Eczema	Phlegm-dampness	Rash moist and oozing, signs of phlegm
	Heat	Red face, hot child, rash is bright red
	Qi and blood deficiency	Pale weak child, rash is less red
	Lingering pathogenic factor	Swollen glands, skin dry, powdery
	Accumulation disorder	Digestion impaired
	Accumulation with Stomach heat	Big appetite, greedy
Failure to thrive	Spleen qi deficiency	Poor appetite
	Lingering pathogenic factor	Swollen glands
	Unwanted child	Appears lost

	Pattern	Distinctive Symptoms
Mental retardation	Spleen and Kidney deficiency	Low ears, poor bone structure
	Qi and blood deficiency	Weak, exhausted, poor appetite
	Phlegm-dampness	Signs of phlegm, slippery pulse
	Heat affecting the Heart	Restless, cannot sit still
Hyperactivity	Heat	Strong, but no signs of phlegm
	Mania	Obscene behavior
	Overstimulation	Weak, thin
	Heat in the Intestines	Always drinking
Crossed eyes	Congenital	
	Lingering pathogenic factor	Swollen glands, appears after a fever
	Overstimulation	Variable, excitable, and attractive
	Paralysis	Squints when looking in one direction only
Convulsions (acute)	Wind	With a fever
	Phlegm-heat	Signs of blockage and phlegm
	Damp-heat	Acute diarrhea
	Fright	Blue-green color somewhere on the face
Convulsions (chronic and petit mal)	Spleen yang deficiency	Pale face, dribbling
	Spleen and Kidney yang deficiency	Pale face, cold, floppy, weak constitution
	Liver and Kidney yin deficiency	Heat signs
Epilepsy	Fright	Blue-green color somewhere
	Phlegm	Much phlegm
	Blood stasis	Brain damage

	Pattern	Distinctive Symptoms
	Spleen and Kidney yang deficiency	Pale face, cold, floppy, weak constitution
	Liver and Kidney yin deficiency	Heat signs
Enuresis	Lower gate cold from deficiency	Dreamy, not 'with it'
	Spleen and Lung qi deficiency	Easily upset, obviously ill
	Damp-heat	Red face, sore urinary tract
	Lingering pathogenic factor	Swollen glands
	Emotional	Family disturbance, better away from home
Acute urinary tract infection	Damp-heat in Bladder	Acute, urgent cystitis
	Damp-heat in Liver channel	Irritation, soreness
	Damp-heat in Stomach and Intestines	Irritation, soreness, fever
Chronic urinary tract infection	Spleen and Kidney deficiency	Flabby child, pale face, poor appetite, lethargic (or occasionally hyperactive)
	Kidney yin deficiency	Thin child, irritable, red tongue, restless
Glandular disturbance	Lingering pathogenic infection	History of infection (child)
	Liver qi stagnation	History of frustration (teenager)
	Yin deficiency	History of frustration and over-work (adult)

❖

7 ❖ Constipation

Many babies and children become constipated. Hence, it is commonly seen in the clinic, either as the presenting complaint or as an additional symptom in another illness. Often just regulating the digestive system and causing the bowels to open regularly can be enough to clear the presenting condition in such disorders as abdominal pain, insomnia, eczema, asthma, and many others. It is also fairly simple to diagnose (see Appendix 1).

WHAT IS CONSTIPATION?

There is not complete agreement among practitioners as to what constipation is. Babies should pass a stool twice or even three times a day. So if a baby misses a day, we consider it constipated. If it misses a day just occasionally, as a symptom it may not be worth treating, but we would still classify the condition as constipation. This applies up to about the age of seven, after which the occasional missed day counts for nothing.

One of the reasons that constipation is seen so often is that it is one of the manifestations of accumulation disorder or of Spleen qi deficiency, depending on whether the child suffers from excess or deficiency, respectively. There is also a third pattern, Intestinal cold from deficiency.

EXCESS PATTERN

Etiology & Pathogenesis

There are many causes of excess-type constipation:

- overfeeding
- demand feeding
- irregular feeding
- unsuitable foods at weaning
- weaning too early
- temporary stress put on the child
- immunizations
- not drinking enough water

These etiological factors are identical to those for accumulation disorder, the exception being not drinking enough water. Some children do not really know that they are thirsty and may forget to drink in hot weather. As a result, the body fluids become a bit depleted, and the stools become hard. There is a delightful saying in traditional Chinese medicine, "A boat cannot float without water." Since this condition is identical to accumulation disorder, its pathogenesis is also the same as discussed in Chapter 3.

Symptoms

- stools can be hard, or more commonly, constipation alternates with diarrhea: one day no stools are passed, while the next day the stools are runny and vile smelling
- red cheeks
- strong child
- green nasal discharge
- irritable
- swollen abdomen
- may feel hot

Pulse: if you can take it, the pulse is sometimes full at both middle positions, expressing stagnation in the middle burner.

Treatment

In children under the age of four, use:

si feng (M-UE-9)

In older children, use points from the following list:

S-25 *(tian shu)*	Alarm (mù) point of Large Intestine
TB-6 *(zhi gou)*	Moves qi in the Intestines
CV-12 *(zhong wan)*	Moves qi in the Intestines
G-34 *(yang ling quan)*	Moves qi in the middle and lower burners
LI-4 *(he gu)*	Moves qi in the Intestines
B-57 *(cheng shan)*	Moves qi in the anus

Method: a moving technique is used at all the points. Typically, three points are enough in all but the most severe cases. A prescription that we use frequently includes TB-6 *(zhi gou)*, G-34 *(yang ling quan)*, and S-25 *(tian shu)*.

Prognosis: the reaction to the treatment in children under three can be quite dramatic. If given in the morning, it is common for the child to pass really vile smelling stools three or four times during the day. If given in the after-noon, the stools may be passed during the night, and sleep will be very disturbed. Often, the child is rather irritable for a day or two before calming down. Warn the parents of these reactions, otherwise they may be un-necessarily alarmed. With older children, the results are not usually as dramatic.

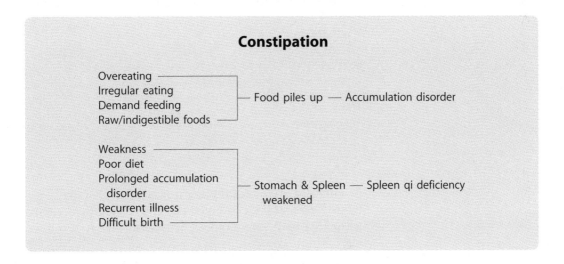

Constipation

Overeating
Irregular eating
Demand feeding
Raw/indigestible foods
— Food piles up — Accumulation disorder

Weakness
Poor diet
Prolonged accumulation
  disorder
Recurrent illness
Difficult birth
— Stomach & Spleen — Spleen qi deficiency
  weakened

DEFICIENCY PATTERN

Etiology & Pathogenesis

- long-term presence of accumulation disorder
- recurrent illnesses
- immunizations
- poor constitution
- anesthetics during childbirth or later, depressing the qi
- weak qi of the mother (overworking while pregnant)
- long childbirth
- anemia of the mother

We just saw that excess-type constipation and accumulation disorder have the same etiology and pathogenesis. Similarly, deficiency-type constipation and the Spleen qi deficiency pattern (discussed in Chapter 3) share the same etiology and pathogenesis. The qi of the child has been weakened, so there is simply not enough qi to move the food through the intestines, leading to constipation. In other words, the transportive function of the Spleen is too weak. Weak Spleen energy will also lead to a poor appetite and give rise to the formation of dampness and phlegm in the body. This, coupled with the fact that there is not enough qi to fight off external pathogenic factors, lays the child open to recurrent illnesses, such as coughs and colds, which will further weaken the qi.

Symptoms

- may be constipated for days at a time
- passes stools with difficulty
- stools may be loose or hard when passed, but usually not smelly
- lethargic
- floppy
- pale
- prone to coughs and colds

Pulse: weak
Tongue: pale

NOTE

Commonly, children suffering from deficiency-type constipation go much longer without passing stools than is the case with excess-type constipation. Five to seven days is quite common, and one baby we saw did not pass a stool more often than once every two weeks!

Treatment

Treatment principle: tonify the digestive system and the Spleen. Typical points include:

S-36 *(zu san li)*
CV-12 *(zhong wan)* ⎫ Tonifies Spleen qi
Sp-6 *(san yin jiao)* ⎭
B-20 *(pi shu)*   Back associated *(shū)* point of the Spleen

Method: all the points may be needled, but it is common to just use indirect moxibustion at CV-12 *(zhong wan)*. Avoid using B-20 *(pi shu)* in the first few treatments, and only use it if the child is extremely exhausted, since children hate points on the back.

Prognosis: gradually, the child's qi increases and the digestion and stools become regular. Ten treatments are typically required, especially if the child is taking some Western medication—for example, antibiotics—because they can deplete the Spleen qi even more. They are, therefore, working against you. It is rare to get any strong reaction to the treatment.

NOTE

Do not use *si feng* (M-UE-9) in treating deficiency-type constipation as this point disperses the qi. If it is used incorrectly, the constipation is often made worse, and the child may not pass a stool for more than a week.

INTESTINAL COLD FROM DEFICIENCY PATTERN

Etiology & Pathogenesis

• eating ice-cold foods
• drinking ice-cold drinks

There may be other factors that contribute to the etiology of this condition, but diet is the most obvious. It may be compounded by eating a generally poor quality diet containing many cold energy foods.

The qi of the Stomach is weakened by eating cold energy foods, as well as those served at cold temperatures. The digestion is weakened, and there is not enough qi to move stool through the Intestines. In addition, cold accumulates in the Intestines and prevents the bowels from moving.

This pattern differs from Spleen qi deficiency in that the overall qi is strong: children with Intestinal cold from deficiency may even have pretty good appetites and lots of energy. The problem is localized in the Intestines.

Symptoms

• pale face
• good energy
• appetite can be poor or acceptable
• usually a high proportion of cold and junk foods in the diet
• stools usually every other day, but may be constipated for days
• stools may be dry and hard to pass
• possibly abdominal pain

Pulse: may be weak or tight; sometimes full and slippery at both middle positions
Tongue: often pale

Treatment

Treatment principle: tonify the Intestines, even though the overall qi is good. Points should include:

S-36 *(zu san li)*
CV-12 *(zhong wan)*

Method: use a tonifying technique at these points as well as moxibustion at CV-12 *(zhong wan)*. In addition, advice must be given on diet: regular meals, and no cold or junk foods, are essential to effect a cure.

Prognosis: three to five treatments are usually enough to get the Intestines working. What you may then find is that the condition transforms into accumulation disorder if the child is an excess-type in other respects. If this should happen, treat for that disorder.

ADVICE FOR EXCESS AND DEFICIENT PATTERNS

It is important to advise parents when treating constipation, especially about diet. For the excess pattern, normally a simple change in diet will ensure that the problem does not return, for example, avoiding whole or raw foods. For the deficiency pattern, it is important to advise the parents to give easily digested foods and to avoid those which put strain on the Spleen, such as bananas, cow's milk, and peanuts. For both patterns, a regular diet is important, as is avoiding too much food, which overloads the system. In addition, make sure that the child is taking enough fluids (especially in hot weather). Again, the main points include:

• regular feeding (which means no snacks)
• avoid overfeeding
• give easily digested foods

If in doubt, delay introducing new foods, and in times of illness, reduce the food intake and go back to an earlier feeding pattern.

Constipation is often a problem during weaning. Some babies find that the change in diet is a real problem, and they may need to include something that helps the bowels to move. We suggest they add a mild 'food supple-ment' such as prune juice. A stronger one is syrup of figs. When there is a problem with constipation, we prefer the simple food-based remedies over those based on medicinal herbs, which we tend to save for the really obstinate cases.

NOTE

• For a case history involving constipation, see Case 10 in Chapter 47.

❖

8 ❖ Diarrhea

INTRODUCTION

Diarrhea is potentially a very dangerous disease in babies. In serious cases, diarrhea can develop into chronic convulsions (see Chapter 39) and can even lead to death. In developing countries, diarrhea (usually as dysentery) is the major cause of infant mortality. Set against this gloomy picture are the positive effects of acupuncture in curing diarrhea of all kinds. The use of acupuncture in the treatment of bacterial dysentery was one of the turning points in the acceptance of acupuncture, both inside China during its civil war, and outside China by the World Health Organization. Many studies have shown that acupuncture is at least as effective as Western medicine or Chinese herbs in the treatment of this disorder.

We depart from the traditional method of discussing diarrhea by dividing the subject into acute and chronic varieties. In the acute form, a child who does not normally get diarrhea suddenly suffers an attack. The stools are generally watery and frequent, possibly many times a day. Acute diarrhea is divided into three stages, the last of which being the most serious. In its chronic form, the problem has been going on for several weeks or months. There is not such a feeling of urgency associated with this type of diarrhea, and the symptoms may come and go.

ACUTE DIARRHEA

Acute diarrhea occurs suddenly. It is often the result of an epidemic, that is, a 'bug' going around or a serious disease such as typhoid or dysentery. It may be accompanied by severe pains and fever. There is a great feeling of urgency associated with acute diarrhea. You feel that something is very wrong and it must be put right or there will be serious consequences. This is true, because left untreated, a child may die from a severe attack.

There are three stages in an acute attack of diarrhea, progressing in severity. These are discussed below.

Stage one

Invasion of dampness. This is caused by the invasion of an external pathogenic factor and includes the Western medical category of infection as well as eating contaminated food or food which simply does not agree with the child (such as curry or melons). It is divided into two subpatterns, one being cold and the other hot.

In both patterns, there is an element of dampness. There are two sayings in traditional Chinese medicine that are appropriate to this pattern: "Without dampness there is no diarrhea" and "Excessive dampness leads to the five types of diarrhea." Since the Spleen is better suited to dryness and has difficulty with dampness, the damp pathogenic factor readily obstructs Spleen yang. When this occurs, the Spleen's ability to transform fluids is impaired, and water and dampness accumulate and pass downward in the form of diarrhea.

The cold-damp pattern is the manifestation of food poisoning, enteritis, eating too many cold energy foods, or simply getting chilled. The hot pattern is the manifestation of dysentery, becoming too hot in the summer (i.e., sunstroke, or in Chinese parlance, 'summer heat'), or the consumption of spicy foods such as curry. These are not rigid distinctions, however, and attention must be paid to the actual manifestation.

Stage two

Spleen qi deficiency is regarded as the second stage in an attack of diarrhea. In the Chinese texts and in all the traditional Chinese medical books that we have seen, there is no distinction made between the Spleen qi deficiency pattern during an acute attack and a chronic condition. We, however, feel that it is worth separating these out, for although the treatments are basically the same, the situations are very different. *Above all, in the acute attack there is a pathogenic factor present as well as Spleen qi deficiency.* Therefore, as we will see, it is possible to have bad smelling stools during Spleen qi deficiency.

During an attack by an external pathogen, the child is rapidly weakened by the continuing loss of stool and body fluids, and the condition progresses to that of Spleen qi deficiency in a matter of days or even hours if the child was weak in the first place. The condition is a mixed pattern of excess and deficiency, with the deficiency dominating. The condition has the element of deficiency because the child is exhausted, and the element of excess because the pathogenic factor is still there. As a consequence, the symptoms retain the characteristic of the original pathogenic factor. For example, if the original attack was that of damp-heat with hot smelly stools, then although the condition is now that of Spleen qi deficiency, there will still be hot smelly stools because the pathogenic factor remains. It is important, in these cases, to treat for Spleen qi deficiency, for to disperse may further weaken the child.

Stage three

Kidney and Spleen yang deficiency is the third and most severe stage of the illness. The child has become so depleted by the diarrhea that the yang qi is injured. If untreated, it will lead to death.

Etiology & Pathogenesis

Stage one

Dampness can arise from many sources, most commonly from damp weather and damp-forming foods (e.g., dairy products) or an external pathogenic agent such as contaminated water. Dampness readily obstructs the Spleen yang and impairs its function of transforming the fluids. Water and dampness accumulate and sink downward, leading to diarrhea.

Dampness may combine with heat or cold to form a damp-heat or cold-dampness disorder. When dampness combines with cold, there are characteristic signs of cold such as a white face, chilliness, and cramping pains. When it combines with heat, there will often be fever, and the stools become foul-smelling and burning.

COLD-DAMPNESS

There are three primary causes of diarrhea associated with cold-dampness:

1. Cold wind attacking uncovered tummies. Young children do not seem to notice how cold they are getting. They happily run around in the cool of the evening, blue and with goosebumps, yet quite unaware of being cold. Children's clothes are often ill-fitting or pulled off in quite unsuitable climates, allowing the exposed area to become chilled. Wind-cold may thus enter the body and pass to the Intestines and Stomach. The yang qi is thereby weakened, and the regulation of the entire qi mechanism becomes disrupted. The digestion is soon affected, leading to diarrhea.

2. Bad food is often cold in nature, leading to cold-damp-ness diarrhea, which is to say, food poisoning. Salmonella poisoning, as well as cholera, give rise to this pattern.
3. Food that is itself cold in temperature or has a cold energy (see Appendix 2), if consumed in large quanti-ties, can lead to this pattern, for example, eating a large tub of ice cream or a lot of plums. Cold invades the Stomach and the Intestines, and obstructs the flow of qi. The function of the Spleen is impaired, and the entire qi mechanism is disrupted, leading to diarrhea.

DAMP-HEAT

There are likewise three primary causes of damp-heat diar-rhea:

1. Summerheat arises when the child becomes severely overheated, which occurs often in the summer after a child becomes sunburned or has sunstroke. In theory, however, it can arise whenever the child becomes over-heated, for any reason. Summer and autumn weather is hot in China. The blazing heat may cause profuse sweating, which consumes the body fluids. Replacing these fluids imposes a great demand on the Spleen, such that the water balance is disturbed, giving rise to violent diarrhea.
2. Eating too many hot foods may also give rise to this type of diarrhea.
3. Again, contaminated food or water, typhoid, or dysen-tery may manifest as damp-heat diarrhea.

Dampness and heat, which can arise from various sources, accumulate in the body. The Stomach and Spleen functions of rotting and ripening the food is disrupted, and the food quickly turns putrid. As a consequence, not only are there loose stools, but the stools smell foul as well. Finally, heat gives rise to burning pain and fever.

Stage two

After an attack by an external pathogenic factor, the child can quickly become exhausted and the digestion disturbed since the Spleen is weakened and its function thereby impaired. Often, this is aggravated by taking antibiotics during the attack, which, being cold and damp in nature, aggravates the condition and further weaken the Spleen qi.

All of this can happen in a very short time, depend-ing on:

• the severity of the attack. The stronger the pathogenic factor, the quicker the progression to stage two.
• the strength of the child or baby. If the child was weak

before the attack, it will quickly evolve to stage two and even three, if not treated properly.

The external attack by damp-heat or cold-dampness injures the Spleen, which thereby becomes deficient in energy. Once its function of transporting and transforming the fluids is disrupted, water and dampness begin to accumulate, leading to diarrhea. Finally, since the pathogenic factor is still present in the child, the symptoms in this stage retain the characteristic of the original pathogenic factor, which is to say, either damp-heat or cold-dampness.

Stage three

This stage follows the second, after the Spleen qi has become deficient. The third stage is very serious and will lead to death if not treated immediately. It is very unusual to see this stage in the clinic as these children are usually put in the hospital for emergency rehydration.

The diarrhea has continued and weakens both Kidney and Spleen yang. This pattern may arise in a matter of days in a small baby if the original attack of diarrhea was very violent, or if, before the attack, the child was weak either constitutionally, or from a prolonged illness. As a consequence, the fire of the gate of vitality *(mìng mén)* becomes exhausted and fails to warm the Spleen. Undigested food transforms into dampness, and there is a general feeling of cold as well as diarrhea. The diarrhea is severe and worsens when the child is tired.

Symptoms

Stage one

General signs include the following:

- sudden onset
- usually a history of an epidemic at school
- may have been exposed to damp weather (e.g., caught in the rain)

COLD-DAMPNESS

- stools hardly smell
- stools are watery, copious, and pale colored or green
- cramping pain in abdomen (borborygmus)
- white colored face
- feels cold
- possibly a history of eating cold energy foods (bananas, cucumbers)
- possibly a low fever
- possibly nasal discharge with clear, watery fluid and mild cough
- absence of thirst

Tongue coating: white, moist

Pulse: floating
Finger vein: broad, red

DAMP-HEAT

- stools smell foul
- stools are painful to pass, and the child may cry out as a result
- stools are watery and barely formed, containing particles of undigested foods or pockets of fluids
- may continue for as long as ten days, during which the anus becomes red, inflamed, and sore
- possibly a fever
- urine may be scanty and yellow

Tongue body: red
Tongue coating: yellow, greasy
Finger vein: thick, purple ·
Pulse: floating, rapid

Stage two

- lethargy
- pale face
- no appetite
- child appears exhausted, likes to sleep during the day
- eyes sunken
- dehydrated
- muscles on arms and legs are flaccid
- in severe cases, diarrhea appears every time food or milk is taken
- whites of eyes are visible during sleep
- stools are watery and contain either undigested food and water, white lumps in the diaper, or food particles and dregs

Tongue body: pale
Tongue coating: thin, white
Pulse: deep, forceless

As mentioned previously, the pattern of Spleen qi deficiency can present with different symptoms, depending on whether the first stage of the attack was that of damp-heat or cold-dampness. Therefore, following an attack of cold-dampness:

- stools hardly smell and are copious and watery
- there are cramping pains in the stomach
- child feels cold, with a white face

Following an attack of damp-heat:

- stools smell foul and are painful to pass
- there are signs of heat such as a red face, possibly a fever

Stage three

- chronic diarrhea which continues nonstop, often with a prolapsed anus
- immediately after taking food, there is an attack of diarrhea containing undigested food
- face and limbs are cold; there is an aversion to cold
- spirit is tired and weak
- 'three white eyes' (whites of the eyes are visible to the left, right, and below the iris), and the whites are also visible during sleep; this is a sign of Kidney deficiency, known as sanpaku in macrobiotics

Tongue body: pale
Tongue coating: thin, white
Pulse: minute, fine

In extreme cases, either the yin or the yang, or both, can be injured. Characteristic symptoms for injured yin include the following:

- eyes sunken
- skin dry and hot
- spirit very weak and feeble, or irritable
- scanty urine
- thirst
- diarrhea has yellow color
- lips red

Tongue: thin, dry
Pulse: minute, rapid

Characteristic symptoms of injured yang (collapse of yang) include:

- watery stools
- pallid face
- limbs extremely cold
- spontaneous cold sweats

Tongue body: pale, colorless
Pulse: deep, fine

Characteristic symptoms of injured yin and yang include:

- ashen-white face
- limbs extremely cold
- vomiting increases and diarrhea lessens
- tends to sleep more and more, even to the point of coma
- twitching, convulsions
- cries without tears

Tongue body: bright red
Pulse: deep, fine

Treatment

MAIN POINTS

The main points for treating all diarrhea are the following:

S-25 *(tian shu)*	Alarm *(mù)* point of Large Intestine
S-36 *(zu san li)*	Harmonizes the Intestines and tonifies the Spleen

Other commonly used points include the following:

CV-12 *(zhong wan)*	Benefits the Spleen and stops diarrhea
LI-11 *(qu chi)*	Regulates the Intestines
B-20 *(pi shu)*	Both points benefit the Spleen
B-21 *(wei shu)*	and resolve dampness
B-25 *(da chang shu)*	Associated *(shū)* point of the Intestines
GV-1 *(chang qiang)*	Sends qi upward and stops diarrhea

Method: use even technique for stage one diarrhea, and tonifying technique for stage two diarrhea

COLD-DAMPNESS

Treatment principle: disperse the cold, transform dampness, and expel the pathogenic factor

This pattern usually passes anyway, unless it is unusually violent, in which case it must be treated quickly. Use the main points listed above, plus:

CV-6 *(qi hai)*

Method: use both moxibustion and needles on the points.

A combination of CV-6 *(qi hai)* and S-25 *(tian shu)* with both moxibustion and needles is effective in this case. It is often helpful to use both abdominal and distal points with a combination of moxibustion and needles. For example, consider using acupuncture at S-36 *(zu san li)* plus two to three minutes per point of indirect moxibustion at S-25 *(tian shu)* and CV-12 *(zhong wan)*. Even technique is typically used, unless the pain is very intense.

Prognosis: this condition will often pass quickly without treatment. If it is unusually violent, however, it must be treated quickly. In a reasonably healthy child, a change should be seen within three treatments.

DAMP-HEAT

Treatment principle: clear the heat and transform the dampness. In addition to the main points listed above, use:

S-44 *(nei ting)*	Benefits the Spleen, resolves dampness, and clears heat
Sp-9 *(yin ling quan)*	Clears damp-heat
GV-1 *(chang qiang)*	Stops the diarrhea and pain in the anus
GV-10 *(ling tai)*	

If there is a high fever, use:

GV-14 *(da zhui)*
LI-11 *(qu chi)*

Method: all points are reduced to clear heat, and moxibustion is not used. Treatments should be given daily, even twice a day if the symptoms are very severe. A sample prescription might include S-25 *(tian shu)* and S-44 *(nei ting)*. In case of very high fever, bleed the well *(jĭng)* points once or twice a day.

Prognosis: the progress of the diarrhea depends very much on the cause. If it is due to an epidemic infection, then no rule can be stated for the number of treatments required, as some epidemics are mild and some violent. In cases of dysentery and typhoid, the main symptoms should be controlled within three days, but the treatment should continue for ten days.

IN THE CLINIC

In real life, I am afraid that the children seen in the clinic do not always present as clearly as these stage-one patterns would suggest. Very often the child is neither very hot nor very cold, but somewhere in the middle. In these cases, just treat the diarrhea using points like S-25 *(tian shu)* and S-36 *(zu san li)*. You should use moxibustion on the abdominal points, which should be enough to stop the attack. If the child subsequently develops a hot or cold pattern, treat accordingly.

Stage two

Treatment principle: for all patterns, nourish the Spleen and stop the diarrhea. In addition, for cold-dampness, tonify the Spleen, scatter cold, and stop diarrhea; and for damp-heat, tonify the Spleen, stop diarrhea, and clear the hot pathogenic factor.

This is a serious disorder requiring urgent treatment. If the child is dehydrated, then rehydrate using a salt solution obtainable at pharmacies.

You can use the main points listed above with acupuncture to tonify the Spleen but be very careful with your needle technique. You must use a *tonifying* technique. If you disperse the qi, it can be dangerous.

Feel the stomach. If it feels cold to the touch, moxibustion may be used either alone or with ginger to great advantage. However, if the stomach feels hot to the touch, use acupuncture without moxibustion. A sample prescription would be S-36 *(zu san li)*, S-25 *(tian shu)*, and CV-12 *(zhong wan)*, with moxibustion on the latter, especially if the abdomen feels cold.

Prognosis: if the body is severely depleted, it may take a long time (10 to 20 treatments) to build up its strength.

Stage three

Treatment principle: regardless of the pattern, always tonify the Spleen and warm the Kidneys. In addition, for injured yang, warm, tonify, and restore the yang. For injured yin, clear the heat and enrich the yin. For injured yin and yang, either augment the qi and shore up collapse, dispel the cold, and restore the yang, or alternatively, warm and reinforce the Spleen and Kidneys.

Acute diarrhea generally injures the yin because the fluids are so quickly depleted, but it can also injure Kidney yang. Because it can occur so rapidly and with such severity, it can quickly lead to both yin and yang deficiency. This is a very serious condition, especially in a young baby. It must be treated with great urgency.

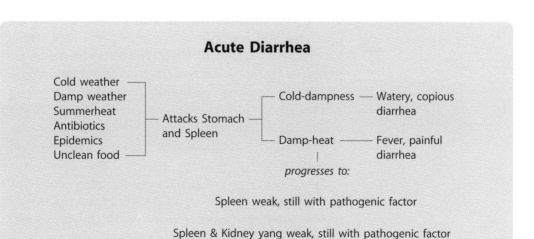

Acute Diarrhea

Cold weather
Damp weather
Summerheat
Antibiotics
Epidemics
Unclean food

Attacks Stomach and Spleen

Cold-dampness — Watery, copious diarrhea

Damp-heat — Fever, painful diarrhea

progresses to:

Spleen weak, still with pathogenic factor

Spleen & Kidney yang weak, still with pathogenic factor

Acupuncture is not the treatment of choice for this condition. In every pattern it is important to rehydrate and restore the body's electrolytes since this condition is life-threatening if the fluids are not replaced. The simplest way is with water containing salt and sugar. (If the child is too weak to drink this liquid, then the Western medical treatment of intravenous drip is excellent.) One might use moxibustion at the abdominal points listed above. In case of both yin and yang deficiency, acupuncture can be of supplementary benefit in restoring consciousness, with such points as GV-26 *(ren zhong)*, CV-1 *(hui yin)*, P-6 *(nei guan)*, and S-36 *(zu san li)*.

Chronic Diarrhea

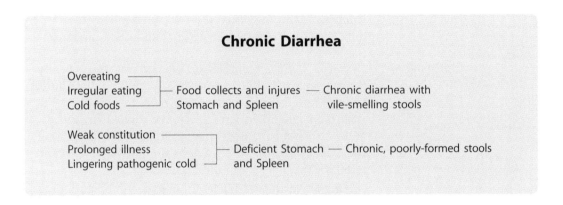

CHRONIC DIARRHEA

Introduction

Chronic diarrhea is marked by its long duration. It has several presentations. Either it is variable—sometimes better, sometimes worse—or it continues in a mild form for weeks without much change. In addition, there are two types of chronic diarrhea, depending on the pattern. The first is the excess pattern, where the child is strong and has a lot of energy. In this case the stools are vile and runny. The second pattern is one of deficiency, where the child is deficient in energy. Here the stools are loose and have little smell.

Because of the chronic nature of the illness, the child will be weakened by the attacks. Nevertheless, there is not the same feeling of urgency as with acute diarrhea. Both types of chronic diarrhea can be treated very effectively with acupuncture and diet.

Excess Pattern

INJURY FROM FOOD

This is the most common cause of chronic diarrhea. It is seen in strong children with good appetites, red cheeks, and the like. It is actually a minor variation of the accumulation disorder pattern, and is therefore a condition of excess.

The pattern is given the name 'injury from food' rather than 'accumulation disorder' because the principal symptom is diarrhea, rather than constipation. As a consequence, food does not accumulate in the same way, and there are slightly different signs and symptoms. In babies, this pattern is very often aggravated by teething.

Deficiency Pattern

SPLEEN AND STOMACH QI DEFICIENCY

This pattern is one of deficiency, that is, the child does not have the energy to digest food properly. Consequently, the food passes through as diarrhea. This deficiency can stem from anything that depletes the qi of the Spleen and Stomach, for example, the use of antibiotics in the treatment of acute diarrhea, a weak constitution, or recurrent illness.

Deficiency Pattern

HYPERACTIVE SPLEEN QI DEFICIENCY

This is a variation on the above pattern of Stomach and Spleen qi deficiency, the difference being that the child appears to have a lot of energy. The etiology and pathogenesis are the same as the previous pattern, with the additional factor that the child has found ways to absorb energy from those around it (see Chapter 3).

Etiology & Pathogenesis

Injury from food

This pattern is virtually identical to accumulation disorder, with just a few differences. The most common causes of this pattern are:

- irregular feeding
- too much food
- inappropriate foods, including cold and damp energy foods such as fruit, fruit juice, and whole foods

All mothers like to see their children eating well, and it is very common for them to give their babies or children too much food, or food which they believe to be good for them, but which may actually be quite unsuitable. Other causes include:

- mothers eating inappropriate foods while breast feeding
- overfeeding bottle-fed babies
- formulas that are too rich for bottle-fed babies

The most common cause of this pattern can be summed up in the saying, "Food and drink in excess attack the Intestines and Stomach" (*Basic Questions,* Chapter 43). Giving a child too much to eat overloads the digestive system. The Stomach and Spleen are overtaxed and their energies are depleted. They then do not 'rot and ripen' the food nor transform or transport the food. The food is not properly digested, and the undigested food moves to the Large Intestine and is expelled as diarrhea.

Similarly, if inappropriate foods are taken either directly or through the mother, then the Spleen can be injured, impairing its function. Food is not properly digested and is expelled as diarrhea.

Spleen and Stomach qi deficiency

There are several causes of this pattern:

- it can arise from a previous bad attack of diarrhea, which leaves the child exhausted and with disturbed digestion
- any severe or long-term illness, such as fevers or asthma
- immunizations can deplete the qi
- a very common cause is the inappropriate use of antibiotics, as they are cold and damp in nature, and the use of anesthetics in childbirth
- another common cause is overconsumption of fruit juice
- it can also occur as a result of a growth spurt, in children who grow very quickly, or in children who have many late nights. All of these factors deplete the qi, possibly only temporarily, but enough to impair the function of the Spleen and thus cause diarrhea.
- in older children, it can arise if too much time is spent on schoolwork, as this diverts the energy from the Spleen to the head, with the consequence of depleting the Spleen energy
- it is common in children who have been weak from birth or an early age

Any of the above factors can deplete the Spleen qi and thus interfere with the Spleen's transportation and transformation of food and fluids, resulting in the formation and accumulation of dampness. In addition, the Stomach function of rotting and ripening the food is impaired, such that food remains undigested. The accumulation of dampness and undigested food results in diarrhea.

Hyperactive Spleen qi deficiency

The etiology of this pattern has been discussed in Chapter 3. It is the same as that of Spleen qi deficiency, with the additional factor that the child has no boundaries and so can draw on the energy of those around it. The pathogenesis likewise mirrors that of Spleen qi deficiency.

Symptoms

Injury from food

- stools are foul-smelling and often green; in mild cases, they may only smell sour
- possibly abdominal distention and pain or feeling of fullness
- before passing a stool, the child can be in pain and may cry out
- foul breath
- days of diarrhea may be interspersed with days of constipation
- child is typically strong, with red cheeks, and a greenish tinge around the mouth if the stools are passed up to twice daily; if more frequent, the child is more likely to have green around the mouth, but without red cheeks
- often has nasal discharge
- possibly vomiting

Tongue coating: thick and greasy, or thin, yellow or normal
Pulse: slippery

The symptoms listed here are mostly those of accumulation disorder. However, there are some differences, which depend on the frequency that stools are passed. If on some days the child only passes stool once or not at all, then there is time for the food to accumulate. As a consequence, there will be signs of excess, with the abdomen really swollen like a drum, and the cheeks red. On the other hand, if there are stools more than two or three times a day, the condition is not entirely one of excess. The abdomen is not as swollen simply because a lot of the excess food has passed out as stool. Also the cheeks are not red because the accumulated food has not had time to transform into heat.

Spleen and Stomach qi deficiency

- loose stools that do not smell. They may be watery or contain undigested food and water. There may also be white lumps of curdled milk in the nappy, or the stools may consist of food particles and dregs.
- in severe cases, there is diarrhea every time food or milk is taken
- facial color is pale
- child likes to sleep during the day, but wakes frequently at night

- no appetite
- spirit is weak, and the child may appear exhausted
- only a slight thirst, and then for warm drinks
- can range from mild to serious: the child may have bad attacks of diarrhea many times a day, or it may present as a child who does not strictly speaking have diarrhea, but may never have had formed stools either

Tongue: pale
Tongue coating: thin, white
Pulse: deep, forceless
Finger vein: faint or nonexistent

Hyperactive Spleen qi deficiency

In this pattern, although the child presents with many of the signs of Spleen qi deficiency, it appears to have a lot of energy. Symptoms include:

- loose stools that do not smell
- pale facial color
- poor appetite, picky about foods
- appears to have a lot of energy, runs around a lot, does not complain of the cold, and does not seem to need to sleep that much
- parents are often exhausted
- often drinks lots of juice
- can be very manipulative

Treatment

Injury from food

Treatment principle: reduce the food stagnation, transform the blockage, harmonize the middle burner, and stop the diarrhea. The main points are the same as for acute diarrhea.

In babies under three years old add the following points:

Sp-4 *(gong sun)*   Regulates the Spleen
si feng (M-UE-9)   Clears the retention of food

Method: if all the food has been evacuated with the diarrhea, then it is probably best to use Sp-4 *(gong sun)* alone, with even technique. But if you feel that the child is still full of food, then *si feng* (M-UE-9) may also be appropriate.

In older children, add the following points:

S-25 *(tian shu)*   Alarm *(mù)* point of Large Intestine
CV-12 *(zhong wan)*   Tonifies Spleen qi
Sp-4 *(gong sun)*   Regulates the Spleen

Method: even technique (i.e., obtain qi)

Prognosis: if treated promptly, three to five treatments are sufficient. If the diarrhea has persisted for a month or more, it can take a surprisingly long time to treat, which is to say, ten or more treatments.

NOTE

To effect a cure it is essential, in appropriate cases, to change the diet or otherwise reduce the quantity of food that is eaten. If the child is breast feeding, then question the mother carefully about *her* diet.

Spleen qi deficiency

Treatment principle: nourish the Spleen and stop the diarrhea. The main points to use are:

S-25 *(tian shu)*	Alarm *(mù)* point of Large Intestine
S-36 *(zu san li)*	Tonifies the Spleen

Method: both points should be tonified

Other points which tonify the Spleen can also be used:

Sp-6 *(san yin jiao)*
CV-12 *(zhong wan)*
B-20 *(pi shu)*

Method: use moxibustion, or moxibustion with ginger

Prognosis: usually it will take from ten to twenty treatments, but more may be needed if the child is severely depleted. In cases of deficiency like this, it just takes time for the qi to be replenished, so a long course of treatment is necessary, over a longer period of time.

The child must be encouraged to rest and to eat warming and nourishing foods. All cold foods—cold both in temperature and in energy—as well as difficult to digest foods, should be avoided.

Hyperactive Spleen qi deficiency

From the point of view of acupuncture, the treatment is the same as for Spleen qi deficiency. The advice given, however, is different. You need to advise the parents to set up clear boundaries for the child—such as going to bed on time—and to stick to them.

The prognosis is also different. These children are very hard to treat because they rather enjoy not having to make their own qi! As you try to change this situation, they put up a fight—with wailing, howling, and many tears. As the parents are often exhausted, battling with their child each time they come for treatment may prove to be more than they can cope with, and so they give up.

NOTES

• The primary cause of death from dysentery is the depletion of body fluids. A dramatic reduction in infant mortality can be achieved by replacing fluids and electrolytes. Many pharmacists have sachets of suitable electrolyte fluids. If these are not available, make up a solution of a third of a pint (200ml) of boiled water with one heaping teaspoon of sugar, a generous pinch of sea salt, and two generous pinches of bicarbonate of soda.

• It is not uncommon in Western children to see a combined pattern of heat in the Stomach with Spleen qi deficiency. The Stomach heat causes the child to overeat, leading to diarrhea. In treating such children, first clear the Stomach heat with such points as S-44 *(nei ting)* and LI-4 *(he gu)*.

• It cannot be overemphasized that for babies, 'long-term' diarrhea may be as short as two or three days, as they quickly become exhausted from a violent attack of diarrhea.

• For case histories dealing with diarrhea, see Case 15 and Case 16 in Chapter 47.

❖

9 ❖ Teething

INTRODUCTION

Teething is a major event for babies. Quite suddenly and out of the blue, a placid and happy child can be transformed into an angry and miserable one who keeps everyone awake at night. The parents are also distressed: seeing their baby in such pain and agony, they feel as if there is nothing that can be done. As well as the pain to the gums, there are a multitude of other possible symptoms—diarrhea, cough, and insomnia, among others. In fact, the list of symptoms is so large that almost any problem encountered by a baby can be attributed to teething!

Although some parents feel helpless watching their screaming baby, there are many folk remedies that are renowned for helping a child through this time. We still recommend many of these because they are very effective and can be given by the parents at home every hour or so. Acupuncture is also very effective if given during this time, as it is good at taking heat out of the gums. However, it is probably better at preventing the problems from arising in the first place.

Teething is not a recognized pattern in traditional Chinese medicine. For although the trials and tribulations associated with teething are commonly seen in the West, they are not often seen in China. The reason for this is that teething is a digestive problem, that is, the common pattern of accumulation disorder. Although one does see this problem in China, it is generally not as severe, as the Chinese tend to feed their babies in a more sensible way.

THE TCM POINT OF VIEW

Normally, the teeth are associated with the Kidneys, and it is certainly true that late or poorly formed teeth are an indication of Kidney deficiency. It is also true that the rising energy needed to push the teeth out comes from the Kidneys. Yet the severe symptoms which are associated with the teeth pushing through the gums are related to the Stomach and Intestines. This is because of the channels that pass through the gums. What seems to happen is that, as the teeth come through, they influence the flow of qi in the Stomach and Intestine channels, causing irritation and stagnation of qi. This in turn causes the flow of qi in the organs themselves to slow down and stagnate slightly.

Teething only causes problems
if there is accumulation disorder.

In many children, this does not matter—if the digestion is functioning normally. A slight stagnation is easily overcome. Similarly, in deficient children the qi just slows down a bit more and becomes somewhat weaker, but not much is noticed. It is in strong children, however, that the problems occur because they are prone to accumulation disorder. If a young baby has accumulation disorder before it starts teething, then, as long as this disorder persists, there will certainly be much distress associated with the teeth coming through. Interestingly enough, many babies go off their food just before and while a tooth starts to come through—a natural reaction to clear out the digestion.

Unfortunately, however, even for strong children who do not present with accumulation disorder, teething can be a big problem. For very often these babies have the beginnings of accumulation disorder all the time, although they are reasonably healthy, tend to enjoy life, and have good appetites. They tend to have slightly rosy cheeks, eat slightly too much, and occasionally get some diarrhea—nothing to worry about in the normal frame of things, but a problem when they start teething. The heat associated with the teeth coming through, causing the qi to stagnate in the Stomach, even just that little bit, can turn a slight accumulation disorder into a full-blown case. The extra heat generated by the stagnating food aggravates the heat in the gums, resulting in the agony of the teething process.

Teething aggravates accumulation disorder.
Accumulation disorder aggravates teething.

Complications Associated with Teething

Most cases of teething just cause mild discomfort to the baby, and some disruption to the family in the form of sleepless nights and uncomfortable days. It is unusual for anything serious to happen. But in the minority of cases, the heat generated by accumulation disorder is so great that the child develops a high fever and suffers an attack of febrile convulsions. It is for this reason that severe symptoms of teething should be taken very seriously. (Treatment of convulsions from teething is discussed in Chapter 38.)

The heat generated during teething can
become so great as to cause convulsions!

Common Symptoms of Teething

Most of these symptoms are identical to those of accumulation disorder:

• one cheek red
• sore gums, dribbling
• irritability and restlessness
• pain in the gums
• insomnia
• diarrhea with foul-smelling stools
• swollen abdomen
• nasal discharge, often yellow or green
• possibly phlegmy cough
• sometimes poor appetite just before and during teething

Treatment

Despite the simplicity of diagnosis, teething problems are not always that simple to treat. The trick is to bring down the heat and clear the accumulated food which is causing the heat, without giving rise to any complications.

The point, of course, that springs to mind when treating accumulation disorder is *si feng* (M-UE-9). But using this point can actually release a lot of heat and phlegm into the system, making the heat already there from the teething even worse in the short term. This added heat may cause a fever to rise too fast and too high, with the real danger of convulsions.

―――――

Si feng (M-UE-9) may increase heat in the body, especially when teething. If you use this point, there is a risk of causing convulsions.

―――――

In some cases, it is still possible to use *si feng* (M-UE-9). These are usually mild cases where the accumulation disorder is not severe, or is just developing. The important thing is that the child is *not very hot!*

To avoid the complications of using *si-feng* (M-UE-9), however, use the following point combination instead:

LI-4 *(he gu)*
S-44 *(nei ting)*

This combination is effective in all cases of teething. It takes the heat out of the gums, Stomach, and Intestines without causing too much movement.

Another useful prescription is 'without heat' moxibustion or point stimulation therapy. Powdered *Evodiae rutaecarpae (wu zhu yu)* is made into a paste with vinegar and placed on LI-4 *(he gu)*. It is covered with a waterproof plaster and left on for six to twelve hours or overnight. The plaster is then removed, and the process repeated. Keep the point stimulated for the duration of the teething period. You can make a similar powder with ground cloves. This is a gentle but quite effective method to reduce fever and irritation without causing further aggravation.

What to Expect from Treatment

Acupuncture is very effective at reducing heat and inflammation in the gums, and in all but the most severe cases, one or two treatments can relieve much of the suffering. In those babies with very severe accumulation disorder or badly swollen and inflamed gums, acupuncture may not give immediate relief because once the gums are inflamed, it takes time for the pain to die down. This is because the gums are being continually aggravated by the new teeth coming through. However, acupuncture does lessen the discomfort by taking some of the heat out of the gums, and it cannot be stressed too strongly that any relief that can be given is welcome and should be offered. Then, in subsequent treatments, you can go on to clear the accumulation of food.

Prevention

"Prevention is better than cure." A cliché, but most definitely true in the case of teething problems. Offer the following tips on diet to prevent the recurrence of accumulation disorder:

• regular meals
• at least two hours between each meal
• easily digested foods

General advice to the parents for when the next lot of teeth start coming in:

• lighten the diet; give more water if the baby is on milk
• if the child is being weaned and starts to get distressed while teething, go back to simpler foods such as baby rice or even milk until the problem passes
• especially avoid giving any meat and other high protein foods

Occasionally, even after one lot of teething problems has been resolved and you have given the appropriate advice on diet, you will still need to treat with acupuncture. For some children, it takes a little more than just a change in diet to rid themselves of accumulation disorder. At this stage, it is safe to use *si feng* (M-UE-9). If the child is greedy, also use S-44 *(nei ting)* to reduce the Stomach heat.

How Often to Treat?

In mild cases, only one treatment should be necessary to see the child through the teething. In addition, give the appropriate advice on diet so as to clear the accumulation disorder. In more severe cases, you may have to treat every day. If the child is very hot and there is a risk of convulsions, treat twice a day.

Remedies to Use at Home during Teething

There are certain "home remedies" that all mothers should know about to help them through the trials of a teething baby:

• homeopathic Chamomilla teething granules help reduce the heat and discomfort
• biochemic tissue salts are also used for teething

Both of these are easily obtainable from pharmacists and can be given every two hours. Other self-help remedies include:

- Bonjela (a remedy available in Britain) can help cool down the gums
- chamomile tea can be given to sip
- oil of cloves is cooling and alleviates the pain
- essential oil of chamomile: put one to two drops of essential oil of chamomile in a cup of ice-cold water, stir, and then rub on the inflamed gums
- gin or brandy rubbed on the gums with the forefinger can help reduce the pain

Comment

Teething is, in fact, one of the 'gateways' of life (see Chapter 43), a transition where one's health takes a turn either for the better or the worse. It is now rare for health to be injured at this time, but it can happen that the uprising of Kidney energy needed to push the teeth out can be a decisive time in clearing out cold and dampness that has been there since birth.

❖

10 ❖ Abdominal Pain

INTRODUCTION

Abdominal pain of one sort or another is extremely common in children, so much so that one Chinese doctor told me, "Children only have digestive problems." Below we will outline eight causes of abdominal pain, the last three of which, being less common, will not be discussed further in this chapter.

External cold (excessive exterior cold). The most common cause of this pattern is the consumption of cold energy foods. However, there are two additional etiologies: catching a chill and food poisoning or enteritis. The clinical manifestations and prognosis of these three disorders vary slightly, but the broad picture is the same, as is the treatment, whether with acupuncture or herbs.

Milk and food causing accumulation disorder (interior excess with or without heat). This is the common pattern of accumulation disorder. The Intestines and Stomach become blocked with food, which causes pain. The blockage may begin as a cold pattern, but the obstructed food may subsequently transform into heat.

Organs cold from deficiency (interior cold from deficiency). This pattern usually arises over a period of time, often after a long or serious disease when the child's qi has been weakened. In practice, however, it is rare to find a purely excessive or deficient pattern upon the first presentation. You may, therefore, see this deficient pattern during the course of treating another disease after the excessive aspect has been cleared.

Qi obstruction and blood stasis (interior excess). This pattern is more commonly seen in hospitals than in outpatient practice.

Roundworms (interior excess). Roundworms are commonly seen, but in the West it is rare for them to develop to the stage where they cause abdominal pain.

Retention of phlegm (interior cold from excess). If the digestion is weakened for a long time (the third pattern above) and the child consumes many phlegm-producing foods, or is treated frequently with antibiotics, it is possible for phlegm-dampness to accumulate in the middle burner. This can give rise to mild abdominal pain. Further discussion of this pattern is provided in the chapter on vomiting, which is usually a more pronounced symptom than abdominal pain.

Lingering pathogenic factor (interior excess). A lingering pathogenic factor can cause swelling of the lymph glands in the abdomen, which results in pain. The pain is dull and has no specific pattern.

Intestinal prolapse. This usually occurs after another illness, especially diarrhea. True intestinal prolapse (as opposed to anal prolapse) is an acute disorder which may require surgery.

The first five patterns above cover most situations where abdominal pain is the main presenting symptom. They include the following biomedical diseases, all of which can be effectively treated with acupuncture:

- appendicitis (usually associated with either the first or second pattern)
- colic (usually associated with either the first or second pattern)
- dysentery, diarrhea, enteritis
- colitis

It is our opinion that cases of uncomplicated, acute appendicitis should be treated with acupuncture first, where this is possible. If acupuncture is unavailable or unhelpful, such patients will require emergency surgery.

ETIOLOGY & PATHOGENESIS

Attack of External Cold

Etiology

- periumbilical area is exposed to cold wind or left uncovered in cold weather
- contaminated food or drink introduce a pathogenic factor
- overconsumption of fruit or cold foods and beverages. (This refers both to food whose temperature is cold and to food of a cold nature, such as bananas.) Also

indigestible foods, foods to which the child is allergic (see "Notes" below), and cold medicines, such as antibiotics.

• in very young babies, the cold may come from the mother taking anesthetics during childbirth

We have found in our practice that this pattern is frequently caused by a *combination* of weak digestion and the consumption of foods that are difficult to digest, for example, raw carrots or whole foods. By themselves the foods are not cold in nature, but this combination gives rise to the cold pattern.

Pathogenesis | Cold invades the Intestines and, owing to its contracting nature, causes spasms, which in turn leads to obstruction. This causes the qi to stagnate and results in severe, violent pain.

Milk and Food Causing Accumulation Disorder

Etiology | Irregular feeding, demand feeding, overfeeding, or over-drinking injures the Spleen and Stomach. Indigestible foods, failure to burp after meals, or sleeping immediately after feeding may all cause stagnation.

Pathogenesis | Too much food blocks the middle burner, which obstructs the flow of qi and causes pain.

Organs Cold from Deficiency

Etiology | Owing to general yang deficiency or a long illness, the Spleen and Stomach become deficient and cold. In newborn babies, the cause may be a difficult birth or anesthetics given during childbirth.

Pathogenesis | The yang of the middle burner is insufficient, inhibiting its transportive and transformative functions. The Spleen yang is unable to digest food and water, leading to the formation of interior cold and dampness. There is likewise a breakdown in the functioning of the qi mechanism, which gives rise to dull and deep abdominal pain.

Qi Obstruction and Blood Stasis

Etiology | This pattern arises from traumatic injury or surgery.

Pathogenesis | The flow of qi and blood is impaired due to trauma, injury, or surgery. This causes pain.

Roundworms

Etiology

This pattern is associated with contaminated or unwashed food, or the failure to properly wash one's hands.

Pathogenesis

Eggs hatch in the small intestine, and the larvae migrate to the lungs. They then ascend through the respiratory tract and are swallowed. The worms mature in the jejunum. In severe cases, there may be many mature worms, 25-35cm in length, which block the intestines.

The primary cause of roundworms is the ingestion of roundworm eggs via the mouth, but they will not develop and hatch in a body with well-regulated digestion. If a child keeps getting roundworms, it is an indication of underlying accumulation disorder. This should be treated accordingly, in addition to giving vermifuges.

Abdominal Pain

Exposure to cold —
Contaminated food — Cold accumulates — Sudden pain (often colicky)
Cold food —

Overeating —
Wrong food — Accumulation disorder — Pain and distention
(often with heat)

Illness —
Exhaustion — Spleen qi deficiency — Intermittent pain

Injury —
Surgery — Qi obstruction and blood stasis — Fixed and knife-like

Worms — Block intestines — Pain and swelling

PATTERNS & SYMPTOMS

Attack of external cold

- onset of abdominal pain is sudden and rushes violently up and down; pain is often colicky, as though a battle is raging inside
- patient curves spine backwards and shouts out
- facial color is bright white, with blue-gray between the lips and nose
- often sweating in upper half of body because of the pain
- pain is relieved by warmth and aggravated by cold
- cold hands and feet
- cyanosed lips

- abdominal area very tender
- borborygmus.

In addition to these signs and symptoms, there may also be:

- infrequent vomiting and diarrhea, with watery and unformed stools
- clear and copious urine
- if due to cold food, the symptoms are more pronounced for up to two hours after feeding, and may recur during the night

Tongue coating: thick, white
Pulse: deep and strong or wiry
Finger vein: red or hidden (invisible)

Note: this pattern is readily differentiated from the deficient pattern by the violence of the child's reaction to the pain, and from accumulation disorder by the white facial color.

Treatment principle: regulate the qi and disperse the cold

Milk and food causing accumulation disorder

- abdomen is distended, full, and painful; the pain is severely aggravated by pressure
- facial color is green, especially around the mouth, and there are often red cheeks
- foul breath
- absence of appetite or thirst
- burping with regurgitated food and foul smell
- flatulence with foul smell
- stools are often irregular, with very foul smell or undigested food
- possibly abdominal pain preceding diarrhea, with the pain relieved by passing stool
- possibly pain preceding vomiting, with the pain reduced by vomiting
- restless at night, with much crying

Tongue coating: greasy
Pulse: wiry, slippery
Finger vein: purple, full

Treatment principle: reduce the food stagnation and remove the obstruction, move the qi, and harmonize the middle burner

Organs cold from deficiency

- intermittent abdominal pain which comes and goes and is relieved by warmth; when the pain is present, the child moans and groans
- patient is choosy about food and often gets a dull pain after eating

- facial color often dull white
- body wasted and tired
- spirit is weak
- cold limbs
- poor appetite
- weak digestion
- watery stools

Tongue coating: thin, white
Pulse: fine, soft
Finger vein: thin or invisible

Treatment principle: warm the middle burner and tonify the deficiency, nourish the Spleen, and stop the pain

Qi obstruction and blood stasis

- pain is fixed, continuous, and knife-like
- lumps, which do not move when pressed
- any pressure causes extreme aggravation of the pain
- pain is more severe at night
- color of lips is dull
- history of traumatic injury

Tongue body: purple dots
Pulse: fine and irregular, or wiry and slippery

Treatment principle: move the blood and transform the clots, move the qi, and reduce the pain

Roundworms

- abdominal discomfort and swelling, slight pain
- poor appetite and pica (craving) for dirt, candles, coal
- disturbed sleep—dreams of battles, grinds teeth, wakes up shouting
- easily startled, clings to mother
- cough due to the worm larvae migrating to the lungs
- black spots on sclera of eyes
- white, unpigmented patches on cheeks

Note: this pattern is sometimes difficult to distinguish from that of milk and food blockage

In severe cases:

- nausea, vomiting (perhaps of roundworms)
- intestinal blockage, diarrhea
- severe cough, even pneumonia; blood-stained phlegm
- urticaria
- fierce pain from gallbladder or pancreas
- muscles weak and wasted

TREATMENT

Main points	CV-12 *(zhong wan)*	Alarm *(mù)* point of the Stomach
	S-25 *(tian shu)*	Alarm *(mù)* point of the Large Intestine
	S-36 *(zu san li)*	Tonifies the Spleen and Stomach and clears the excess
	Sp-4 *(gong sun)*	Master point of the penetrating vessel, clears the excess, and regulates the middle burner
Additional points that are frequently used	LI-4 *(he gu)*	Although more often used for disorders of excess, this point can also tonify with appropriate needle technique
	Sp-6 *(san yin jiao)*	Meeting point of three leg yin, and regulates the abdominal area, specifically for abdominal pain
	B-20 *(pi shu)*	Tonifies and regulates the Spleen

According to Symptom

P-6 *(nei guan)*	Vomiting
Liv-3 *(tai chong)*	Violent pain

According to Pattern

Attack of external cold

The main points listed above are sufficient and are used with the reducing technique. The abdominal points may be warmed with moxibustion.

PROGNOSIS

Weather chill: one to three treatments

Food poisoning: one treatment in mild cases; in severe cases treatment should be given every two hours until patient recovers

Enteritis: one to three treatments

Cold food: this disorder has usually been present for a long time before the patient comes for treatment; consequently, it has often developed into a pattern of excess complicated by deficiency. Requires one to three treatments to clear the excess, but longer to tonify the deficiency.

Anesthetics in childbirth: possibly five to ten treatments

Milk and food causing accumulation disorder

In babies under the age of four, the main point might be: *si feng* (M-UE-9), which clears the blockage. An additional point is:

LI-4 *(he gu)* — Clears the blockage from the Stomach and Intestines

Some sources add:

S-43 *(xian gu)* — Clears the blockage in the Stomach area (point's name can be translated as "descend food")

Method: all the points are treated with a reducing technique

Prognosis: in genuine cases of excess, one treatment is usually enough. In patterns of excess complicated by deficiency, first treat the excess, and when it has cleared, then treat the deficiency. May require three to six treatments to provide sufficient tonification. Following treatment the child may be irritable for one or two nights and discharge foul-smelling stools.

Organs cold from deficiency

S-36 *(zu san li)*
CV-12 *(zhong wan)* — Tonifies the Spleen and Stomach
CV-8 *(shen que)*

Method: in patients who are still reasonably strong, both acupuncture (tonifying method) and moxibustion may be used. In really weak patients, only use indirect moxibustion or moxibustion on ginger. Pay attention to the needle technique: accidental reducing can further weaken the qi and cause more diarrhea.

Prognosis: five to ten treatments are common. Even if treatments are given every day, it may still take two to three weeks to cure in very deficient cases. With older children in whom the condition has been present for a long time, it may take six months to a year before the child is really healthy.

Note: it is important to pay attention to the diet. Make sure the child does not become overtired and that it gets enough sleep.

Qi obstruction, blood stasis

The main points listed above are not used. Instead, use *ashi* points, points which lie on the same channel as the area of pain, and the following points:

Liv-2 *(xing jian)*
Liv-3 *(tai chong)* — Transforms blood stasis
B-17 *(ge shu)*

Method: all the points are treated with a reducing technique

Prognosis: one to three treatments to clear the excess; in very severe cases, treat every two hours

Roundworms

Roundworms are better treated with herbs or herbal derivatives than with acupuncture. If herbs are not available, or if for any reason the child cannot take them, then acupuncture may be substituted. The following treatment is described in *Collection of Clinical Experiences with Acupuncture (Zhen jiu lin zheng ji yan)*, but I have no experience with its use. Always remember that unit measurements are relative to the size of the patient's body. Deep needling in the treatment of worms should be performed only with great caution.

Sp-15 *(da heng)*	After insertion, the needle is directed toward the umbilicus to a depth of 2 to 2.5 units; apply strong manipulation with lifting and thrusting
CV-12 *(zhong wan)*	Needle to a depth of 1.5 to 2.5 units; lift and thrust
CV-6 *(qi hai)* *ashi* points Sp-4 *(gong sun)*	Needle to a depth of 1 to 1.5 units

Continue lifting and thrusting the needles at the above points until the abdominal pain is reduced, then treat the following points with the dispersing method:

S-36 *(zu san li)*	1 to 2 units deep
LI-4 *(he gu)*	0.5 to 1 unit deep

Prognosis: treat once a day. Most of the roundworms should be eliminated in three to five days.

If there are roundworms in the bile duct, use the following points:

G-34 *(yang ling quan)*
CV-15 *(jiu wei)*
ashi points

NOTES

• Pay attention to the diet. Take care especially to give cooling foods for warm disorders and warming foods for cold disorders. Traditional Chinese medicine teaches that the temperature of a food affects the Stomach, while the nature of the energy of a food affects the Spleen. Also watch for difficult-to-digest foods taken by the baby or the mother. Commonly eaten foods in this category include onions, turnips, cabbage, leeks, brussel sprouts, green peppers, and generally any food with a lot of fiber, such as brown rice, brown bread, and raw vegetables. Regularity of meals is also very important for children. Eating too much or too often ('grazing') is a common cause of accumulation disorder and abdominal pain in young children.

- Look out for food allergies. Among the most common culprits are the following: bananas (very cold), cow's milk (also produces phlegm), peanuts (also produces phlegm), tomatoes, and gluten. Almost any food, however, can cause an allergic response in some children. For example, we had one patient who was allergic to honey and another to chicken.

- Pay attention to weaning. It should be done gently, on foods that are easy to digest. Rough foods such as whole wheat bread and brown rice should be avoided at the beginning.

- Pay attention to the state of the mother. If she is anxious or angry, or has gall stones, her milk can be very bitter and cause abdominal pain.

- For a case history involving abdominal pain, see Case 11 in Chapter 47.

❖

11 ❖ Vomiting

INTRODUCTION

Vomiting is very common in babies and children because their digestive systems are weak and only gradually strengthen with age. In Shakespeare's seven ages of man, the baby is depicted as "mewling and puking in its mother's arms." It is the normal function of the Stomach to send food down to the Small Intestine, and vomiting occurs when, for some reason, it is prevented from doing so.* In children there may be a substantial physical blockage, such as accumulated food, or there may be a less substantial factor, such as accumulated heat. (This contrasts with the adult disorders, where one of the most common patterns of vomiting is due to Liver qi invading the Stomach.)

Four basic patterns of vomiting are described here, with the second pattern subdivided into three parts. This subdivision is not commonly made in Chinese textbooks, but is included here because we have found it to be quite helpful, especially in areas with a damp climate and where much cow's milk is consumed.

1. Retention of food and milk (interior excess). This pattern appears in strong, healthy children. It is often a temporary phenomenon from overeating, or as a result of overexcite-

---

*The proper direction for the movement of Stomach qi is downward, that is, it should descend. When the qi moves the wrong way, it is said to rebel. In such cases there will be symptoms like vomiting, burping, and heaving. This condition is expressed in traditional Chinese medicine by the word *nì*, which is usually translated as 'rebellious'. However, it can also simply mean 'ascending' or 'rising up'. We use the words 'rebellious' or 'rising' interchangeably, as suits the situation.

ment. If it keeps recurring, one may suspect accumulation disorder.

2. Spleen and Stomach deficiency. This pattern can be divided into three patterns, which may blend into each other. In all three patterns the Stomach and Spleen are weak and cold. It is therefore a condition of deficiency. However, for vomiting to occur there must be some factor of excess, in this case cold. The cold may be internal or an external pathogenic factor.

The degree of deficiency in the three patterns ranges from a mainly deficient condition, with the emphasis on weak digestion, to a more excessive condition, with the emphasis on cold or phlegm. In all three patterns the vomit may contain undigested food because the Stomach is cold and cannot digest it properly.

In the first pattern, *Stomach cold*, the child is predominantly deficient with a weak Spleen and some cold from excess in the Stomach, often due to the diet.

In the second pattern, *Stomach water*, the child may appear remarkably healthy in all other respects because the cold is localized in the Stomach and Spleen. Therefore, the overall qi of the child may be quite good; it is just that the Stomach and Spleen are cold.

In the third pattern, *phlegm obstruction*, the child is full of phlegm. This pattern is an extension of either of the two previous ones. It may develop either because the Spleen is weak, allowing phlegm to form (an extension of Stomach cold), or because the child is relatively healthy but simply eats lots of cold and phlegm-forming foods (an extension of Stomach water), or because it has a history of taking many antibiotics.

3. Accumulated heat in the Spleen and Stomach (interior heat from excess). This is a condition of excess, where heat from excess accumulates in the Stomach. These children are usually hot and have red faces. In addition, the heat may make them irritable and restless. This condition is the nearest equivalent to the adult pattern of Liver invading the Stomach, but in children, it is not due to emotional causes. Rather, it is more commonly associated with overeating, especially of hot, spicy foods, or with a lingering pathogenic factor that has been left behind after an immunization.

In some cases the cause may be traced back to 'womb heat'. A glance at the mother is usually enough to determine if this is the cause, for she will have a red face. This pattern includes the symptom of projectile vomiting.

4. Insufficient Stomach yin (interior heat from deficiency). This pattern is not commonly seen in the West because febrile diseases are usually treated promptly with antibiotics.

There is one other pattern that is not discussed in this chapter, but which may cause vomiting: pathogenic wind-heat. Because heat has a dispersing nature, pathogenic wind-heat usually causes diarrhea as well as vomiting. However, the vomiting is usually so short-lived that it is not worth treating.

Both vomiting and diarrhea are common problems when babies are weaned from the breast and started on regular food. This is a very important period in the development of a child, and problems that start here may last a lifetime. When weaning, new foods should be introduced gradually to give the Stomach time to adapt. Rough, fibrous foods in particular, such as bran, brown rice, brown bread, and raw vegetables, should be avoided if there is any sign of accumulation disorder.

ETIOLOGY & PATHOGENESIS

Retention of Food and Milk

Etiology

Usually due to overeating, eating when overexcited, or eating oily, greasy, or indigestible foods. If it is a recurring phenomenon it is usually due to accumulation disorder, which itself is caused by an inappropriate diet.

Pathogenesis

In children, the Spleen and Stomach are weak. The Stomach has difficulty 'ripening and rotting' the food, and the Spleen has difficulty 'transforming' it, especially when it is oily or greasy. The Stomach becomes too full, and the Spleen's ability to transport and transform is impaired. Undigested food thereupon obstructs the Stomach passage; unable to descend, it rises up as vomit.

Spleen and Stomach Deficiency

Etiology

All three of the followng patterns have their root in deficiency, which varies from mild to severe. There is nearly always the added factor of a cold or dampness-forming diet on top of an already weak, cold Spleen.

Pathogenesis

In all three patterns the Stomach and Spleen are deficient in energy and cannot transform, transport, or rot and ripen the food, which is then only partly digested. When the Stomach qi rises up and causes vomiting, there is often partly-digested food in the vomit.

Stomach Cold

Etiology

This pattern is seen in children who are obviously Spleen qi deficient. It may be present from birth if it was long and traumatic, or if anesthetics were used in the delivery. It is also seen after a long or severe illness, or if the child has been weakened by immunizations. The problem is often compounded by a cold-energy diet.

Pathogenesis

Cold food obstructs the Stomach, which is too weak to warm it, or external cold causes cold qi to rise up, causing vomiting.

Stomach Water

Etiology

These children tend to have more qi and look comparatively healthy; the problem is localized to the Stomach, which is cold. The cause is an external attack by cold on the Stomach, most commonly when too many dairy products, fruit, or other cold and dampness-forming foods are eaten. It is also seen after exposure to cold and dampness. Hence, this pattern is very common in regions which are cold and damp and where a lot of dairy products are eaten.

It is also common in young babies that are breastfed when the child is greedy or when the mother's milk flows abundantly and the energy of the mother is cold. Another contributory factor is the tendency of these babies to fall asleep while feeding. This compounds the already existing problem.

Pathogenesis

The long-term presence of cold in the Stomach weakens the Spleen yang so that cold-dampness accumulates in the Stomach. There is insufficient yang to 'rot and ripen' the food, thus some food and/or a thin watery fluid is vomited.

Phlegm Obstruction

Etiology

This is a chronic pattern where the Stomach and Spleen are somewhat deficient and there is the added factor of phlegm. The pattern may be caused by a variety of factors, including:

- history of illnesses treated with antibiotics
- diet of phlegm-forming foods
- illness that has weakened the Spleen and given rise to much phlegm in the body
- immunizations (e.g., for pertussis or polio)

Pathogenesis	The Spleen yang is deficient, cold-dampness accumulates, and the fluids readily stagnate, all leading to the formation of phlegm. The phlegm obstructs the Stomach qi, which results in vomiting.

Accumulated Heat in the Spleen and Stomach

Etiology	This pattern can arise from:

- eating too much fatty, oily, or spicy foods
- possibly the accumulation disorder
- womb heat
- a hot lingering pathogenic factor that is left behind after an immunization
- a febrile disease

Pathogenesis	Heat accumulates and obstructs the middle burner. Qi rises up and causes vomiting.

Insufficient Stomach Yin

Etiology	This pattern is usually the result of a long-term febrile disease. For this reason, it is rarely seen in the West.
Pathogenesis	During febrile diseases the qi and yin are weakened, and internal heat dries out the body fluids and injures the yin. The Stomach becomes disharmonious and is unable to moisten and digest food. Vomiting ensues.

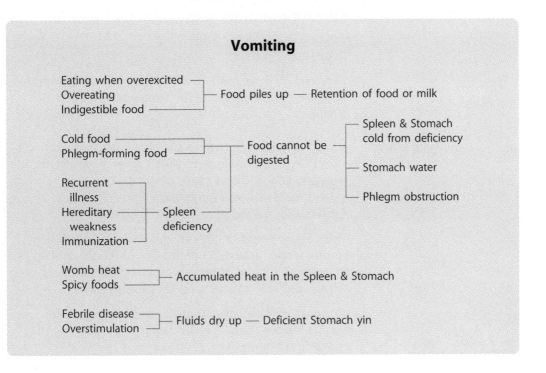

PATTERNS & SYMPTOMS

Retention of food and milk

- vomiting of curdled milk or undigested food; vomit has a sour smell, and the breath smells foul
- abdominal pain
- child weeps and is restless

If this continues for any length of time, accumulation disorder may develop, with the following symptoms:

- red cheeks
- irregular stools with diarrhea alternating with constipation
- stools are foul-smelling or smell like apples

Tongue coating: thick, gray
Pulse: slippery

Treatment principle: harmonize the digestion and resolve the obstruction, reduce the food stagnation, and stop the vomiting

Stomach cold

- vomiting of undigested food and milk
- aversion to cold, limbs are cold
- lack of vitality
- pale face
- dull eyes
- blue above the lips
- tends to sleep a lot during the day
- stools contain particles of undigested food

Tongue coating: sticky, white
Pulse: small, forceless

Treatment principle: regulate the Spleen and strengthen the middle burner, harmonize the Stomach, and direct the rebellious qi downward

Stomach water

- healthy-appearing (strong and cheerful) child with milk trickling out of the mouth for about an hour after eating
- occasionally vomits a clear, watery fluid
- vomit contains partly digested food
- dribbles at the mouth

This pattern continues day-in and day-out, sometimes getting worse, sometimes better. The child does not appear to be deficient, and, if herbal tonics are used, is likely to have vomit with mucus soon after ingestion.

Treatment principle: regulate the Spleen and warm the middle burner, transform the dampness, and direct the rebellious qi downward

Phlegm obstruction

- vomiting of phlegm and clear, sticky fluid or vomiting food mixed with watery phlegm
- vomit may become yellow or green in prolonged attacks
- may have mucus in the stools
- often has other signs of phlegm

The child may vomit phlegm only once a week or less, and usually feels better after vomiting. The phlegm then gradually builds up again, and the child becomes increasingly irritable and loses its appetite before vomiting again.

Tongue coating: yellow, greasy
Pulse: slippery

Treatment principle: regulate the Spleen and transform the phlegm

Accumulated heat in the Spleen and Stomach

- vomiting follows eating
- vomit has a foul smell or yellow color
- projectile vomiting
- thirst
- good appetite
- irritability, restlessness
- poor sleep
- clingy
- body hot, face red

The vomiting associated with this pattern may be very violent, with food being thrown over the room (projectile vomiting). Soon after vomiting the child feels better and often asks for more food. This pattern may develop suddenly if there is a sudden attack of heat, or it may come in waves of a few days duration interspersed with periods of no vomiting.

Tongue body: red
Tongue coating: yellow
Pulse: slippery, rapid

Treatment principle: clear the heat and harmonize the Stomach, direct the rebellious qi downward, and stop the vomiting

Insufficient Stomach yin

- vomit contains little fluid
- throat and mouth are dry, but no desire to drink
- cheeks are red, palms and soles are hot

Tongue body: red and dry, with very little coating
Pulse: fine, rapid, forceless

Treatment principle: clear the heat and enrich the yin

TREATMENT

Acupuncture is usually very successful in the treatment of vomiting in children.

Main points

P-6 *(nei guan)*	Coupled point of the penetrating vessel; the main point for controlling vomiting (the Pericardium channel passes through the Stomach)
S-36 *(zu san li)*	Regulates and harmonizes the Stomach
CV-12 *(zhong wan)*	Alarm point of the Stomach; a local point
Sp-4 *(gong sun)*	Moves the qi in the abdomen; master point of the penetrating vessel; when combined with P-6 *(nei guan)*, especially effective for relieving fullness in the middle burner

If there is very violent, uncontrolled vomiting, do one of the following:

- needle the 'Stomach and Intestines' hand point, located 0.5 unit distal to P-7 *(da ling)*
- prick and bleed *jin jin* and *yu ye* (together known as M-HN-20), which are located on the underside of the tongue on either side of the frenulum

These points should only be used when other methods fail.

According to Pattern

Retention of food and milk

Use the main points listed above, but select CV-10 *(xia wan)* instead of CV-12 *(zhong wan)*; this point is more effective in causing food to descend. In addition, add the following points:

CV-22 *(tian tu)* CV-23 *(lian quan)*	Both of these points have the action of causing food to descend

OR—

S-43 *(xian gu)*	The name of this point literally means "descend food"

OR—

S-41 *(jie xi)*	Strengthens the Spleen, transforms the dampness, clears the Stomach, and directs the rebellious qi downward

In babies, if there is any sign of accumulation disorder, use:

si feng (M-UE-9)   Clears accumulation disorder

For lower abdominal pain, add:

S-25 *(tian shu)*   Alarm *(mù)* point of Large Intestine

Prognosis: this condition often resolves by itself. If not, one to three daily treatments should be sufficient.

Spleen and Stomach deficiency

For all three patterns, use the main points listed above, plus the following:

B-20 (pi *shu*)   Associated *(shū)* point of the Spleen
B-21 *(wei shu)*   Associated *(shū)* point of the Stomach
CV-6 *(qi hai)*   Tonifies the qi of the body
S-25 *(tian shu)*   Promotes movement in the Intestines

Method: indirect moxibustion or moxibustion on ginger at CV-12 *(zhong wan)* may be used

Stomach cold

The main points and those listed immediately above are sufficient. Use a tonifying technique as well as moxibustion.

Prognosis: if due to a pathogenic factor, the vomiting is usually resolved in one or two treatments even though the pathogenic factor may still remain. If due to weakness it may take five to ten treatments to restore the child to health, depending on how weak the child has become. In some cases of severe deficiency it may take up to fifteen treatments.

Stomach water

Use the same points as for Stomach cold, especially P-6 *(nei guan)* and S-36 *(zu san li).* It is also helpful to add the following:

Sp-9 *(yin ling quan)*   Both points strengthen the Spleen
Sp-6 *(san yin jiao)*   and resolve dampness

Prognosis: if the child has a poor appetite but is reasonably healthy, this disorder is easy to cure and takes only three to five treatments. If, however, the child has a good appetite, the disorder cannot be cured *if* the mother persists in letting it breastfeed too much. This may be hard to change, as such children often have strong dispositions.

Phlegm obstruction	Use the same points as for Stomach cold plus S-40 *(feng long)*, which acts to transform the phlegm. Moxibustion on garlic may be used.

Prognosis: this disorder usually takes five to ten treatments to cure unless the patient has become very weak, in which case more treatments will be needed. Often the phlegm is voided through the stools. |
| *Accumulated heat in the Spleen and Stomach* | Use the main points listed above plus S-44 *(nei ting)* and Ll-4 *(he gu)*, which clear the excessive heat from the Stomach and Intestines. If there is extreme heat, with danger of convulsions or delirium, add P-9 *(zhong chong)* and LI-1 *(shang yang)*.

Prognosis: this disorder can take from five to ten treatments to clear completely |
| *Insufficient Stomach yin* | Use the main points listed above, plus the following: |

S-43 *(xian gu)*	Clears heat from the Stomach
CV-4 *(guan yuan)*	⎫
K-7 *(fu liu)*	⎬ Tonifies the yin of the entire body
K-6 *(zhao hai)*	⎭
B-20 *(pi shu)*	Associated *(shū)* point of the Spleen; regulates the yin and yang of the Spleen
B-21 *(wei shu)*	Associated *(shū)* point of the Stomach; regulates the yin and yang of the Stomach

Prognosis: depends on the severity of the disease and how depleted the patient is. Yin deficiency in children is very rare in the West, primarily because of the early use of antibiotics in treating febrile disease.

NOTES

• Vomiting is sometimes seen as the only side effect of immunization against pertussis.

• In breastfed babies, always consider the state of the mother. If she is anxious and nervous, the milk may be indigestible and give rise to accumulation disorder. If she is tired and exhausted, the milk may be insufficiently nourishing or too watery, which may give rise to patterns of Stomach cold from deficiency or Stomach water.

• In bottle-fed babies, check the composition of the milk and the frequency of feeding. Cow's milk and artificial milk are usually richer than human milk, and can easily lead to accumulation disorder or to phlegm obstruction.

• For case histories involving vomiting, see Cases 12, 13, and 14 in Chapter 47.

❖

12 ❖ Childhood Nutritional Impairment

INTRODUCTION

Childhood nutritional impairment *(gān)* used to be one of the four great scourges in pediatrics, along with measles, smallpox, and febrile convulsions. With improved living standards and intravenous feeding, it is now no longer the fatal disease it used to be in the Western world, although in developing nations it takes as large a toll as it ever did. The condition is only really encountered in the West as 'celiac disease' (gluten allergy) and certain other food allergies, and even then it rarely reaches the stage of severe malnutrition. As a result, the whole of this chapter is based on translations from the Chinese, and we have no experience of our own to offer. One thing that emerges from the Chinese doctors who do have experience in treating childhood nutritional impairment is that acupuncture is extremely effective and is even the therapy of first choice in clearing accumulation.

The etiology and pathogenesis of the principal types of childhood nutritional impairment are quite clearly presented in the textbooks as being a further progression of accumulation disorder. What is not so clear is the description of the complications. Only the more important complications are listed, but in older Chinese books upwards of a dozen different patterns are associated with childhood nutritional impairment. While each pattern has its specific treatment, the priority in all cases is to cure the childhood nutritional impairment. Any sequelae can then be dealt with.

The pattern of most interest to Western practitioners in this category is 'tooth childhood nutritional impairment' *(yá gān)*, which is the nearest thing in Chinese texts to the common Western problem of teething. Chinese children do not appear to have any comparable problems when their teeth erupt, so the Chinese texts have little to offer. I am unsure why this is so. It may be a genuine difference in physiology, but I suspect that it is more a cultural difference. Chinese in general keep their children quieter than we do in the West, and less stimulated.

In addition, they seem to take more care with their diets. Tooth childhood nutritional impairment has many symptoms which are common to teething, but is generally a much more severe disease, progressing rapidly with really black gums. (For further discussion of teething, see Chapter 9.)

ETIOLOGY & PATHOGENESIS

Food and Drink not Digested, Spleen and Stomach Attacked and Injured

Etiology

It takes energy for children to digest milk or food. This type of childhood nutritional impairment is caused by overconsumption of fatty or sweet foods, or simply overeating.

Pathogenesis

If the consumption of food exceeds the tolerance of the Spleen and Stomach, the food becomes cold and obstructs the middle burner, which further affects the Spleen and Stomach. Digestion is then unregulated, and accumulation disorder occurs. Over a long period of time, the accumulation disorder becomes more and more severe. Without proper digestion, the organs, qi, and blood become weak and exhausted, the body is emaciated, the qi and fluids are consumed, and childhood nutritional impairment ensues.

Inadequate Food: the System of Nourishment Becomes Unregulated

Etiology

Insufficient mother's milk, too early weaning, or eating unsuitable food.

Pathogenesis

Lack of proper nutrition for an extended period of time provides inadequate support for the Spleen and Stomach. When these organs are injured, water and food cannot be transformed, and exhaustion and further malnourishment occur. Traditionally, this is referred to as a failure of support for the "yin organs, yang organs, flesh, four limbs, and hundred bones." The body is emaciated, tired and feeble, the qi and blood are weak and collapsed, and childhood nutritional impairment ensues.

From Other Diseases

Etiology

The result of prolonged vomiting, diarrhea, dysentery, abdominal pain, tuberculosis of the intestines, parasites, and similar problems.

Pathogenesis

Prolonged illness injures qi and blood, the Spleen and Lungs are weakened, and the digestion becomes unregulated and is without foundation. As a result, the basal qi becomes deficient, and bone marrow is not created. Extreme injury to the yang affects the yin, and yin fire from deficiency flares up, consuming body fluids and wasting the body away. The yin organs are thereby injured, and childhood nutritional impairment ensues.

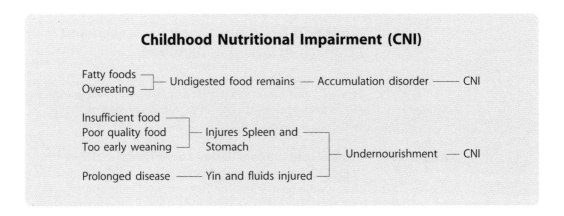

Childhood Nutritional Impairment (CNI)

Fatty foods / Overeating —— Undigested food remains — Accumulation disorder —— CNI

Insufficient food / Poor quality food / Too early weaning — Injures Spleen and Stomach

Prolonged disease —— Yin and fluids injured — Undernourishment — CNI

PATTERNS & SYMPTOMS

Accumulation disorder injures the Spleen

• yellow facial color
• emaciated flesh
• thirst
• restless sleep
• stools unformed or constipation
• urine yellow, turbid, or milky

Tongue coating: dirty, greasy
Pulse: slippery, fine
Finger vein: thin

Treatment principle: clear the obstruction and regulate the Spleen

Spleen qi deficiency

• dull-yellow face
• body emaciated
• spirit weak and withered
• eyes without luster
• abdomen feels full of food and is distended

- whites of eyes are revealed when asleep
- possibly mild fever
- stools contain undigested food or resemble thin milk
- lips pale

Tongue body: pale red
Tongue coating: greasy
Pulse: soggy, fine, or slippery
Finger vein: thin, purple

Treatment principle: augment the qi, strengthen the Spleen, and reduce accumulation

Both qi and blood deficient

- bright-white facial color
- skin yellow and dry
- lips dry, thirst
- head big with thin neck
- body becomes emaciated and wasted
- scaphoid (boat-shaped) abdomen
- spirit tired and worn out
- sleeps with eyes open
- voice without strength
- stools unformed

Pulse: fine, forceless
Finger vein: thin

Treatment principle: reinforce the qi, support the blood, and strengthen the Spleen

Complications

CORNEAL OPACITY

- eyes become red in the wind and shed tears
- at other times, the eyeballs are blue, the cornea are opaque, and there is visual difficulty and pain in the eyes. In the past, this was known as Liver (related) childhood nutritional impairment *(gān gān).*

Treatment principle: support the Liver and brighten the eyes

EDEMA

- lower limbs and ankles have edematous swelling, and there is irregular urination. In the past, this was known as edema (related) childhood nutritional impairment *(gān shuǐ).*

Treatment principle: warm the yang and harmonize the water

BLEEDING GUMS

• gums bleed, and the mouth and lips are pale; this is often accompanied by purpura

Treatment principle: augment the qi and contain the blood

TOOTH CHILDHOOD NUTRITIONAL IMPAIRMENT

• starts as hard, red, and painful swelling of the gums or cheeks and quickly develops into gum or mouth ulcers; these may be rotten and purulent, or turn black and exude a purple-black fluid
• facial area around the mouth and on the jaw and nose is a dull-brown color
• urine is scanty and yellow
• irritability and restlessness
• in severe cases the lips are rotten, teeth fall out, and the bridge of the nose collapses; in the past, this was known as horse-tooth childhood nutritional impairment

Treatment principle: enrich the yin, clear the heat, and expel the toxin

TREATMENT

Main point

si feng (M-UE-9)

Method: the four points are pierced with a triangular needle and a few drops of yellow fluid are withdrawn. Most texts advise treating every other day, alternating the hands. However, in a study done at a hospital in Guilin, China, both hands were treated on the analogous points to *si feng* (M-UE-9) in the distal phalangeal and metacar-pophalangeal joints daily for ten days. (They called these points upper and lower *si feng*.) Every patient who completed the course of ten treatments was cured!

Additional points

CV-12 *(zhong wan)*	
S-25 *(tian shu)*	Tonifies the Spleen yang and clears blockage
B-20 *(pi shu)*	
B-21 *(wei shu)*	
S-36 *(zu san li)*	
B-18 *(gan shu)*	Tonifies the Spleen yang and Liver yin and clears blockage
B-19 *(dan shu)*	Tonifies the Spleen yang and Liver yin and clears blockage
B-23 *(shen shu)*	Tonifies the Kidney yin

According to pattern

ACCUMULATION DISORDER INJURES THE SPLEEN

S-25 *(tian shu)* is especially well-suited, in addition to *si feng* (M-UE-9).

Method: even method
Prognosis: one to three treatments

SPLEEN DEFICIENT, QI WEAK

Si feng (M-UE-9) plus the following points that tonify the Spleen qi and clear the blockage: CV-12 *(zhong wan)*, S-25 *(tian shu)*, B-20 *(pi shu)*, and S-36 *(zu san li)*

Method: tonifying method; moxibustion may be used, and especially moxibustion on garlic

Prognosis: five to ten treatments

BOTH QI AND BLOOD DEFICIENT

Si feng (M-UE-9) plus the following points that tonify the qi and blood: B-18 *(gan shu)*, B-20 *(pi shu)*, B-23 *(shen shu)*, CV-12 *(zhang wan)*, and *er bai* (M-UE-29)*

Method: tonifying method is used, also moxibustion on garlic or ginger

Prognosis: ten to twenty treatments

Complications

CORNEAL OPACITY

After clearing the childhood nutritional impairment, Liv-3 *(tai chong)* and G-20 *(feng chi)* are used to regulate the Liver and brighten the eyes.

Method: even method is used; the sensation from needling G-20 *(feng chi)* should reach the eyes

EDEMA

After clearing the childhood nutritional impairment, B-23 *(shen shu)* and K-3 *(tai xi)* are used to tonify the Kidneys.

Method: tonifying method; add moxibustion at B-23 *(shen shu)*

BLEEDING GUMS

After clearing the childhood nutritional impairment, LI-4 *(he gu)* is used to regulate the qi and blood in the gums.

Method: even method

---

*Location of *er bai* (M-UE-29): four units proximal to the middle of the transverse crease of the wrist on the palmar aspect. One point is between the tendons of palmaris longus muscle and the flexor carpi radialis muscle, and the second is on the radial side of the tendons. These are points which have been shown to be useful for intestinal prolapse.

TOOTH CHILDHOOD NUTRITIONAL IMPAIRMENT

After clearing the childhood nutritional impairment, LI-4 *(he gu)* is used to regulate the qi and blood in the gums and expel the toxin, and K-3 *(tai xi)* is used to tonify Kidney yin and clear heat.

Method: even method

❖

13 ❖ Oral Thrush and Mouth Ulcers

INTRODUCTION

Oral thrush (infection of the oral tissues with *Candida albicans)* and mouth ulcers are common in a mild form in children of all ages, from breastfed babies to school children. In severe cases the mouth can be so inflamed and painful that the child no longer wants to eat and its sleep is disturbed. It is often a result of improper diet, especially overconsumption of sweets, chocolates, and so-called 'junk' foods, overconsumption of warming foods, or heat accumulating inside. In breastfed babies it is often due to heat rising from blocked digestion, a hot condition of the mother, or medicines (especially antibiotics) that she is taking. Oral thrush and mouth ulcers can also arise as a complication of another disease, in which case that disease should be treated first.

The differentiation of patterns and treatment regimens discussed in this chapter are those for thrush. However, because mouth ulcers are nearly the same, a separate chapter devoted to that disorder is unnecessary. The first two patterns are those given in the Chinese books and are still seen in the West. However, recently in England and in the United States, a new pattern has arisen, one that is more cold and damp.

ETIOLOGY & PATHOGENESIS

Traditional Patterns

According to the Chinese, there are two interior patterns: full heat in the Stomach and Spleen, and fire from yin deficiency. In both patterns, heat rises up to the mouth, which then becomes infected. In the West another pattern has arisen, cold-dampness.

Full heat in the Stomach and Spleen

In babies that are breastfed, the common causes are:

- the mother has hot energy
- the mother is eating hot and dampness-producing foods
- the baby has accumulation disorder

In older children the cause can usually be traced to a diet containing a lot of hot, spicy, and rich foods, junk foods, or lots of sugar. All of these contribute to the formation of heat. When heat accumulates in the Stomach and Spleen, it can rise up and transform into pathogenic toxin, which 'smokes and steams' in the mouth and tongue, manifesting in white spots surrounded by areas of red. The white spots may spread to the larynx, trachea, and esophagus, causing difficulty in breathing and swallowing food. Fire also rises up, causing a red face and red lips. Fire may spread to the Heart, leading to irritability and restlessness, and scanty, yellow urine. The heat excess in the Spleen and Stomach gives rise to halitosis and constipation.

Fire from yin deficiency

This is rarely seen in the West. When it is, it is usually due to being overtired and overstimulated. In China it is more frequently due to the yin being injured by a febrile disease. When a child's yin is injured, water can no longer control fire, and the fire from deficiency floats upward. External pathogenic heat then readily enters the mouth and causes white patches, which are surrounded by areas of red in severe cases. With insufficient Kidney yin and heat from deficiency trapped inside, symptoms characteristic of heat from yin deficiency may appear: heat in the five centers, malar flush, and a red tongue with little coating.

Cold-dampness

This usually results from either the child or mother taking antibiotics or from any other factor that causes cold and dampness to accumulate, such as overconsumption of cold fruit juice, ice cream, or sugar. The accumulation of cold-dampness in the Stomach and Spleen causes cold and dampness to accumulate in the mouth, giving rise to oral thrush.

PATTERNS & SYMPTOMS

General

White spots surrounded by areas of red appear in the mucous membranes of the mouth and may spread to the gums and lips. In severe cases there is bleeding. Often the

Oral Thrush

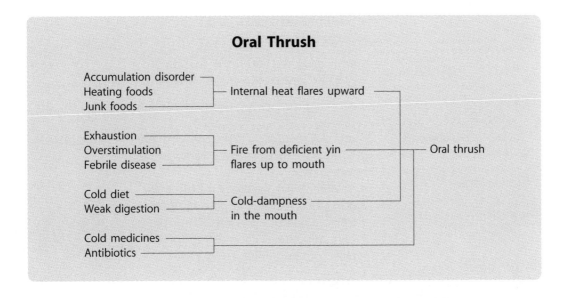

child is whimpering and clings to its mother, is restless, and does not want to eat or refuses the breast. In severe cases the white spots may spread up the nasal passages and down the throat, trachea, and esophagus, causing difficulty in swallowing and breathing. The facial color is then bluish-purple, and there is a gurgling noise on breathing.

Full heat in the Stomach and Spleen

- mucous membranes of the mouth are covered with many white spots surrounded by areas of deep red
- mouth is painful
- face and lips are red
- irritability and restlessness
- refuses milk and clings to mother
- constipation
- urine scanty, yellow

Tongue body: red
Tongue coating: white, thick, and greasy
Finger vein: purple, broad
Pulse: slippery, or slippery and rapid

Treatment principle: clear the heat, resolve the toxicity, and drain the fire

Fire from yin deficiency

- mucous membranes of the mouth have a few white spots, and the surrounding area is slightly red
- child is rather weak
- facial color is white, cheeks are red
- heat in the five centers (chest, palms, and soles)
- absence of thirst

- possibly aversion to warmth
- possibly night sweats

Tongue body: red with little coating
Pulse: fine and rapid, without strength

Treatment principle: enrich the yin and bring down the fire

Cold-dampness

- mucous membranes of the mouth are covered with white, yellowish white, creamy patches
- face is pale
- possibly loose stools with little smell
- possibly screaming at pain in night
- signs of dampness, such as runny nose, puffy face
- poor appetite or choosy over food
- feels cold and damp to touch

Tongue body: pale
Tongue coating: white
Pulse: slippery or weak

TREATMENT

Main points

Three pairs of points are used, each of which is comprised of one local and one distal point which has a direct connection with this area:

1. CV-23 *(lian quan)* with H-6 *(yin xi)*
2. S-5 *(da ying)* with S-36 *(zu san li)*
3. S-7 *(xia guan)* with LI-4 *(he gu)*

Method: treat once every day, using the first pair the first day, the second pair the second day, and so on

According to Symptom

If there are just one or two large ulcers, these may be pricked with a triangular needle. (At least that is what it says in the Chinese books, but in some countries it may take some time to persuade the mother that this is the best course of treatment!)

According to Pattern

Full heat in the Stomach and Spleen

Use the main points listed above, and add:

S-44 *(nei ting)*	Clears heat in the Stomach
LI-4 *(he gu)*	Clears heat in the Stomach, benefits the mouth

In young children where there is accumulation disorder, you may use:

si feng (M-UE-9)

Prognosis: one to three treatments are usually sufficient

Fire from yin deficiency

In addition to the main points listed above, points to tonify the body's yin should be added, such as the following:

K-3 *(tai xi)*
CV-4 *(guan yuan)*

Prognosis: depends on the origin of the disease and the severity of the condition; where another disease has caused the mouth problem, it too must be treated

Cold-dampness

In addition to the main points, use the following:

S-36 *(zu san li)*
CV-12 *(zhong wan)*
Sp-6 *(san yin jiao)*

Method: needle with even method and use moxibustion on CV-12 *(zhong wan)*

Prognosis: treat every day to clear the thrush; a few treatments should be enough if the child has stopped taking antibiotics. If the child is still taking antibiotics and sweet foods, then the treatment will only be supportive, not curative.

NOTES

- Oral thrush and mouth ulcers are sometimes encountered as a side effect of Western chemotherapy. Acupuncture is usually successful in controlling this side effect, which allows the therapy to continue.

- It is always worth including at least one local point. Children do not like points near the mouth, but using these points makes a big difference.

❖

14 ❖ Fevers and Influenza

INTRODUCTION

In this chapter we outline the treatment of fevers in children. The fundamentals are the same as fevers in adults, but there are some additional complicating factors special to babies and children.

The Chinese word for influenza *(gǎn mào)* encompasses a range of conditions from a cold in the head to a bad cough to influenza with high fever. It is often translated as 'common cold', but this is misleading, especially when one considers the meanings of the two characters. The word *gǎn* here can be understood as an effect or influence, in this case of the weather. The word *mào* shows a picture of a man unable to see because his hat is pulled down over his eyes; it means moving about wildly or reckless behavior, causing susceptibility to influence by the weather. The two words together may thus be said to mean the 'influence of reckless behavior'.

This can be compared with our own word 'influenza', which derives from Renaissance Italy, when it was regarded as being caused by the 'influence' of the elements (used here in its broader sense to mean both the elements of weather and the constituent elements of the universe). Returning to the differentiation of patterns, we can see that the Chinese also included a weather aspect to the cause of influenza, and thus we see how very close the traditional Western view of influenza is to that of the Chinese.

For the etiology, pathogenesis, and pattern differentiation, I (JPS) have translated the pertinent section from the 1979 edition of *Traditional Chinese Pediatrics (Zhong yi er ke xue)* without any alteration, for I feel it clearly expresses how influenza affects basically healthy children. But there is another factor at work in Western children, who are not nearly as robust and healthy as Chinese children, and who are treated with antibiotics at the first sign of fever. This factor is the beneficial effect of fevers in expelling accumulated heat. We have, therefore, included a section on the beneficial aspects of fevers, and how they strengthen the immune system. Thus, the section on internal factors and on lingering pathogenic factors is based on our clinical experience.

ETIOLOGY & PATHOGENESIS

Etiology

EXTERNAL FACTORS

An attack by pathogenic wind-cold or wind-heat, especially at times of change in the weather, can lead to influenza. Rapid temperature changes are particularly common in winter and spring, and the disease accordingly attacks most frequently during these seasons. Internally, the child's body is weak, allowing the pathogenic factor to readily enter. As noted in an 18th-century work entitled *Explaining the Puzzles of Pediatrics (You ke shi mi),* "The origin of influenza is weakness of protective qi."

INTERNAL FACTORS

Accumulated heat can lead to fever, which can be beneficial to a child. Heat can accumulate for a variety of reasons, for example, the heat may be from a lingering pathogenic factor. In this case, the heat may have been there for quite a long time—months or even years—and the fever may be the manifestation of the body finally expelling the pathogenic factor.

A second internal factor is termed 'latent heat of spring'. We use the term 'latent' to translate a traditional Chinese medical term *(yú),* which also means hidden. Latent is a slightly better term because it conveys the sense of potential to do something, to wreak havoc![1]

Latent heat can be a problem at any time of year, but it is especially a problem in springtime, because it is the Liver which "is the official in charge of making things go smoothly." Thus, any problems in adaptation to change in

---

1. In traditional Chinese medicine it means heat in the system which is hidden, so you do not know it is there. The person may not feel, look, or act hot, but heat is nonetheless present. There may or may not be heat signs on the tongue. So what is it?

the weather relate to the Liver and are thus more likely to arise in springtime. So one way of looking at the epidemics of influenza that sweep through communities in spring is that the fevers are needed to burn off the residues of Christmas pudding and turkey that the Liver could not transform at that time.

The term is used to describe and explain fevers in springtime, and its basis is as follows. When winter comes we prepare for the cold. In November and December (in the northern hemisphere) we eat warming foods such as roast meat, Christmas puddings, and mince pies. We do this in order to adjust the basic metabolism of the body to produce more heat. Thus, we do not feel the cold, shiver, or need to wear hundreds of layers of clothes in order to keep warm.

With the arrival of spring the weather becomes warmer, and if we are still producing the same amount of heat as we did in winter, we will be too hot. This is the basis of latent heat. One aspect of latent heat is simply the overproduction of heat.

In fact, there is more than just heat production involved, for there are also reservoirs of heat in the body. All the tissues of the body are filled with warming substances (mainly fats) that can be called on to provide heat at short notice, if needed. Sometimes people eat so much warming foods (in the form of fried, roasted, or greasy foods) that these reservoirs overflow, and boils and other eruptions appear on the skin.

When spring comes the system has to find a way to get rid of these reservoirs of heat. There are quite a number of ways. The most straightforward is for the Liver to transform the heat. It can be assisted by reverting to a lean diet (such as the traditional Lent fare). It could also come out as boils, but if this fails, it may come out as fevers.

Pathogenesis	The Lung system unites with the skin and hair and opens through the nose. The external pathogenic factor can therefore enter via the mouth, nose, and skin. It is then met by the Lung protective qi, resulting in the disruption of the superficial circulation of protective qi. This in turn affects the Lung qi, with such symptoms as aversion to cold, fever, nasal discharge, and cough.
Heat transformation	Children are said to be the 'embodiment of pure yang', and often have insufficient yin. After the influenza pathogenic factor has entered it readily transforms into heat, giving rise to typical symptoms of heat from excess such as thirst, red face, red lips, dry and irritated mouth and nose, and constipation.

Summerheat

During the summer, the summerheat pathogenic factor is common. Summerheat can attack the qi and obstruct the Spleen. Typical symptoms include high fever, aversion to cold, heaviness in the body, vomiting, and diarrhea.

Accumulated heat

The fever is caused by the body expelling the accumulated heat. In general, it is not easy to distinguish between the fever from accumulated heat and fever from external attack. Fortunately, however, it is not necessary to do so!

Latent heat and lingering pathogenic factor (Western children)

There is not really a great difference between the fever resulting from latent heat and that caused by a lingering pathogenic factor. Both are likely to be hot. Both need to come out for the child to be healthy. The major difference is that all children are subject to the change of seasons and need to clear out in spring the heat generated over the winter. Healthy children will get rid of it naturally, without illness. Less healthy ones will get rid of it by means of a fever. Really unhealthy ones cannot get rid of it at all, and will be rather ill during the summer.

Complications

PROGRESSION TO COUGH

The Lungs of children are especially fragile: they like clean, pure air and dislike stuffiness, too much heat, or too much cold. For this reason, an attack of wind-cold can easily develop into a serious cough. The Lung qi becomes depressed and retarded and the qi mechanism is disrupted. The body fluids are not properly dispersed and are transformed into phlegm, which obstructs the passages of the Lungs and results in cough, severe at times, with gurgling noises in the throat. This is called 'influenza complicated by phlegm'. In extreme cases, it can develop into pneumonia.

PROGRESSION TO THE DIGESTIVE SYSTEM

The Spleen yang in children is often insufficient, and as a result of the attack by an external pathogenic factor, the transportive and transformative functions of the Spleen can be adversely affected. It is easy for food to build up and remain in the abdomen and Stomach passages. Blockage of the middle burner results in abdominal distention and fullness, aversion to food or drink, vomiting, and diarrhea. This is known as 'influenza complicated by accumulation disorder'.

PROGRESSION TO THE NERVES

The spirit and qi in children are weak, which makes them vulnerable to fright and nervousness. During influenza it is common to see the pattern of heat in the Heart affecting the clarity of the spirit, with such symptoms as troubled sleep, fright, and much loud coughing. In extreme cases the pattern can transform into Liver wind with heat, leading to convulsions or Heart fire. This is known as 'influenza complicated by fright'.

In short, children's yin and yang are both readily thrown out of balance. Children easily become hot, cold, deficient, or excessive, and one pattern may transform into another. It is important to pay attention to the clinical picture and its changes.

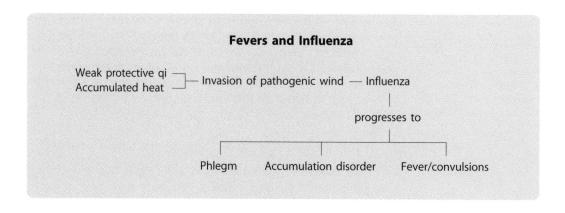

PATTERNS & SYMPTOMS

General signs of attack by wind
- fever
- child is very floppy, like a rag doll
- no appetite
- onset is very sudden, well one day and ill the next; in some cases, the temperature may go up within a few hours

Pulse: rapid

Wind-cold
- pale face
- shivering, feels cold
- fever without sweating
- dribbling of saliva
- violent sneezing, with nasal discharge
- cough
- vomiting of phlegm or clear liquid
- headache
- itching, ticklish throat

Tongue coating: thin, white
Pulse: floating, tight, rapid
Finger vein: superficial, red

Treatment principle: release the exterior (i.e., cause sweating), direct the Lung qi downward, and scatter cold

═══

**The pulse is always rapid in cases of wind-cold.
This sign sometimes leads the unwary into
mistaking wind-cold for wind-heat.**

═══

Wind-heat
- red face
- high fever
- mild aversion to cold
- sweating
- headache
- yellow nasal discharge
- coughing and sneezing
- vomiting yellow phlegm
- throat red, swollen, and painful
- mouth dry, thirsty

Tongue body: red
Tongue coating: thin and white or thin and yellow
Pulse: floating, rapid
Finger vein: superficial, obvious, deep red

Treatment principle: release the exterior, direct the Lung qi downward, and clear heat

When these children show any sign of cold (e.g., chills or aversion to cold) they should also be warmed. This is because it is especially important to keep the digestion functioning properly (i.e., warm) in babies and very young children.

Discussion

These basic categories are the ones generally provided in the Chinese textbooks. In clinical practice, however, one often sees the wind pattern without especially strong heat or cold signs. It is also common to see signs of deficiency, both at the beginning of a fever and at later stages. This is characterized by low-grade fever and inability to sweat, and is due to the qi being so weak that there is not enough energy for a good fever to develop.

Generally, the wind-cold pattern seems to affect weaker children. In order to expel wind-cold, some tonification and warming is necessary. This is not the case for wind-heat, which usually responds very quickly to treatment.

TREATMENT

The primary aim of treatment should be to clear the wind and secondarily to relieve the dominant symptoms. If the wind is not cleared, the other symptoms will remain, but if no attention is paid to relieving the symptoms, then the cure will take longer.

According to Pattern

Wind-cold

GV-14 *(da zhui)*
LI-4 *(he gu)*
G-20 *(feng chi)* } Clears wind-cold and nasal obstruction
L-7 *(lie que)*
TB-5 *(wai guan)*

Method: these points are needled with a dispersing method

If the child is shivering or shows very few signs of heat, add the following points:

S-36 *(zu san li)*   For both points, use the tonifying
CV-12 *(zhong wan)*   method, then moxa

Method: tonify, then moxa. Alternatively, cupping may be applied to the back. According to the textbooks, B-12 *(feng men)* and B-13 *(fei shu)* should be cupped, but it is often more effective to search for tender points on the upper back and cup these instead. Tenderness in the upper thoracic area is a strong indication that cupping will be helpful. Apply up to three cups on either side.[2]

Management: the child should be kept warm and encouraged to sweat. (This is contrary to the conventional wisdom of Western medicine.)

Prognosis: acupuncture is usually extremely effective for this disorder; the stronger the symptoms, the easier it is to cure. One treatment is often enough, and it is rare that more than three treatments are needed unless the patient is very depleted.

Wind-heat

G-20 *(feng chi)*
GV-14 *(da zhui)* } Clears wind
LI-11 *(qu chi)*
LI-4 *(he gu)*

Method: these points are needled with the dispersing method

---

2. It is our experience that a new generation of children is growing up which is more fearful: they are even afraid of cupping. For such children, needling is also frightening but has the advantage that it is over much more quickly.

Together, the last three points are very effective in clearing heat from the body. As in the case of wind-cold, cupping may be used, but acupuncture is generally more effective with hot disorders.

Prognosis: one to three treatments are required to clear wind-heat from the body. Further treatments may be necessary to assist in the child's recuperation.

Frequency of Treatment

It is rather hard to say how often to treat, because it depends very much on the severity of the condition and the child's response. Treatments can be given as often as once every two hours if the fever is very high and you are worried that convulsions are likely to occur. In slightly less severe cases, two or three treatments may be given over twenty-four hours, depending on how the child reacts. If the perspiration changes and comes pouring out, you may not need to do any more treatments.

Likely Results of Treatment

Very frequently, one treatment is enough to transform the situation, so that the fever breaks and the natural healing process may occur. Further treatments may be needed to tonify qi in the recuperation stage.

Problems in Treatment

Feverish children are very distressed and often fearful. The last thing that they want at this time is for a huge monster of an acupuncturist sticking great big nails in them! Not surprisingly, you will find a strong resistance to treatment. However, do not be put off. The actual pain to the child is much less than the child fears, and the benefits far outweigh the discomfort that you may cause.

Clinical Observations

Use of S-36 (zu san li)

There is a school of thought which says that the effect of S-36 *(zu san li)* is too tonifying to be used in treating fevers. We think this is quite mistaken. Perhaps this point of view arises because in some situations S-36 *(zu san li)* works in much the same way as ginseng, and ginseng is certainly contraindicated in fevers.

Our experience is that it is usually beneficial to use this point in treating wind-cold disorders because the child is usually deficient as well as cold. Put another way, the child is only likely to catch a cold when it has become tired and run down, so it is appropriate to use points that tonify as well as points that expel wind.

We have also found that S-36 *(zu san li)* can be used in treating wind-heat disorders provided that points are included in the prescription for expelling the pathogenic factor. In this respect, acupuncture seems to be quite different from herbal medicine.

Use of moxibustion

Following the herbal tradition, it is often taught that moxibustion should not be used in the treatment of hot disorders. However, it is our experience that moxibustion can often be used safely in any situation where the skin surface feels cold, irrespective of whether the overall condition is hot or cold. Moxibustion can also be used safely when the patient likes the sensation of warmth. It is particularly beneficial in treating hot disorders where the hands or feet are cold, when moxibustion should be applied to the hands or feet. This treatment has the effect of drawing the heat out toward the extremities.[3]

Cold to heat transformation

It may happen that a fever starts out as wind-cold, then transforms into wind-heat. These changes can take place very quickly, and you must take account of what is actually happening at that moment when you give a treatment. For example, when a hot child catches a cold (say from a brother or sister), the pathogenic factor may evolve in a space of about twelve hours from a cold disorder to a hot disorder.

Deficiency before the onset of fever

It is well known that pathogenic factors attack when a child is run down. This means that the child is a little bit tired already. This can affect the development of a fever. If the child is really weak (one of those skinny, undersized, deficient children), then there is not enough qi to generate a decent fever. The child may be weak and exhausted, but with only a very low-grade fever. This is important to recognize, for the treatment at this stage should be to tonify the qi. It is often appropriate to use moxibustion, for the condition may manifest as wind-cold.

Deficiency during and after the fever

Once the fever has really got going, the protective qi is fully involved in fighting the pathogenic factor. This is an exhausting process, and the child may get tired. When this happens the temperature may go down and perspiration

---

3. There is a parallel in the treatment of uterine hemorrhage, when moxibustion is applied to Sp-1 *(yin bai)* even though the condition is one of heat.

may subside. However, the fever may continue for some time, and it may be necessary to continue giving mild, tonifying treatment to keep up the temperature and the sweating.

After the fever is over the child may again be very exhausted. At this stage it is appropriate to give gentle, tonifying treatment to assist the recovery. This is summarized by the saying, "Any long illness injures the qi."

Normal ebb and flow of fevers

It is normal for fevers to be lower in the morning and higher in the evening. In some children this is so pronounced that the temperature goes right down to normal in the morning, then rises quite high by the time evening arrives. This should not be confused with the 'tidal fevers' of yin deficiency. These can be distinguished by the floating, rapid pulse and the exhausting nature of the night sweats.

TREATMENT OF DEFICIENCY DURING FEVERS

Weakness before onset of fever

If the child is very weak—very thin and pale—when a fever strikes, the protective qi may not be strong enough to put up a good fight and generate a good fever. Treatment is then aimed at warming the child and tonifying the qi. Use points such as:

S-36 *(zu san li)*
L-9 *(tai yuan)*

Be prepared to perform follow-up treatments, possibly even the same day or the next day, to expel the pathogenic factor.

Weakness during fever

Generally, you shouldn't have to treat this. If the child rests and takes honey and lemon to drink, usually the struggle will soon resume. Treatment is only necessary if the fever has continued for some days without resolution.

COMPLICATIONS

The description of fevers given so far is more or less the same as for adults. Children have, in addition, several common complications. These are not complications in the sense of further development or greater danger. Rather, they complicate the straightforward picture by not allowing you to plunge in and treat the wind-cold or wind-heat. You must first do something else. The main complications are:

- phlegm
- accumulation disorder
- fright or fear

Fright or Fear

Babies and young children often get very anxious and fearful when they have a fever. The traditional explanation is that the heat rises up to the Heart and disturbs the spirit *(shén),* but it seems to us to be more than that. They are actually afraid of the fever itself. This fear definitely hinders the cure of the disease, partly because fear has a heating effect (fueling the fever), and partly because fear is contracting in nature, preventing the expulsion of the pathogenic factor. So watch for fear in children who have fevers. It is particularly damaging if the child is prone to asthma, for the fear may precipitate an attack.

Symptoms

- clinging, shouting, and crying
- troubled and restless sleep
- grinding teeth
- possibly delirium in severe cases

Tongue tip: red
Pulse: wiry, rapid
Finger vein: blue-violet

Treatment

Treatment is very simple since there are many points which can be used to calm the spirit. Even the point GV-14 *(da zhui),* which you are likely to use, has the effect of soothing the fear. The point most commonly used for this purpose is:

H-7 *(shen men)*

There are, however, many others.

As far as home remedies are concerned, the Bach flower remedy 'Rescue Remedy' is very helpful. In my opinion, this remedy should be in the medicine chest of any home where there are young children because they will so frequently need it.

Results of treatment

It is usually quite safe to treat the fear pattern, and the results are purely beneficial. The child quickly becomes calmer and less agitated, and often falls into a deep sleep.

Accumulation Disorder

Here is our old friend again! Accumulation disorder commonly accompanies fevers. In fact, the heat generated by accumulation disorder is often the very reason why the fever develops in the first place. Without the accumulation the child might have had perhaps no more than a sniffle cold.

Symptoms

- abdominal distention and fullness
- cheeks are bright red
- no appetite
- vomiting sour bile
- bad smell from mouth
- stools sour and foul-smelling
- possibly abdominal pain and diarrhea or constipation
- possibly yellow, scanty urine

Tongue coating: greasy, white, or yellow
Pulse: slippery, forceful
Finger vein: violet, broad

Treatment

Be careful in the treatment. As we explained previously, when you clear out the accumulated food, a lot of heat can be released. During a fever, this is a potentially dangerous situation and would be adding fuel to the fire. A suitable treatment during the fever stage would be:

GV-14 *(da zhui)*
LI-4 *(he gu)*
S-44 *(nei ting)*

These points should clear the heat and expel the pathogenic factor, but will not have too strong an effect on moving the accumulated food.[4]

Results of treatment

If you use the points above, the heat should clear quite quickly. The child should become calm and sweat in its sleep. However, the effect of these points is somewhat unpredictable. There can be a huge discharge of stool over the next twelve hours, and a real risk at this time of the fever rising further.

Phlegm

The third complication is phlegm. It is often found that fevers go in epidemics, and while the other members of

---

4. If the child is actually constipated, this must be relieved. Otherwise the accumulated food will continue generating heat. In such cases, we advise a mild laxative, rather than acupuncture, which can be rather unpredictable in its effect. One that is especially indicated is Senna *(Cassia angustifolia)*, which is available at most pharmacies. This has a gentle effect on moving the bowels and has a cold energy.

the family just get a fever, the younger members often get a cough as well.

Treatment

If the fever is still the significant factor, use the following points:

GV-14 *(da zhui)*
LI-4 *(he gu)*

with the addition of either L-7 *(lie que)* or S-40 *(feng long)*. Other points which may be useful include:

Sp-9 *(yin ling quan)*   Clears dampness
CV-6 *(qi hai)*   Clears dampness and tonifies
                           the qi

On the other hand, if the cough is a real problem, then more attention should be paid to the cough than to the fever. Rather than describe it in detail, we refer you to Chapter 16 on acute coughs.

Results of treatment

The results of treatment vary. For the majority of children the phlegm simply gets better: the chest feels better and the cough improves a bit. However, there are some exceptions:

• if the cough is very hard, the first effect will be for the cough to loosen and become more productive. At this stage, it may seem to the parents that the cough is a bit worse. In fact, however, it is a good sign. In the past they referred to this as the cough 'breaking'.

• if there is already a lot of phlegm in the system, the cough may continue for a longer time than expected because the child needs to get rid of all the accumulated phlegm. In older children you can determine the presence of this accumulated phlegm by taking the pulse, which will be slippery or even wiry at *all* positions, not just the first position on the right hand.

According to Symptom

Headache: *tai yang* (M-HN-9), *yin tang*
                       (M-HN-30)
Cough with phlegm: CV-22 *(tian tu)*
Neck and spine pain: B-12 *(feng men)*, B-13 *(fei shu)*, SI-3
                       (hou xi)
Whole body aching: Liv-3 *(tai chong)*
Abdominal pain,
   diarrhea: S-25 *(tian shu)*, S-37 *(shang ju xu)*

Nausea, vomiting:	P-6 *(nei guan)*, S-36 *(zu san li)*
Sore throat:	L-11 *(shao shang)* [bleed in severe cases], L-10 *(yu ji)*
Nasal obstruction:	LI-20 *(ying xiang)*
Hoarse voice:	TB-6 *(zhi gou)*, GV-15 *(ya men)*

In very strong children there is another cause of fever, which is entirely beneficial. They seem to lack any infectious agent, and they appear for perhaps as little as six hours at a time. These fevers are simply a manifestation of vigorous Kidney energy.

FURTHER CONSIDERATIONS

Febrile Convulsions

At one time or another, about one child in twenty will have a febrile convulsion. This is a frightening aggravation of a child's fever which justifies the use of drastic measures to bring the temperature down. As we will see in Chapter 38 on acute convulsions, the basic components are easily generated: heat plus phlegm plus fright. With these three components, febrile convulsions readily develop. In this chapter we have focused on the treatment of uncomplicated fevers, but we will see in the chapter on convulsions that they too respond very well to acupuncture.

It should also be mentioned that from the point of view of conventional medicine, febrile convulsions are not caused so much by a *high* fever as by a *rapidly rising* fever. A child can sustain a fever of 40°C (104°F) provided it rises fairly slowly to that level.

When Not to Treat

If you go to a conventional general practitioner, you are likely to be given a prescription. Likewise, if you call in an acupuncturist, you are likely to get needled! Normally, if you are called to the bedside it is because the situation is quite serious. However, there are times when the situation may not be serious, and it may be better not to treat. For example, you may feel that the mother is worrying unduly. This is especially likely in a first-time mother when her child is having its first fever. It may be important for the mother and child to get over the fever with your support, but without your treatment. This may require some courage on your part!

Recuperation

Qi deficiency

The most common post-fever pattern is qi deficiency. Sometimes this takes a dramatic turn, with the child being completely wiped out. They are still floppy like a rag doll, dull-eyed, and with absolutely *no appetite* at all. This is very worrying for the parents, for they know that without eating any food at all, there is no hope of getting better. Fortunately, this state of affairs is easy to cure. Needling or even applying pressure on the point S-36 *(zu san li)* can 'kick start' the digestive system so the child starts eating again.

Lingering pathogenic factor

The second most common post-fever pattern is our old friend, the lingering pathogenic factor. This pattern, as well as its treatment, were discussed previously in Chapter 3.

Yin deficiency

Another pattern, though much less common in the United Kingdom and the United States, is yin deficiency. We do not have any experience in treating this.

OTHER TREATMENTS

Here we have limited our discussion to acupuncture treatments. Many other therapies are helpful, especially herbal medicine (both Western and Chinese) and homeopathy. Some remedies are set forth in my (JPS) book *Natural Medicine for Children.* We strongly encourage parents (and practitioners) to familiarize themselves sufficiently with one of these therapies to administer as first aid in the case of fever. You may find that first-time mothers will not have the confidence to administer such remedies on their own. But by the time they have seen several fevers, they just want something that they can use and that is effective, so they do not need to call anyone in to help unless the situation looks like it is getting really out of hand.

Case History

A 1½-year-old boy had many fevers. Each time he caught a "chill" a fever developed, and nearly always, twelve hours later he developed febrile convulsions. Each time he caught a "cold" he was quickly given antibiotics, and although it stopped the fevers from going high, it had no effect in reducing the convulsions. By the time he came to see us, he had had twenty to thirty fevers, convulsive episodes, and courses of antibiotics! Being of very strong parents, he had not given in to this and still had good spirit.

What was very striking about the boy's appearance was the combination of a very puffy white face, and scarlet lips. The puffy white face indicated Lung dysfunction with accumulation of dampness, while the scarlet lips showed lots of heat inside. On questioning, it turned out that he frequently got fevers and convulsions after racing around and getting "hot and bothered." It also turned out that when this happened, although he felt hot to the touch, he did not sweat at all. His skin was completely dry.

Treatment was not especially easy and is still continuing after some twenty treatments. However, he is beginning to perspire slightly when he gets too hot, and this is beginning to reduce the frequency of the fevers and convulsions. The points we have been using are GV-14 *(da zhui)*, LI-11 *(qu chi)*, LI-4 *(he gu)*, K-7 *(fu liu)*, and others. The combination LI-4 *(he gu)* and K-7 *(fu liu)* is indicated for regulating perspiration.

This story is the sort of nightmare that every parent has. (To make matters worse, both parents are conventional general practitioners.) However, it does illustrate the need for pathogenic factors to be expelled through the skin by perspiration.

ADVICE TO PARENTS

Nursing Their Child

A sick child needs to be nursed and looked after. One of the terrible repercussions of women going out of the home to work, without a compensatory change in men's work patterns so that they can stay at home, is that it is very difficult for a parent to stay at home and nurse a child. One or the other parent has to take time off, and neither is willing! Although a parent may take time off during the fever stage, once the fever is down the child is sent back to school, and there is no time for recuperation. Parents should be advised to keep their children at home for as long after the fever has gone down as the fever lasted. Thus, if the fever lasted three days, then the child should be kept at home for three more days after the fever has gone down.

Diet

Generally speaking, a child with a fever should not eat, for two reasons. First, the food may add fuel to the fever, increasing the temperature. Second, the food takes energy to digest and so draws energy away from fighting the pathogenic factor. However, if the fever continues for a long time or if the child is weak in the first place, then the child must take something to keep its strength up. Generally, honey in water and other sweet drinks are advised.

Sweating

Many parents think that because a child is hot, it should be cooled down. In practice, however, this is usually not the right thing to do, especially in the early stages. During the early stages, when the child is not perspiring, it should be wrapped up as warmly as possible. Even during the perspiration stage in an attack of wind-heat, the child should be kept covered enough to keep the perspiration going.

Thirst

During the perspiration stage the child will lose a lot of fluids. An appropriate drink to keep up fluids and to benefit the qi is warm honey and lemon.

The Need for Children to Have Fevers

Fevers are universally regarded as a "bad thing," so it is usually against the tide of orthodox opinion to suggest that fevers can be beneficial. However, it does seem that fevers are an important part of childhood. Of course, repeated fevers which need emergency treatment cannot be regarded as beneficial, but occasional fevers going as high as 40°C seem to be part of the process of building a strong immune system.

Immunization for Influenza

In this context, it can be seen how misguided are influenza immunizations. The only justification is for people who have become so deficient that an attack of 'flu' and the consequent effort needed to throw out heat would be so violent as to cause death.

NOTE

• For a case history involving fever and influenza, see Case 1 in Chapter 47.

❖

15 ❖ Chronic Cough

INTRODUCTION

Cough in a child is very distressing to witness. It disturbs the whole family's peace by day and their sleep by night. Although most coughs are not dangerous, in a weak child, a mild cough can progress to pneumonia. Thus, if there is any sign of heat as well, the child is usually treated with antibiotics. In many children, taking antibiotics results in the generation of dampness, which then leads to a chronic cough. With repeated treatment by antibiotics, the Lungs and Spleen are further weakened, which may give rise to asthma. This vicious circle of chronic coughs with acute flare-ups being treated with antibiotics can be avoided with acupuncture treatment, for acupuncture (with cupping) is extremely effective in treating both acute and chronic coughs. Even if the point selection and needle technique is not quite correct, acupuncture still has a pronounced effect in treating this condition in children.

The 'external attack of pathogenic wind' in Chinese medicine corresponds broadly to attack by viral or bacterial agents in Western medicine. It is uncommon among breast-fed infants who receive immunity from their mothers, but becomes much more common when children go to their first play group or kindergarten. The causes of 'internal injury' coughs are more varied and include poor diet, damp living conditions, inadequate treatment, pertussis, and immunizations. Poor diet and damp living conditions give rise to phlegm-damp coughs, as does repeated treatment with antibiotics. Pertussis and immunizations for diphtheria, polio, tuberculosis, and pertussis can all give rise to coughs of the phlegm-damp variety. In practice, there seems to be a range of conditions caused by immunizations, including:

- mild, chronic coughs
- tight, chronic coughs with rather thick, ropy phlegm
- glandular congestion of the lingering pathogenic factor type (see Chapter 44)

Measles immunization may also produce a chronic cough or susceptibility to cough, but this is usually of a hot nature and presents in a way similar to the phlegm-heat pattern, although less acute. This type of cough can also be caused by 'womb heat', that is, heat passed on from the mother, either due to her constitution or some other heating factor such as a febrile disease or a hot climate during pregnancy.

Acute Versus Chronic

In Chinese textbooks there is little distinction between acute and chronic coughs. The big distinction that is made is between a cough at the external level and one which has caused internal injury. We feel that this approach is often misunderstood by Western practitioners, so we have adopted a different approach in this chapter. We have decided to discuss chronic cough first and then acute cough (what we might call viral or bacterial) in the following chapter. We have changed the order because we think that it is easier to understand acute cough if you understand the long-term underlying condition. Moreover, most of the coughs that an acupuncturist will see are chronic. It is rare to see an uncomplicated case of acute cough.

We have also departed from the Chinese texts in other ways: the patterns here are somewhat different from those set out in Chinese books, and also from those provided in earlier editions of this book. This is because over the years we have found that children coming to the clinic really do have different patterns. Thus, what is given here is based on what we actually see in our clinic. We hope our observations are helpful. It is possible that you, who may be living in a different culture and different climate, have children who exhibit yet different patterns! At least what we give here will be a start. For the sake of completeness, we have also set out the yin deficiency pattern which appears in every Chinese textbook, even though we have never seen it in clinic in the form described.

ETIOLOGY & PATHOGENESIS

Etiology

Children frequently get coughs. Their skin is soft, and the activity of the protective qi is comparatively weak.

Moreover, children often go out without sufficient clothing and are unaware of changes in the weather and of
becoming cold. It is therefore easy for the pathogenic
factors of wind-cold or wind-heat to invade and give rise
to cough.

Pathogenesis

*External attack by
a pathogenic factor*

The Lungs are known as the 'fragile' yin organ and are
related to pure essence. They rise up to the throat, open
through the nose, and govern respiration. Externally, they
unite with the skin and hair. The Lung qi should descend
and disperse the pure qi throughout the body. If the protective qi is weak, it is easy for the six pathogenic factors
to invade via the nose and skin. They then obstruct the
interior and invade the Lungs such that the qi mechanism
of the Lungs in descending is impaired. The Lung qi
becomes obstructed and fails to descend, resulting in qi
rising up rebelliously. This causes coughing.

Internal weakness

If a child's body is tired and weak, or if external pathogenic factors remain in the body for a long time without
being resolved, the normal or upright qi is consumed.
The body is then readily attacked by a mild pathogenic
factor which quickly turns more severe. The Lungs' power
of recuperation is impaired, and the pure essence of the
Lungs is restored only with difficulty. This can give rise to
insufficiency of Lung yin or deficient Lung qi, which
correspond to the 'internal injury' types of cough.

Phlegm

Phlegm can arise because a child's Spleen and Stomach are
'thin and soft' and easily affected by food and drink. As a
result, the Spleen is unable to transform food and drink,
which ferment and become turbid phlegm. The phlegm
rises up into the Lungs and obstructs them so that the
Lungs can no longer direct the qi downward, giving rise to
cough. Hence the saying, "The Spleen is the originator of
phlegm, and the Lungs are the container of phlegm."

WHAT IS CHRONIC COUGH?

When we talk about chronic cough we mean one that
continues for a long time, or that keeps coming back. The
term includes the perpetual catarrhal cough that some
children have, the croupy cough that others get when
they are tired, and also the condition where a child keeps
getting one 'infection' after another.

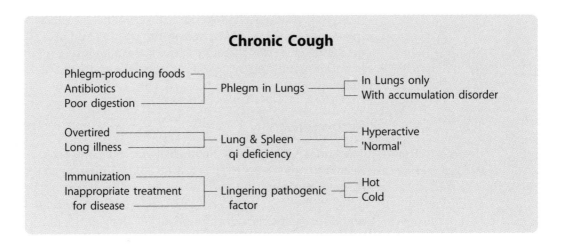

Chronic Cough

Phlegm-producing foods
Antibiotics ⎯⎯ Phlegm in Lungs ⎯⎯ In Lungs only
Poor digestion ⎯⎯ With accumulation disorder

Overtired ⎯⎯ Lung & Spleen ⎯⎯ Hyperactive
Long illness ⎯⎯ qi deficiency ⎯⎯ 'Normal'

Immunization ⎯⎯ Lingering pathogenic ⎯⎯ Hot
Inappropriate treatment ⎯⎯ factor ⎯⎯ Cold
for disease

There are three main patterns of chronic cough:

- phlegm
- Lung and Spleen qi deficiency
- lingering pathogenic factor

You will notice that these patterns are exactly the same as those seen after an attack of a pathogenic factor. The reason for this is straightforward: a chronic cough is one which either goes on and on or which comes back many times. A cough always starts somewhere, and a chronic cough is one which started as an acute cough, but never completely stopped.

The three patterns listed above can be further subdivided:

Phlegm

- in the Lungs only
- originating in accumulation disorder

Lung and Spleen qi deficiency

- normal
- hyperactive

Lingering Pathogenic Factor

- hot
- cold

We will now discuss the etiology and symptom pictures for each of these six patterns.

PHLEGM

Phlegm in the Lungs only

This pattern does not appear in the Chinese texts. At least it is not distinguished from Lung and Spleen qi deficiency (or in other texts, from Lung and Kidney deficiency), where the sputum is dilute and watery. A child with a pattern of phlegm in the Lungs is not as weak as a child with Lung and Spleen qi deficiency. Moreover, the phlegm is not dilute and watery. Rather, it is thick and viscous. Of course, there is some Lung weakness, otherwise there would not be a cough at all. What is happening is that the child is reasonably strong, but is overwhelmed by a large amount of sticky phlegm, and this phlegm is mostly in the Lungs. Although the child has some energy, it does not have enough to get rid of all the phlegm, because, being so sticky, it is very difficult to expel. Typical symptoms include:

- croaky, rattly cough
- thick nasal discharge
- gray face
- possibly swollen glands[1]
- appetite variable, that is, may eat a lot, but is picky about food

Pulse: full and slippery, especially in the Lung position, and maybe less slippery in other positions

Treatment principle: clear phlegm from Lungs

Phlegm with accumulation disorder

Here again the child is strong. This time, however, the digestive system as well as the Lungs are impaired. The digestion is impaired by the now familiar accumulation disorder. Because of one of the reasons underlying accumulation disorder—overeating, irregular eating, or unsuitable foods—the digestion becomes overloaded and the food stagnates. The stagnation of food leads to stagnation of fluids, which in turn transform into phlegm.

As can be seen, this pattern is significantly different from the previous one. When it comes to treatment, it is essential to treat the digestion, for it is from the bunged-up digestion that the phlegm is being formed; and as long as phlegm is being formed, the cough will continue. This is in contrast to the previous pattern where the main focus of treatment is to clear the phlegm from the Lungs only.

Typical symptoms of phlegm with accumulation disorder include:

- croaky, rattly cough
- thick nasal discharge
- red cheeks
- swollen abdomen (like a drum)
- irregular stools (green and sour, or foul-smelling) or constipated

---

1. See Chapter 4 for a discussion of glands.

Treatment principle: resolve the phlegm and clear the accumulation

Treatment of Phlegm

When there is a lot of phlegm, certain precautions must be taken when treating this pattern. For example, the child could have serious difficulty breathing when there is too much phlegm in its throat; there is thus a danger of suffocating on its own phlegm. For this reason, we recommend starting with the following treatment if there is the slightest doubt in your mind about the safety of aggravating the condition:

CV-22 *(tian tu)*   Clears the bronchi

Just use this one point, which has the effect of opening the bronchi. If you feel that is not quite enough, add:

CV-17 *(shan zhong)*   Opens the chest

Do not use any more points in the first treatment. Explain what you are trying to do to the parents, and tell them that there may only be a slight improvement from this treatment, but that you would rather it were like this than to get a dramatic worsening of the condition. Once you have explained this, parents will be reassured. There is an old saying in traditional Chinese medicine that addresses this situation, "Better too little medicine than too much medicine."

For the next treatment, you may branch out to points on the Lung channel, such as:

L-5 *(chi ze)*   Drains water from the Lungs
L-7 *(lie que)*   Clears phlegm from the Lungs

These points do have some effect in stirring up phlegm. So again, if there is any doubt about the stability of the child's condition, add:

CV-22 *(tian tu)*   Clears the bronchi

Once you are sure that there is no danger of aggravating the condition, you are much freer in your choice of points. In particular, you may now proceed to use:

S-40 *(feng long)*   Resolves phlegm

This point is left until last, for although it is the supreme point for transforming phlegm over the long term, in the short term it has the effect of stirring up phlegm, and increasing the amount that needs to be coughed up.

Method for needling CV-22 (tian tu): in adults this point is needled obliquely, threading the needle about one unit under the sternum. In babies and children up to (at least) seven years of age, the point is needled perpendicularly, to a depth of about 5mm. You must not needle under the sternum because the thymus gland is still quite large; moreover, it is unnecessary. It is quite enough to just obtain the qi and direct it downward into the chest with your needle technique.

According to Pattern

Phlegm in Lungs only

A typical prescription includes:

B-13 *(fei shu)*	Benefits the Lungs
L-5 *(chi ze)*	Clears fluid from the Lungs
L-7 *(lie que)* or	Clears phlegm from the Lungs
L-9 *(tai yuan)*	Clears phlegm from the Lungs

These points are generally enough. Occasionally, you may feel that the following point is also indicated:

S-40 *(feng long)*	Transforms phlegm and encourages the Spleen's transportive and transformative functions

Number of treatments: this depends on the thickness of the phlegm and the strength of the child; typically, ten to twenty treatments are given

---

Sometimes, once the phlegm has been cleared, this pattern evolves into the lingering pathogenic factor pattern.

Advice to parents: avoid cow's products (milk and cheese), peanut butter, and bananas

Phlegm with accumulation disorder

Although the root cause is the digestive disturbance, there has to be some weakness in the Lungs for the cough to occur. Therefore, always use a point which benefits the Lungs such as L-7 *(lie que)* or L-9 *(tai yuan)*. In addition, treat the accumulation using *si feng* (M-UE-9).

Results of treatment: there may be a huge explosion of stool, and the child is likely to have one or two very bad night's sleep. Also, it is quite likely that the cough will get much worse. Only after three or four days will an improvement be noticed. Once again, warn the parents about the likely results of treatment. If you do not warn the parents, they may lose confidence in you.

Number of treatments: about five or six is usually enough in a straightforward case. Occasionally the treatment reveals something else underneath, and sometimes the straightforward phlegm pattern evolves into the lingering pathogenic factor pattern.

Advice to parents: impress on the parents the need to regulate their child's eating habits. Encourage them to offer less food, simpler foods, and easier-to-digest foods. Also encourage them to sit the child down for regular meals and to avoid giving snacks in between.

Summary of Treatments

If the child is drowning in phlegm, in the first treatment use CV-22 *(tian tu)* and CV-17 *(shan zhong)*. For the next treatments use L-5 *(chi ze)* and L-7 *(lie que)*. Add CV-22 *(tian tu)* and CV-17 *(shan zhong)* if there is any doubt about the stability of the child's condition.

For later treatments, and for the first treatment when there is less phlegm, use:

- B-13 *(fei shu)*, L-5 *(chi ze)*, and L-7 *(lie que)* for the pattern of phlegm in the Lungs only
- L-7 *(chi ze)* or L-9 *(tai yuan)* plus *si feng* (M-UE-9) for the pattern of phlegm with accumulation disorder

LUNG AND SPLEEN QI DEFICIENCY

Normal

This is the traditional pattern set forth in Chinese textbooks and is identical to the adult pattern. It arises because both the Lungs and the Spleen are weakened. Because of weakness in the Spleen, the fluids do not circulate properly and so transform into phlegm, which is then sent upward to the Lungs. If the Lungs were strong, they would transform the phlegm and there would be no problem, but because the Lung qi is weak, the phlegm accumulates in the Lungs and has to be coughed up. Typical symptoms include:

- weak and wet cough
- watery nasal discharge
- pale face
- undersized child (or else growing rapidly)[2]
- poor appetite or choosy over food

2. In some cases the child is undersized because not enough nourishment is absorbed by the Spleen. In other cases, the Spleen is weakened by all the energy that is used in the rapid growth.

- easily tired
- wakes many times at night
- dull eyes
- possibly dark rings under eyes
- possibly copious dribbling

Common causes of Lung and Spleen qi deficiency were set out in Chapter 3. They include:

- exhaustion after a difficult or long labor
- anesthetics during childbirth
- exhaustion of mother after birth
- repeated illnesses of the child, especially if they were treated with antibiotics
- neglected child

Hyperactive

This pattern, described in Chapter 3, is becoming more common. As previously explained, the pattern does not seem to occur in China where very strict and very quiet upbringing is the norm. In the West, however, upbringing is much less strict and boundaries are less clearly defined. As a consequence, children in this culture can easily become overstimulated without parents thinking that there is anything abnormal. Also, there is a tendency to overstimulate children with constant amusements and exposure to television. Other factors contributing to over-stimulation are:

- sugar in the diet
- artificial additives in the food
- drinking too much fruit juice, especially orange juice

The symptom picture is the same as that of Lung and Spleen qi deficiency:

- weak and wet cough
- watery nasal discharge
- pale face
- undersized child
- poor appetite or choosy about food
- easily tired
- wakes many times at night
- dull eyes
- possibly dark rings under eyes
- possibly copious dribbling

However, the child's behavior is quite different from the previous pattern:

- child is restless
- alternates between shyness and boldness
- coy
- may show signs of extreme distress or fear toward the practitioner

- willful
- manipulative

Spleen qi deficiency with cold

We are now seeing yet another pattern emerge, Spleen qi deficiency with cold. This pattern is especially common in the West, where the consumption of large quantities of ice-cold fruit juice is the norm. The symptoms are very similar to conventional Spleen qi deficiency, but the pulse may be full and slippery, which you would not expect to see in a deficiency pattern. Also, these children are very ticklish and rather fearful of treatment, even moxibustion.

Treatment of Lung and Spleen Qi Deficiency

The basic treatment of the two patterns is the same. The principle is to tonify the Lung and Spleen qi, with points such as:

L-5 *(chi ze)*	Drains fluid from the Lungs
L-9 *(tai yuan)*	Tonifies the Lungs
S-36 *(zu san li)*	Tonifies Spleen qi
CV-12 *(zhong wan)*	Tonifies and warms the Spleen

Method: use a tonifying method with indirect moxibustion at CV-12 *(zhong wan)* only

Results of treatment: in treating the straightforward Lung and Spleen qi deficiency pattern the results are generally good, provided there is enough energy around the child, which is to say, that the parents are not too exhausted and the child gets enough rest. The child will gradually improve and become stronger in about ten treatments.

In treating the hyperactive pattern, however, the case is quite different. The child may possibly get well in about ten treatments, but the results are very unpredictable. One certain result is that the child will make a great fuss over needling: wailing, screeching, and implying that you are torturing it. This will play both on you (if you are not ready for it) and on the parents. After two or three treatments, the mother may well start to question whether the treatments are too traumatic for the child. There is no answer for this. You will have to decide for yourself, and if you want to continue treating the child, you will then need to do some persuading. What the mother is in fact saying is that the treatments are too traumatic for *her,* for the child makes the mother experience the pain.

In really bad cases, it may be worth using moxibustion alone. For example, start with just indirect moxibustion at CV-12 *(zhong wan)*. Then proceed to moxibustion on the governing *(shū)* points of the back.

Evolution of the Pattern

This pattern may be cured in about ten treatments, or it may evolve into that of lingering pathogenic factor. Having cured the basic Lung and Spleen qi deficiency pattern and gotten rid of the watery phlegm, you may come down to the hard bedrock of congealed phlegm, which is characteristic of the lingering pathogenic factor pattern.

Advice

See the general advice about how to handle hyperactive Spleen qi deficiency in Chapter 3. You should also suggest regular meals, no ice-cold drinks, and no food straight from the refrigerator, salads, or other cold energy foods.

LINGERING PATHOGENIC FACTOR

This pattern is perhaps the one most commonly treated in the clinic because both the phlegm pattern and the Lung and Spleen qi deficiency pattern naturally evolve into this one. After getting over the initial cough, most children recover to a certain extent, but not completely, leaving a lingering pathogenic factor behind. Likewise with treatment: after clearing the phlegm or tonifying the basic deficiency, this is the pattern that remains. Basically, this pattern is the sequela of repeated infections.

The other cause of this pattern is immunizations, especially for pertussis or polio. The cough may appear very soon afterward and stay unchanged for months and months.

This pattern is characterized by phlegm that is very hard and 'knotted'. In the straightforward phlegm pattern, the phlegm is rather thick; here, it has thickened up even more and is viscous to the point of being hard. Consequently, there are often no external signs of phlegm: no nasal discharge, and the cough does not sound gurgly. The phlegm is simply too thick to flow.

Symptoms

- hard, hacking cough, which worsens when tired
- swollen glands in the neck and under the jaw

Treatment of Lingering Pathogenic Factor

Before getting into the details of treatment we must emphasize that this pattern is a later stage of cough. In the early stages of chronic cough the pattern is either that of phlegm, or of Lung and Spleen qi deficiency. To put it another way, if there is obviously a lot of phlegm, treat this first. There is no point in softening and loosening a large amount of phlegm if the child is already struggling to clear its chest of phlegm. Likewise, if the qi is weak, there simply will not be enough qi to soften the phlegm.

If this is the first treatment, then use straightforward points to start with. The following prescription is often very helpful:

L-5 *(chi ze)*	Clears phlegm from the Lungs
L-9 *(tai yuan)*	Tonifies the Lungs
S-40 *(feng long)*	Resolves phlegm
G-34 *(yang ling quan)*	Resolves phlegm

In many cases, these simple points are enough to start the healing process. More often than not, you will reach this stage of thick phlegm after a series of treatments and you will feel that you are not making any progress. In that case, you have to turn to the governing *(shu)* points on the back. (Do not use them in the first treatments, as children hate to have needles inserted in the back. They much prefer needles which they can see.) The following points have the effect of softening very hard phlegm:

bai lao (M-HN-30)	Softens thick phlegm and clears glandular congestion
B-18 *(gan shu)*	Softens thick phlegm
B-20 *(pi shu)*	Softens thick phlegm

Method: choose one or two of these points and needle bilaterally with the tonifying method or the moving method. B-18 *(gan shu)* and B-20 *(pi shu)* are generally regarded as tonifying points. If they are used with the moving method, that is, relatively stronger stimulation, they have the effect of softening thick phlegm. In addition, tonify B-13 *(fei shu)* to clear the chest.

Results of treatment: if the child is coming to you for the first time, you may not get very marked results. The child will likely just feel a little better. However, the effect is cumulative, so that after a few treatments the child starts to feel a lot better. Very often the catarrh which was causing the hacking cough starts to soften so that the child starts to bring up phlegm. This will be especially noticed first thing in the morning. Sometimes the loosened phlegm will result in a nasal discharge or at least in 'bogey men', that is, little pieces of hardened phlegm in the nose.

In some children the effect of using the governing *(shū)* points on the back is quite strong and a huge amount of phlegm is released. If this happens, the pattern has temporarily reverted to that of the phlegm pattern, and should be treated accordingly the next time the child comes to the clinic.

Prognosis: it is quite variable. It may require as little as ten treatments, or as many as thirty or more.

Note: when treating such a deep disorder, you must always pay attention to what is happening on the day of the treatment. For example, if the child also has an acute cough, this must be treated. Likewise, if the child is exhausted, because of sports or overworking at school, then the principle of treatment must be changed to tonifying qi.

Complications

Heat

If the lingering pathogenic factor is hot in nature, the child may be hyperactive and irritable after treatment, as heat is released. The bad behavior and attendant misery can be relieved to some extent by needling Liv-3 *(tai chong)* with the dispersing method.

Vomiting

If the lingering pathogenic factor was originally whooping cough or an immunization for whooping cough, then the phlegm may collect in the Stomach and Lungs, and the child may be prone to attacks of vomiting, especially of phlegm. The obvious points to use are P-6 *(nei guan)* or S-36 *(zu san li)*. Sometimes these points are effective, but in my experience, the vomiting may continue until most of the phlegm has been cleared from the system.

Thick gray phlegm

Some children suffer from a particularly thick kind of gray phlegm. This is often seen after polio immunization. Acupuncture does have some effect on this condition, but sometimes, after initial improvement, there seems to be a plateau in the treatment. In these cases, a nosode[3] may be indicated, after consultation with a homeopath.

Signs and Pointers Along the Way

Giving as many as thirty treatment demands energy and commitment on the part of the parents, and they will

---

3. A nosode is a homeopathic preparation made from the secretions of a person suffering from the disease in question.

often need reassurance about progress in the case. In other words, you will need to give them an idea of how things are going. There are some obvious pointers which parents can observe for themselves but may have overlooked, or may need you to confirm, such as the child's energy level, spirit, and resistance to disease.

Energy level | The child's energy should gradually increase. It will need less sleep, will get up earlier in the morning, go to bed later at night, and will not become as exhausted as it was before.

Spirit | The child is more enthusiastic and complains less.

Behavior | Often the child's behavior becomes very difficult and obstinate after about five treatments. Should this happen, it is a very good sign, and an indication that the treatments are really being successful.

Resistance to disease | As treatment proceeds, the repeated coughs that the child used to get are fewer and further between. The child manages to get over the acute attacks more quickly, and towards the end of treatment, the child may not get a cough from other members of the family.

OTHER SIGNS

Signs which you can observe, but which parents may not, include facial color, pulse, and the condition of the glands.

Facial color | Often the faces of these children are gray or yellow when they come. This gray color gradually disappears. At first there is improvement in color in parts of the face, especially the cheeks. As treatment continues, the overall facial color improves. If there were bags or dark patches under the eyes, these also gradually disappear; the green-yellow color around the mouth goes, as does the white color on the forehead. The pathological colors are replaced by glowing pink over the entire face.

Pulse | Changes in the pulse are harder to measure and harder to explain. Very often, the child starts this pattern with a wiry, slippery pulse. It is slippery because of phlegm, and wiry because the phlegm causes stagnation. Gradually, this pulse may become soft or even soggy, as there is an over-reaction, and the phlegm which was previously hard is now softened. Then the pulse slowly returns to that of a healthy child.

Glands | The glands change only very slowly. As treatment progresses, the glands should become smaller (although at first they may become larger). Above all, they should become softer as the hard phlegm softens. The hardness of the glands is an indication of the hardness of the remaining phlegm. Sometimes (especially in children with weak constitutions) it is impossible to clear the swollen glands completely. In these cases, the best you can do is to improve their health, energy, and resistance to disease.

The Role of Infections

During the course of treatment it is common for the child to suffer an acute attack of cough; after all, a course of thirty treatments may last thirty weeks. It would be surprising if a child did not get a cough during this time.

In the early stages of treatment, before its effect has really accumulated, these infections are not at all beneficial and may set the treatment back, especially so if the cough is treated with antibiotics. However, in the later stages, an attack of cough from outside can be beneficial, especially if the child gets over the attack unaided or with natural therapies. What seems to happen is that the external pathogenic factor has the effect of mobilizing the protective qi, which recognizes the lingering pathogenic factor as alien and expels it. The result is that after such an attack, the child may be left with really quite a bad cough from all the phlegm being loosened at once; but the deep, hard phlegm has been softened and is no longer there. The way is then open for a complete cure.

Dietary Advice

For all coughs, but especially chronic ones, the diet should be modified. Foods which generate dampness or phlegm (e.g., cow's milk, cheese, peanuts, peanut butter, bananas, and sugar) should be avoided. Some children are also strongly affected by bitter oranges. Children suffering from cold disorders should be encouraged to eat warming foods, including ginger. Children with hot disorders should be given cooling foods. Children with phlegm disorders should be given garlic.

YIN DEFICIENCY COUGH

This pattern is always described in Chinese textbooks, but we have never seen it in the clinic in this form. You do occasionally see coughs due to Kidney yin deficiency, but they are rarely due to prolonged fever. Rather, they are due to long-term use of steroids, or simply to overwork and late nights. (We had one eleven-year-old brought to us who regularly went to bed at 2 A.M.) However, it is possible that this pattern may return in the future, when antibiotic-resistant bacteria become more common, and when tuberculosis returns.

Symptoms

- dry cough with little if any sputum (what sputum there is comes in flecks and is difficult to expectorate)
- thirst with dry throat which is not relieved by drinking
- itchy throat
- hoarse voice
- hot palms and soles of feet
- child is frightened and distressed

Alternatively, there may be symptoms characteristic of severe yin deficiency affecting the Lungs, including blood-streaked sputum, afternoon fevers, and night sweats.

Tongue body: red with little or no coating
Pulse: rapid, fine

Treatment principle: clear the Lungs and moisten dryness

K-27 *(shu fu)*	Clears the chest and the Lungs
B-13 *(fei shu)*	Tonifies Lung yin
B-38 *(gao huang shu)*	Tonifies the yin of the entire body
B-23 *(shen shu)*	
K-3 *(tai xi)*	Tonifies Kidney yin
CV-6 *(qi hai)*	

Method: the tonification method is used. Direct moxibustion should be avoided except at CV-6 *(qi hai)*. At other points, moxibustion with garlic may be used.

Prognosis: we have no experience in treating tuberculosis, but reports in the literature and conversations with experienced practitioners indicate that acupuncture is effective. In mild cases, ten to twenty treatments may provide a cure. In more severe cases, fifty to a hundred treatments may be needed. If the tuberculosis germ is not present and the condition is a result of a past febrile disease, five to ten treatments are sufficient. Rest is essential as an adjunct to treatment.

❖

16 ❖ Acute Cough

INTRODUCTION

In traditional Chinese medicine, the cause of acute cough is said to be the invasion of pathogenic wind. In most cases, wind attacks the superficial layer and is generally not a real threat to life. In this way, coughs are very similar to fevers, which are also due to attack of wind at the superficial layer. And, as we saw in Chapter 14, there is not much difference between a cough with a fever and a fever with a cough! Or at least so it would appear from the textbooks, and so it is for healthy people.

However, in your clinical practice, the children who are likely to come to you with a cough are those who already have some respiratory illness, such as chronic cough or even asthma. For these children, an acute cough may pose quite a severe threat to life. Because of this danger, we feel it is important that you be able to treat acute cough attacks because this will enable the child to overcome the pathogenic factor. For a child with a history of chronic cough, this may mean saving it from yet another course of antibiotics. For a child with asthma, you may be able to ward off an asthma attack and so avoid a visit to hospital, with all the attendant trauma. For a child with a multiple drug resistant strain of bacteria, it may mean saving the child's life.

Moreover, a treatment given at this time is worth several treatments given after the time of an acute attack. As the saying goes, "A time of change is a time of opportunity," and if you grasp the opportunity of treating during an acute attack, it can sometimes be a turning point in a long series of treatments.

We have divided our discussion into two parts. The first is a fairly straightforward classical description of acute cough as it appears in textbooks of traditional Chinese medicine. Pattern differentiation and treatment is more or less the same as for adults. In the second part we discuss some of the problems that occur during treatment.

CLASSICAL DESCRIPTION OF ACUTE COUGH

Patterns

The patterns for acute cough are two:

• wind at the superficial level
• phlegm-heat in the Lungs

Put very simply, these two patterns describe a mild cough —for example, one where you, as a practitioner, would continue working—and a severe cough, such as bronchitis or pneumonia, where you would stay at home. The distinction is between cough at the external and internal levels.

The wind pattern can be further subdivided according to the pathogenic factor which rides on the back of the wind. Accordingly, a fuller list of patterns for acute cough would include:

• wind-cold
• wind-heat
• wind-dampness
• wind-dryness
• phlegm-heat

Symptoms

Wind

• sudden onset (within twenty-four hours) and often a result of an epidemic
• at first just a 'tickly' throat
• child is not especially upset by the cough
• possibly a slight fever
• generally an air of whining, irritability

Tongue: unchanged
Pulse: floating (sometimes only at the Lung position), rapid

Wind-cold

• child feels chilly
• clear nasal discharge
• no sweating

- pale face
- tight chest
- harsh cough

Pulse: tight, floating, rapid

Wind-heat

- child may feel hot, with the forehead feeling hot to the touch
- cough is hard and may be painful
- nasal discharge is yellowish
- mild perspiration
- sore, painful throat
- face is flushed (red)

Pulse: rapid, maybe slippery, floating

Wind-dampness

- child feels heavy and tired
- thick gray nasal discharge
- watery cough
- no perspiration, but skin may feel damp and puffy
- face looks pale and puffy

Pulse: slippery-soggy, floating, rapid

Wind-dryness

- child is a bit irritable
- cough is tickly and dry
- no nasal discharge
- usually no perspiration
- skin is dry

The traditional explanation of cough due to wind is that the wind lodges in the skin and superficial layer. The skin is associated with the Lungs, thus the Lung function of descending and dispersing qi becomes impaired, resulting in a cough. Sometimes the Lung channel is affected, such that there is tightness of the chest and a ticklish feeling in the throat.

The sudden onset is characteristic of wind, and the floating pulse is characteristic of the qi coming out to the superficial level to do battle with the pathogenic factor. Grumpy behavior is typical of a not-too-serious disturbance of qi. The child still has enough energy to be quite annoying, and a drain on the parents' energy.

Fever here is due to the energy released in the battle between the protective qi and the pathogenic factor. This is a point that is often misunderstood. For example, in the pattern of wind-cold, it is important to give the child warming herbs, even though the temperature is high. It must be emphasized that although there are Lung symptoms, at this level they are only Lung channel symptoms, and the pathogenic factor has not yet invaded the Lung organ.

Importance of Differentiating Wind

How important is it to differentiate among all the sub-categories of wind? The answer is that often it is not important at all, while at other times it is really important! The times when it is important to differentiate are when the other pathogenic factors accompanying wind are really obvious.

So, for example, in wind-cold, if the child is really shaky and shivery, and feels really deep cold throughout its body, then you must address that; in other words, the child will already feel a lot better if it is kept warm. Similarly, in wind-dampness, if the child's nose is running like a tap and it seems as though it is drowning, it is obvious that the child will feel a lot better if you can drain some of the dampness. On the other hand, there are many times (the majority in our practice) where these other pathogenic factors are not especially significant, and the main problem is simply the cough.

Phlegm-heat

- child is quite hot and feverish
- usually sweating
- rattly and maybe painful cough
- child cries each time when coughing
- nasal discharge is yellow
- generally an air of anxiety and distress
- may have diagnosis of bronchitis or pneumonia

Tongue: may be red with yellow coating[1]
Pulse: full, rapid, slippery

Phlegm-heat represents a further development in the cough and is due to the pathogenic factor penetrating to the interior of the Lungs, where it transforms into heat (even if it started out as a cold pathogenic factor). This means that the lining of the Lungs and the bronchi are inflamed. Most of the symptoms are characteristic of heat in the interior. The symptom of crying out when coughing occurs because it is painful to cough. There is generally much more anxiety surrounding this pattern.

In the past, one could confidently assign the conventional diagnosis of pneumonia—or worse—to the phlegm-heat category. Pneumonia was a very dangerous disease which could proceed rapidly to death. However, like so many other things, this currency has become devalued.

---

1. The tongue does not always change.

So, although the label pneumonia may mean this danger-ous disease, more often than not it refers to 'viral pneu-monia'—rather than lobar or bacterial pneumonia—which is simply a cough due to wind at the superficial layer. This shows once again the need to keep the con-ventional diagnosis and the traditional Chinese medical diagnosis separate in one's mind.

Treatment

Again, following the traditional Chinese medical texts, we will describe the treatment for each of these patterns.

Purpose of treatment

It is not quite the conventional order of things, but let us start first by asking why we are treating, or rather, what is the precise purpose of giving a treatment at this time? In most illnesses, the answer is obvious: to relieve suffering. But in this case there is a more pressing aim. As men-tioned before, it is unlikely that a child will be brought to you merely for a cough which it could overcome on its own. This means that the child will not be able to get over the cough by itself and needs intervention. What are the possible outcomes of acute cough? As we saw, an attack of wind is the first stage. If it goes deeper it will transform into an interior disease, phlegm-heat in the Lungs. If, in turn, this is allowed to progress, it will develop into pneu-monia or asthma, which is life threatening. These path-ways are usually well worn. Usually, past a certain stage, the child is subjected to conventional medication, maybe in the form of antibiotics.

Our aim, therefore, is to prevent a wind pattern from progressing to phlegm-heat, and a phlegm-heat pattern from developing into pneumonia or asthma.

Basic prescription

The treatment of acute cough is really very simple. A prescription such as the following will have quite a strong effect on most coughs:

L-5 *(chi ze)*
L-7 *(lie que)*
B-13 *(fei shu)*

An accurate diagnosis is preferable, but not really neces-sary, in order to give a good treatment for cough. We mention this because the general anxiety surrounding a child with an acute cough affects you, the practitioner, making it hard to think clearly. If there is the time and mental clarity to do a good diagnosis, the following prescriptions will be found to be even more effective.

Wind

L-7 *(lie que)*
LI-4 *(he gu)*
B-13 *(fei shu)* or
B-12 *(feng men)*

Method: strong dispersing technique is needed in order to get any results.[2] Another method is to use cupping at tender areas in the vicinity of B-13 *(fei shu)*.

Prognosis: if you are treating a child who is basically healthy and is not normally prone to coughs, then the results of the treatment are very good. One to three treatments given once a day is usually enough to make a big difference. However, it is unlikely you will be seeing much of this sort of condition unless you are working in the Third World or with very impoverished patients for whom the state of the weather is really important. For patients who have housing with heating or air conditioning, there is a large measure of protection from the weather, and healthy children need little assistance in getting over a cough beyond staying indoors.

What is much more likely is that you will be treating children who already have a chronic cough or even asthma, and the acute attack is an overlay. In these cases, the results of treatment are quite variable and unpredictable. Sometimes wind at the superficial level can be very hard to clear.[3]

Wind-cold

Use the basic prescription to liberate the exterior. Then add moxa at the points to warm up the child:

B-13 *(fei shu)*
CV-17 *(shan zhong)*
CV-12 *(zhong wan)*

---

2. Needle technique is *all important*. Recently we spoke to an acupuncture student who was convinced that acupuncture did not work for acute cough. On questioning it turned out that the student had visited a student clinic, and had been treated for a cough herself. The treatment she received was based on very gentle needling with very fine needles. It was so gentle that she did not actually feel any qi at all. In these circumstances, you cannot expect to do much to disturb a well-established pathogenic factor which has just found a nice new home.

3. The treatment of cough is really quite simple because there are only a few things that you can do. But actually the symptom of cough is very complex with many components. One is the actual pathogenic factor, which may be an epidemic going round the community. Another is the energy level of the child. Others include the amount of phlegm that has accumulated in the child; how the child feels about the weather, family, school, or television programs; and yet another is pollution. If you have been treating a child for a long time, you do eventually start to notice the really important factors in that child's life.

Method: in very young children, use only indirect moxibustion; in older children, you can use direct moxibustion or, better still, moxibustion on ginger. Cupping is also effective. But even these methods may not be enough to warm up the child. Other methods include:

• warm drinks
• hot bath, especially with warming and dispersing essential oils
• ginger and lemon drink
• homoeopathy, especially Aconite or Arsenicum album
• warming herbs

You do not have to use only Chinese herbs. Warming herbs, such as yarrow *(Achillea millefolium)* are also effective.

Prognosis: the results are quite variable. This is because wind-cold is rarely a purely excessive disorder. There is often overall qi and yang deficiency at the same time. That is one of the reasons why it can be so difficult to warm up children.

Wind-heat

The basic prescription is often helpful:

L-7 *(lie que)*
LI-4 *(he gu)*
B-13 *(fei shu)*
L-10 *(yu ji)*   Clears heat & stops pain in throat; can be substituted for LI-4 *(he gu)*

Method: the reducing technique should be used, with or without cupping

If heat is the significant factor, it may be appropriate to use the prescription for wind-heat type influenza:

GV-14 *(da zhui)*
LI-11 *(qu chi)*
LI-4 *(he gu)*

Prognosis: the results in treating wind-heat are generally very good. If a child has this sort of cough, it usually means that its energy is quite good anyway, and the child only needs a push in the right direction to get the body fighting the pathogenic factor.

Wind-dampness

It is more difficult to give a blanket prescription for wind-dampness because the symptoms vary quite a lot. The following points can be used in most situations:

Sp-9 *(yin ling quan)*	Drains dampness
K-7 *(fu liu)*	Drains dampness
B-13 *(fei shu)*	Tonifies the Lungs
S-36 *(zu san li)*	Tonifies qi and benefits the Spleen

If the child is drowning in water, be careful. Be even more careful if the child is drowning in phlegm! You must take care not to aggravate the condition. In such cases, use points like:

CV-22 *(tian tu)*
CV-17 *(shan zhong)*

The main difference here is the need to drain dampness. In some patients this is more important even than treating the Lungs. When I (JPS) was training with Dr. van Buren, I saw a bad cough successfully treated using the following prescription:

K-7 *(fu liu)*
K-9 *(zhu bin)*
K-10 *(yin gu)*

Prognosis: the results are quite variable. This is because wind-dampness is rarely a purely excessive disorder. There is often overall qi deficiency at the same time.

Wind-dryness | The basic prescription is helpful. Other points which moisten the Lungs are:

L-5 *(chi ze)*
K-6 *(zhao hai)*

Prognosis: living as we do in a damp climate, we have never seen this pattern, so we cannot comment on it. We welcome any information from other practitioners.

Phlegm-heat | The following prescription is very helpful:

L-10 *(yu ji)*	Clears heat in the Lungs
L-5 *(chi ze)*	Moistens and cools the Lungs
CV-17 *(shan zhong)*	Opens the chest

Other points which are of use include:

CV-22 *(tian tu)*	Opens the chest
P-6 *(nei guan)*	Opens the chest
L-2 *(yun men)*	Clears heat in the Lungs
B-13 *(fei shu)*	Clears heat in the Lungs

If there is wheezing or difficulty in breathing, add:

ding chuan (M-BW-1)	Clears heat in the Lungs

If there is high fever, add:

GV-14 *(da zhui)*
LI-11 *(qu chi)*

Method: strong reducing method is used at the channel points on the arms. Use a mild reducing method at the chest and back points, since there is real danger of causing pneumothorax if you disperse too strongly.[4]

Once again, this prescription is by way of a suggestion. You must adapt the prescription to your particular situation. CV-17 *(shan zhong)* is helpful if there is pain in the middle of the chest. L-2 *(yun men)* is wonderful if the whole of the chest is sore and inflamed.

Prognosis: strange to relate, the results for this more serious disease are much better than for the less serious condition of wind. Very often just one treatment is enough. Even during the treatment, some of the pain and fever may subside, and with it some of the fear. Antibiotics are usually prescribed in this situation, but they are very rarely needed if you can give two treatments within twenty-four hours.

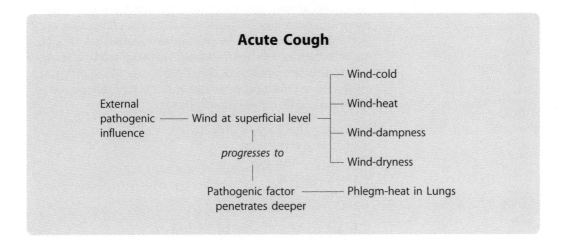

WHAT ACTUALLY HAPPENS IN THE CLINIC

What we have described so far is the ideal situation, that is, the healthy child who has a cough. In practice, it is rare for these children to be brought to the clinic, because if the child is healthy, the mother knows that the cough will go away. The nearest situation you are likely to encounter is the relatively healthy child who cannot quite shake off the cough.

What we see more often in clinical practice is the

---

4. It is believed in conventional medicine that pneumothorax is caused by puncturing the lung cavity. In fact, it is caused by local stagnation and deficiency of qi, which can happen without puncturing the thoracic cavity at all.

pattern of acute cough superimposed on another disorder. The child usually already has chronic cough or asthma and has been coming for treatment for some time. The situation is more complex. In the next few pages, we will try to explain what seems to go on and to suggest some principles of treatment. Unless you see a lot of acute coughs, you do not really need to understand the next section. If you can remember the basic principles of tonifying a weak child and dispersing a strong child, you are unlikely to go far afield.

Problems Encountered

For many patients, the descriptions given above are quite satisfactory. Certainly, if you are treating your own family and they are in reasonable health, you will find that the patterns they have are largely those which have been described above, and the results are broadly in line with what has been described. However, in the clinic, matters are different and can be much more complicated. In fact, there are times when you cannot work out what is going on. In this second half of the chapter, we will review some of the most common problems that we have encountered. They can be summarized as follows:

- clearing the body of phlegm
- making a transition
- Lung qi deficiency
- panic reaction
- submission reaction

Clearing the Body of Phlegm

The unspoken assumption in the description of an attack by a pathogenic factor is that before the attack, the child was healthy. In fact, the truth is often very different. In particular, it is common for a child to have a lot of phlegm in its system. This may be in the form of manifest phlegm, where, even before the onset of the acute cough, the child had lots of catarrh coming from its nose and quite a lot of phlegm in the Lungs. Alternatively, it may be in the form of 'hidden' phlegm: over a period of time, phlegm may have built up in the body (perhaps from low-grade accumulation disorder, or perhaps from eating lots of lovely ice cream in summer), and although there are no obvious signs of phlegm (i.e., no cough or nasal discharge), there is phlegm deep inside the body, waiting to come out. In these children, the presence of phlegm can often be detected in the slippery quality of the pulse, or perhaps as a rough texture of the skin, which is at the pre-eczema state.

The situation here is quite similar to the condition of 'latent heat' of springtime. There is an imbalance which has built up over a period of time, and the body is looking for ways to restore equilibrium and expel the excess. In such cases the external pathogenic factor can be the catalyst for change, and the outcome can be quite beneficial. When a pathogenic factor attacks, it may provide an opportunity for the phlegm to be expelled. However, there is a real danger that the pathogenic factor will take over, and the end result is even worse than before.

Another way this pattern can occur is when the child already has a lingering pathogenic factor and gets an acute cough. What happens is that the invading pathogenic factor 'awakens' the dormant pathogenic factor, and so, no matter the nature of the current epidemic, in the child with the lingering pathogenic factor it will always assume the same pattern. This can cause despair in the parents, who see the same illness appearing again and again. However, if the child comes to you in the acute stage, then you will have an opportunity to throw out the lingering pathogenic factor. The lingering pathogenic factor which had been dormant or sleeping is now awake and visible, and there is the opportunity to expel it!

Symptoms

This pattern has all the signs and symptoms of the wind-damp pattern:

• a cough with lots and lots of phlegm
• phlegm is present before the onset of the acute cough

Pulse: very slippery, or very soggy and large

Treatment

The main difference in treatment is to *avoid stirring up more phlegm.* Therefore, avoid using S-40 *(feng long)* and G-34 *(yang ling quan).* The reason for this is that the body is already deluged in phlegm, and you do not want to make matters worse. So, for once you have to curb the "there is phlegm, so use S-40 *(feng long)*" reflex reaction. Rather, you should take the same cautious approach that we described for the phlegm pattern of chronic cough and needle:

CV-17 *(shan zhong)*
CV-22 *(tian tu)*
B-13 *(fei shu)*

If you really want to be sure of success in treatment (e.g., if antibiotics simply are unavailable), then make every effort to treat at least once a day during the first few days!

Making a Transition

We are so accustomed to the idea of children making major transitions in their lives, and so practiced in preparing children for them, that we hardly notice them when they occur. The major transitions are going to "play school," going to "grown-up school," going to the toilet alone, and so on. There are many other transitions which may even go on inside the child's mind, and so may not have an external manifestation, but which are just as important. An example of such a transition is one where the child realizes that its parents are people, with ups and downs, sadness and happiness, rather than just typical mother and father figures. (This transition commonly takes place at about ten years of age.)

There are many other transitions of this kind, and it is common for them to be punctuated by an illness. Often this is a cough. Sometimes it is one of the childhood diseases like measles.

How can you tell?

With difficulty! You can never be quite sure; there are many similarities with the previous patterns of expulsion of phlegm. There are also some telltale signs, such as:

• the cough is not too severe, but goes on much longer than expected, for example, six to eight weeks
• the child's spirit becomes more open after the change
• it may be followed by a growth spurt

What can you do?

Fortunately, you do not have to know whether the child is or is not going through a transition. All you have to do is support the child through the process, and to treat what you see. So, for example, if there is lots of phlegm, then help the child to clear the phlegm. Also, if the child has become exhausted by the cough, then you may tonify, using such points as:

S-36 *(zu san li)*
Sp-6 *(san yin jiao)*
L-9 *(tai yuan)*

Lung Qi Deficiency

This is the nightmare situation. The child is basically weak, the Lungs are weak, the child has received antibiotics for cough eight times this year, and a particularly vicious epidemic cough is going round the community. You have given the child maybe three or four treatments, but not yet enough to strengthen it sufficiently to overcome such an invasion. What do you do?

The principle of treatment is in fact quite straightforward: since it is primarily a case of weakness, then tonify even though there is an external pathogenic factor. For example, you may select (but not use all of them) from points such as:

B-13 *(fei shu)*
L-1 *(zhong fu)*
L-9 *(tai yuan)*
S-36 *(zu san li)*
CV-17 *(shan zhong)*

Method: use a tonifying method

Prognosis: if you give lots of treatments, at least once a day and possibly even twice a day to begin with, you may well cure the child

Panic Reaction

If a child has had many severe coughs, possibly even leading to asthma, then it may be very frightened of the cough itself. This is a dangerous situation, for the fear and panic can cause all the muscles in the body, and especially the pectoral muscles, to tighten up. Then, what started out as a comparatively mild cough, can quickly transform into a severe cough with a very tight chest.

How can you tell?

One of the telltale signs of this pattern is that the child seems to be quite well. If you take the pulse and look at other signs and symptoms when there is no cough, you may not find anything especially wrong. In particular, the Lung energy will not strike you as particularly weak. Often, you have given the child quite a large number of treatments by now, and the child is much better. With this background, you would not expect a cough to develop quickly or cause much trouble, and yet it does. It is this speed and violence of reaction that is the telltale sign. Another is the look of fear and panic in the child's eyes when it actually has a cough.

What can you do?

One of the main problems here is one of access. The reaction to the cough may be so quick that the child is taken to hospital before even seeing you. If this does not happen and the child is brought to you, then you can usually help. Of course, it is important for you to stay calm and not to enter into the jolly panic-party. This in itself may be enough. You can also supplement it with such points as:

H-7 *(shen men)*
Liv-3 *(tai chong)*

On the other hand, if there is a real problem over access—either because of the speed of the reaction or because the child lives far away—then you have to give the parents something to take. You may have your own remedies for this sort of situation. Personally, we have found the Bach flower remedies especially helpful. These can be given both outside the time of attack and during an attack.

Submission Reaction

The submission reaction is similar to the panic reaction. This may happen in otherwise strong children, and may occur late on in a course of treatments, long after you think the child should be better. What happens is that the child has had so many attacks of severe cough, which have been treated with dramatic intervention, that when another one comes along, the child gives in without a struggle.

What can you do?

Once again, there is the problem of access. If you have free access to the child, then there is no problem. Simple tonifying treatments are usually effective. But if you do not have access, then it can often be helpful to give the parents a concoction of Bach flower remedies to be used in an emergency.

NOTE

• For a case history involving acute cough, see Case 2 in Chapter 47.

❖

17 ❖ Lobar Pneumonia

INTRODUCTION

This chapter deals with lobar, or bacterial, pneumonia. This is what used to be known simply as pneumonia, but must be defined more closely now as there is a disease called viral pneumonia. Viral pneumonia can be a much milder disease, no more than a mild cough. What we are referring to in this chapter is a very serious, life-threaten-ing disease. We have no experience treating pneumonia in children, and very little experience in adults, but even this limited experience has brought such striking results that we have no hesitation in recommending acupuncture as a first treatment for children who are still reasonably strong.[*]

ETIOLOGY & PATHOGENESIS

Etiology

There are two factors which cause pneumonia, one ex-ternal and the other internal. The external factor is wind, which has developed further and penetrated more deeply than in colds or influenza. The internal factor may either be qi deficiency or weakness of the body. Qi deficiency occurs because the production of qi in the child is insuf-ficient, the protective qi is without foundation, and the

---

*The information provided here is based on many sources: the etiology, path-ology, and differentiation of patterns were drawn from *Traditional Chinese Pediatrics* and *Clinical Handbook of Traditional Chinese Pediatrics* by the Shanghai College of Traditional Chinese Medicine; the treatment sections from a variety of textbooks; and the prognosis sections from *Collection of Clinical Experiences with Acupuncture* and *Abstracts of Clinical Experience with Acupuncture*.

Lungs are 'fragile'. Weakness of the body is attributable to a constitutional weakness from birth, or to inadequate nourishment, which weakens the normal qi and diminishes the sustaining force.

Pathogenesis

External pathogenic wind attacks the protective qi, rising up vigorously and obstructing the Lung qi. Pathogenic wind may either be hot or cold, but because a "child's yin does not extend far," and "the six pathogenic weather factors easily transform into heat," then even if the illness begins as wind-cold, it can rapidly transform into heat. The disease often progresses quickly to the stage where the pathogenic factor obliterates the normal qi, leaving the patient in an extremely deficient condition. For this reason, the wind-cold pattern is only rarely seen, and even then, it is mild and of short duration.

Wind patterns

The Lungs govern the qi of the yin organs, unite externally with the skin and hair, open through the cavities of the nose, and control respiration. Pathogenic wind can enter via the skin, mouth, or nose, obstruct the protective qi at the level of the skin, and invade the Lungs internally. The qi is then unable to descend, and the fluids in the middle of the Lungs transform into phlegm, which in turn blocks the bronchi. The Lungs are left unsupported, giving rise to such symptoms as fever, cough, panting, nasal flaring, and wheezing, which are characteristic of the pattern of obstructed Lung qi rising up rebelliously. If fire blazes upward, it distills and thickens the fluids, causing such exaggerated symptoms as hot cheeks, thirst, wheezing, panting, and nasal flaring. If it progresses further, the fire can enter the terminal yin channel where it runs riot, giving rise to loss of consciousness, twitching, and convulsions.

Phlegm-heat, obstructed qi, and blood stasis

The Lungs govern the qi and connect with the 'hundred channels', and the Heart governs the blood and the circulation of nourishment and yin. The qi controls the blood such that when the qi moves, the blood moves, and when the qi is obstructed, so too is the blood. If the pathogenic factor is abundant and the normal qi is deficient, with phlegm-heat depressing the Lungs, the bronchi will be obstructed and the Heart blood will not flow. Obstructed qi and blood stasis give rise to a dark purple color in the face, mouth, lips, and tongue body.

Normal qi obliterated

If the normal qi is unable to overcome the pathogenic factor, the disease may progress to the point that the Heart qi becomes insufficient and the Heart yang is not aroused. If the Heart yang is not aroused, there will be severe blood stasis and obstruction of the Lung qi, giving rise to such symptoms as continuous cough, asthma, gasping for breath, restlessness, green-blue facial color, cyanosed lips, cold limbs, profuse sweating, and a forceless pulse. These are all characteristic of the patterns of obstructed Lung qi and weak and faded Heart yang, or yang qi collapse.

Recuperation

According to traditional Chinese medicine, after the pneumonia has been cured, the pathogenic factor may remain in the body, having only been partially expelled. The child's body is weakened, the qi is damaged, and the yin is injured. With yin deficiency and a lingering pathogenic factor, there are symptoms of sustained fever, much sweating, red face, lips, or cheeks, dry cough with little phlegm, scanty saliva, and dry tongue. In the case of Lung and Spleen qi deficiency, typical symptoms include dull facial color and profuse sweating. If severe, there may be cough without strength, much phlegm, and possibly fever.

Pneumonia in the newborn

In a newborn baby, the qi is extremely weak and the internal aspect of this problem is pronounced. Encountering little resistance, the pathogenic factor can easily enter into the chest cavity. The pattern quickly develops into yang qi deficiency or collapse of yang. This means that, although the normal qi and the pathogenic factor are joined in battle, there are few signs of it.

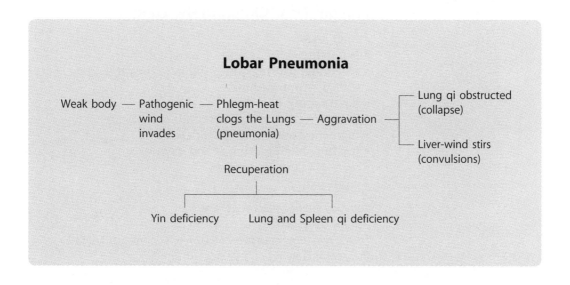

Lobar Pneumonia

PATTERNS & SYMPTOMS

Pathogenic Wind Obstructs the Lungs

Wind-cold

- aversion to cold
- fever without sweating
- absence of thirst
- rough cough, gasping for breath
- sputum white and possibly watery

Tongue coating: thin and white, or white and greasy
Tongue body: not red
Finger vein: purple-red
Pulse: floating, tight, and rapid

Treatment principle: gently warm, release the exterior, direct the Lung qi downward, and transform the phlegm

Wind-heat

- fever with sweating
- cough with thick sputum
- gasping for breath
- nasal flaring
- face, lips, and throat red
- urine yellow
- irregular stools which may be dry or contain specks of phlegm

Tongue coating: yellow
Tongue body: red
Finger vein: purple
Pulse: floating and rapid, or slippery and rapid

Treatment principle: clear the heat, release the exterior, direct the Lung qi downward, and transform the phlegm

Phlegm-Heat Clogging the Lungs

- high fever
- irritability
- wheezing, panting and gasping for breath, and great difficulty in breathing
- nasal flaring
- in severe cases, both sides of rib cage tremble
- high chest and raised shoulders
- writhing and plucking at abdomen
- urine is scanty and yellow
- constipation

Tongue coating: yellow, greasy
Tongue body: red
Finger vein: deep purple, often reaches past 'qi gate'
Pulse: overflowing, slippery, and rapid

Treatment principle: clear the heat, direct the Lung qi downward, break up the phlegm, and stop the cough

Normal Qi Deficiency with Lingering Pathogenic Factor

Yin deficiency, pathogenic factor prevails

• high fever
• much sweating
• face or cheeks red
• dry cough with little phlegm

Tongue coating: bright and peeled, or dry
Tongue body: red, dry
Pulse: fine, rapid
Finger vein: purple, often sunken or fine

Treatment principle: enrich the yin and clear the Lungs

Lung and Spleen qi deficiency

• high fever which comes and goes
• cold limbs
• cough without force
• bright white facial color
• wasting of body
• spirit tired
• dull responses
• stools soft, unformed

Tongue coating: white, slippery
Tongue body: pale
Finger vein: pale color, usually deep

Treatment principle: augment the qi and nourish the Spleen

Complications

Lung qi obstructed, Heart yang deficiency

• panting feebly
• facial color dull white
• mouth and lips cyanotic
• cold limbs
• spirit feeble but restless

Tongue body: dull purple
Pulse: deficient and rapid, or faint and soft
Finger vein: purple, deep, may reach 'life gate'

Treatment principle: open and direct the Lung qi downward, and warm and tonify the Heart yang

Pathogenic factor enters Heart and Liver, heat rises up, and wind stirs

• feeble gasping for breath, possibly breathing stopped altogether for short periods
• high fever
• irritability, possibly delirium and loss of consciousness

- clenched teeth
- both eyes turn upward

Tongue body: crimson red
Finger vein: purple, may enter 'life gate' or even reach the nail

Note: when the pathogenic factor enters the Heart and Liver, it may lead to collapse of yang with the following symptoms:

- facial color ashen
- great sweating (soaked)
- extreme cold in the limbs

Treatment principle: quickly revive the yang and prop up the collapse

TREATMENT

Pathogenic Wind Obstructs the Lungs

Wind-cold

B-13 *(fei shu)*	Clears pathogenic wind from the Lungs
G-20 *(feng chi)*	
L-7 *(lie que)*	Clears pathogenic wind
LI-4 *(he gu)*	

Method: use a dispersing method and treat once or twice a day. Moxibustion may be used. Cupping may be applied at tender points on the back.

Prognosis: three to six treatments

Wind-heat

GV-14 *(da zhui)*	Clears wind-heat
LI-11 *(qu chi)*	Clears heat
LI-4 *(he gu)*	Clears heat
B-13 *(fei shu)*	Clears wind from the Lungs
L-5 *(chi ze)*	Cools the Lungs

Method: use a dispersing method and treat once or twice a day

Prognosis: three to six treatments; after one or two treatments there may be a reduction in the intensity of the heat, leading to a more productive cough

Phlegm-Heat Clogging the Lungs

L-11 *(shao shang)*	Clears excess heat from the Lungs and stops cough
L-7 *(lie que)*	Transforms phlegm and opens the Lungs

S-40 *(feng long)*	Transforms phlegm and benefits the chest
LI-11 *(qu chi)*	Clears heat
CV-14 *(ju que)*	Opens the chest and transforms phlegm

Note: treat L-11 *(shao shang)* with a triangular needle to draw a few drops of blood. The sensation when needling CV-14 *(ju que)* should reach up into the chest, but be very careful: needling too deeply may injure the heart!

If there is red phlegm, add P-7 *(da ling)*, CV-17 *(shan zhong)*, and P-6 *(nei guan)*.

Method: use a dispersing method, treating twice or three times a day

Prognosis: five to ten treatments

Normal Qi Deficiency with Lingering Pathogenic Factor

Yin deficiency

B-38 *(gao huang shu)*	Tonifies the yin of the entire body
B-23 *(shen shu)*	Tonifies Kidney yin
K-3 *(tai xi)*	Tonifies Kidney yin
L-5 *(chi ze)*	Tonifies Lung yin
CV-4 *(guan yuan)*	Tonifies yin of the entire body

Method: use the even method; treat every four to six hours

Prognosis: if treatment is given in the early stages before the patient is too weak, the patient should be out of danger within forty-eight hours; if treatment is given only after the patient is exhausted, acupuncture may be ineffective

Lung and Spleen qi deficiency

B-13 *(fei shu)*	Tonifies Lung qi deficiency
B-20 *(pi shu)*	Tonifies Spleen qi
S-36 *(zu san li)*	Tonifies qi of the entire body
Sp-6 *(san yin jiao)*	Tonifies Spleen qi
CV-6 *(qi hai)*	Tonifies qi of the entire body
CV-12 *(zhong wan)*	Tonifies Spleen qi
L-9 *(tai yuan)*	Tonifies Lung qi

Method: use the even method; moxibustion or moxibustion on garlic may be used at the abdominal and back points

Prognosis: same as for yin deficiency

Complications

Loss of consciousness	S-36 *(zu san li)* P-6 *(nei guan)* GV-26 *(ren zhong)*

Method: these three points should be strongly stimulated to restore consciousness

Lung qi obstructed	GV-20 *(bai hui)*
Heart yang deficiency	CV-6 *(qi hai)*
Collapse of yang	CV-4 *(guan yuan)* CV-8 *(shen que)* CV-12 *(zhong wan)* S-36 *(zu san li)*

These are the most commonly used points for restoring the yang. Moxibustion should be used at all the points. Continuous moxibustion should be applied at the abdominal points until the patient recovers.

Heat rises up and wind stirs

Use strong stimulation at the points for loss of consciousness, that is, GV-26 *(ren zhong)*, P-6 *(nei guan)*, S-36 *(zu san li)*. Also bleed the well *(jǐng)* points or the tips of the fingers, collectively known as *shi xuan* (M-UE-1). Alternatively, bleed L-5 *(chi ze)* and B-40 *(wei zhong)*.

NOTES

- Acupuncture combines well with Western medicine, and the use of antibiotics should always be considered.

- Acupuncture is more effective in treating robust patients.

- It is important to continue treating through the recuperation stage.

❖

18 ❖ Asthma

INTRODUCTION

Asthma is a very serious, life-threatening disease; many adults and children die of it every year. To live with asthma is both physically and emotionally debilitating, especially for a child. The child cannot run and play with friends, which is frustrating, and is often left out of things, which can be really upsetting.

The use of drugs in the control of asthma is of a palliative nature only. Drugs do not cure the condition. From our point of view, the commonly used drugs—bronchodilators and steroids—actually make the problem worse in the long run. Research is being done into the effect of bronchodilators since their long-term use may have increased the mortality rate from this disease over the last few years.

The incidence of asthma is increasing at an alarming rate in the developed world. For example, a pediatrician in Brighton, England told me that asthma is approximately ten times more common today than it was when he started practicing thirty years ago. At that time, he said, the asthma ward in the local hospital (with about forty beds) never had more than a handful of children. By contrast, the diarrhea ward was always full and often overflowed. Now, however, the situation has reversed. There is no doubt that this shift is due at least in part to changes in family and school life, which will be discussed in more detail in the section on etiology.

What is asthma?

The Chinese term for asthma, *xiāo chuǎn*   , literally means "wheezing and gurgling." As such, they refer to dyspnea, or difficulty in breathing, which is not quite the same as asthma. Asthma is generally taken to mean that the child has difficulty in breathing due to an increased responsiveness of the airways. However, many children are labeled as 'asthmatic' even when they may not have that much problem in breathing, but may just get recurrent coughs or have a lot of phlegm on the chest. This makes them a bit rattly in the chest or a bit wheezy, but hardly asthmatic.

Luckily for us, the actual Western diagnosis is not that important: we can make our own diagnosis by pattern differentiation. However, if you read the acupuncture textbooks about asthma you will find differing ideas. There also seem to be many new theories about the disease. What we present here is the treatment of children who have received the Western diagnosis of asthma, and is based on our experience in the children's clinics in London, Brighton, and Seattle. It is different from the descriptions set forth in Chinese textbooks.

Effectiveness of acupuncture

Acupuncture is very effective in the treatment of asthma and is, in our view, the treatment of choice for this disease. However, treatment is not always easy, and many problems are encountered along the way. On a basic level, all you do is tonify the Lungs, resolve phlegm, and strengthen the Spleen: if only life were this easy! Most of the children that we see have been taking various drugs for years. This has two repercussions. First, the organs or *zàng fǔ* are further weakened by the drugs, and second—more serious in some ways—the children are addicted to the drugs. If you watch a child who has just taken some ventolin or becotide, you will see that they get a real kick out of it.

The result of all of this is that treatment takes a long time, many months in some cases. Moreover, the child will still be at risk of attacks during your treatment. This will, of course, happen occasionally, with the result that the parents may become demoralized and stop coming. The child can also find it very hard to come off the drugs, and many reasons can be dreamed up to persuade parents to stop treatment.

However, if you can get through all of this and win the child's and the parents' cooperation—both of which are needed—then you are sure to help that child enormously. It takes patience and care. But perhaps as much as any other disease, if you can treat asthma successfully, you will have saved that child from growing up with a frightening, lifelong disease.

In China, asthma is not yet the scourge that it is here in the West. Consequently, it is not given very much ink in Chinese textbooks. Yet in our clinic, asthma is one of the most common diseases, and we feel it deserves full coverage. We have organized the presentation of this subject as follows:

1. We begin with etiology and pathogenesis, in part translated from the Chinese, and in part based on conditions in the West.
2. This is followed by a discussion of the treatment of an acute asthma attack in a child of any age. Although many practitioners never see this, and others are forbidden by law from treating it, this may well change, for the effects of acupuncture in treating acute asthma attacks are remarkable.
3. The treatment of chronic asthma in the very young (up to about age five) is taken up next.
4. This is followed by a discussion of the treatment of chronic asthma in older children.
5. Finally, we conclude with our observations on clinical problems and advice for parents.

ETIOLOGY & PATHOGENESIS

Etiology

Hereditary factors. Quite often you will find there is a history of lung disease in the family.

Repeated infections. A major cause of asthma is repeated attacks of respiratory tract infections. With the advent of modern antibiotics, these infections take a less serious course, but the antibiotics themselves weaken the Spleen and lead to dampness, thus opening the way for asthma.

Too much phlegm-producing foods. There has been a significant shift in children's diets toward foods which produce phlegm. These include cow's milk, cheese, peanuts, sugar, and orange juice. Cows in this country are regularly given antibiotics, which undoubtedly pass into the milk and further aggravate the situation. (We know of some children whose chronic cough was cured by changing from ordinary milk to organic unpasteurized milk.)

Irregular feeding in babies. The practice of continuously snacking or breastfeeding can quickly lead to deficient Spleen and Stomach qi, which in turn leads to weak overall qi. In strong children, unsuitable foods can easily lead to accumulation disorder. The phlegm that is generated can be a major cause of asthma.

Food additives. More and more foods contain coloring, flavor enhancers, or preservatives, even when sold in their "fresh" state. In some children, these added chemicals give rise to allergic reactions.

Too much television and computer games. Television, computers, and other electronic toys are exhausting as well as stimulating to the senses. Quite often the programs are violent and frightening to children, causing added stress. They also prevent children from running around and using their Lungs. The net result seems to be that both the qi and yin (especially the Kidney yin) is depleted, and the qi stagnates.

Bad posture. Little or no attention is paid to children's posture in the home or at school. In the majority of schools there are no slopes to write on, and children may be seen curled up over their work. This bad posture constricts the chest and gives less space for the lungs, with corresponding effect on the Lung qi.

Lack of exercise. Although living conditions are better, children spend less time out of doors taking exercise. All exercise in moderation strengthens the Lungs and Spleen.

Emotional trauma. According to the recent census in the United Kingdom, it is now estimated that two-thirds of all children are brought up in one-parent families. The traumatic effect of parents separating is overwhelming for many children. Even children as young as three, who may be thought to have little understanding of parental relations, can be strongly affected by the breakdown in marriage.

Corticosteroid creams for the treatment of eczema. Eczema is usually caused by dampness and phlegm accumulating in the skin. The effect of applying corticosteroids to the skin is to return the dampness to the interior of the body. The excess dampness, instead of going outward to the skin, turns inward to the Lungs, leading to the accumulation of phlegm-dampness in the Lungs and asthma.

Allergens. Pollen, crop sprays, exhaust fumes, oil paints, tobacco smoke, animal hair, peanuts, house dust mites, and many other things can all trigger an asthma attack.

Anti-asthmatic drugs. The very use of these drugs tends to weaken the qi of the Lungs and the Kidneys.

These etiological factors have the effect of weakening the body to the extent that asthma is able to develop. Individually, they may not be enough to cause an asthma attack, but in combination, they allow two important changes to occur in the body: they disrupt the Lung qi and allow for the build-up of phlegm in the Lungs. It then only takes a small factor, such as house dust or animal hair, to trigger an attack.

The Trigger

A 'trigger' is some additional ingredient that turns the condition from a bad cough into full-blown asthma. This is on top of everything else we have talked about, that is, the general etiological factors *and* the Lung dysfunction *and* the phlegm. These triggers can be external factors—allergies to animals, changes in the weather, pollution, or other external pathogenic factors—or they can be emotional factors. What seems to happen is that this final straw causes the complete breakdown of the qi mechanism: the Lungs cannot take in qi, the qi cannot circulate and so stagnates, and you have an asthma attack.

Generally, it is unnecessary to treat the trigger, which is the Western medical approach. From our point of view, if you treat the underlying pathology, the trigger will lose its impact.

This highlights a fundamental difference between traditional Chinese medicine and the Western approach to medicine. In Western medicine, all problems are seen as external devils, something outside, so the treatment for asthma often focuses on 'desensitizing' someone to the allergen. In traditional Chinese medicine, by contrast, we recognize that there are both internal and external factors, and in the treatment of asthma, the main emphasis is on treating the internal factors.

Traditional Chinese Viewpoint

Internal factors

Asthma occurs when the qi of the three yin organs—the Lungs, Spleen, and Kidneys—is deficient, the protective qi is not strong enough, and phlegm-dampness accumulates inside. If the Lung qi is insufficient, the protective qi is unable to repel external pathogenic factors, which can invade repeatedly. If the Spleen qi is deficient, it cannot move the Stomach fluids and there will be an accumulation of dampness and phlegm, which rises up to the Lungs. And if the Kidney yang is deficient, it cannot vaporize the fluids, and water and dampness accumulate and transform into phlegm.

In many children, asthma is accompanied by eczema, which is a sign that dampness has accumulated. In other children, the face is bright white and a little puffy, the bridge of the nose is green-blue, the skin is slack and flabby, and there is a gurgling noise from the throat. These are all symptoms of Spleen qi deficiency with accumulation of dampness.

External factors

Changes in the weather, unseasonable heat or cold, the influence of external pathogenic wind, and allergies (e.g., pollen, animal hair, tobacco smoke, shrimp, oil paints, parasites, house mites) are the main external causes which provide the trigger for asthma.

Pathogenesis

Asthma is the result of a combination of external pathogenic factors and internal factors. Internally, the body is weak, with accumulation of phlegm-dampness and poor circulation of qi and blood. Externally, there is contact with cold, other pathogenic factors, and allergens. After this contact, phlegm obstructs the air passages, such that the Lung qi can no longer descend and disperse. This causes the Lung qi to rebel, which is manifested as asthma. If the phlegm remains for a long time, one 'contact' is sufficient to induce asthma.

In the acute stage, there is convulsive breathing, and the focus of the disease is the Lungs. This may be a result of external pathogenic wind-cold or internal injury from cold food; in both cases, the cold weakens the function of the Lungs, and the ensuing accumulation of fluids transforms into phlegm. Alternatively, it may result from internal yang deficiency, which impairs the qi's ability to transform the body fluids, leading to cold-phlegm obstruction internally. These are the two principal causes of cold asthma. For hot asthma, the principal causes are internal yin deficiency, phlegm-heat depressing the Lungs, or cold-phlegm transforming into heat.

Asthma of recent origin is usually excessive in nature, while a chronic disease is typically deficient. If the disease persists for a long time, it can injure the Lungs and scatter the Lung qi. Any chronic disease can affect the Kidneys; thus, Lung disease can progress to Kidney disease, causing Kidney yang deficiency and rendering the Kidneys unable to receive the qi.

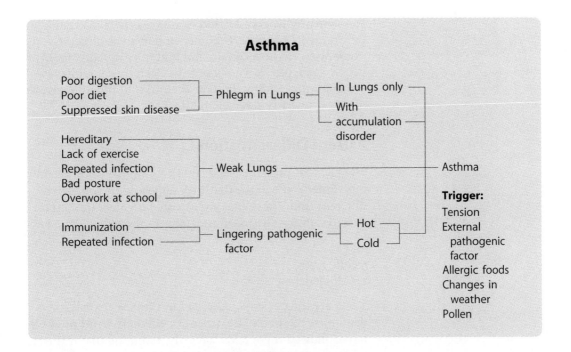

Asthma

Poor digestion
Poor diet ── Phlegm in Lungs ── In Lungs only
Suppressed skin disease ── With accumulation disorder

Hereditary
Lack of exercise
Repeated infection ── Weak Lungs ──────────── Asthma
Bad posture
Overwork at school

Immunization ── Lingering pathogenic ── Hot / Cold
Repeated infection ── factor

Trigger:
Tension
External pathogenic factor
Allergic foods
Changes in weather
Pollen

ACUTE ASTHMA

Introduction

Conventional medicine has taken center stage in the management of acute asthma. As far as relieving the symptoms is concerned—which does save lives—the results are good. However, conventional treatment itself is violent and injurious to health.

The drama and tension surrounding the treatment of asthma, and the rigid doctrine of those involved in administering the treatment, has led to the total exclusion of all other therapies. This is a pity, for other therapies have a lot to offer. Acupuncture in particular has very striking results, often as quick as conventional medicine, just as reliable, and with none of the attendant side effects. It is very much to be hoped that in the future, acupuncture will be part of the routine treatment for acute asthma. As mentioned earlier in this chapter, the treatment of an acute asthma attack is the same regardless of the age of the child.

Other therapies

It is our opinion that acupuncture is the best therapy for treating acute asthma attacks. The success rate seems to be comparable to that obtained with conventional medical treatments, and the treatment itself is simple. There are other therapies which are as effective as acupuncture, but each suffers from some disadvantage. For example, herbal medicine can be very effective, but it takes longer to work and often requires some time to prepare a prescription.

Homeopathy works well and is more easily taken than herbal medicine, but the choice of remedy is difficult. There seems to be a certain "hit and miss" quality about it. The same can be said about the Bach flower remedies, although they definitely have their uses in the home treatment of the early stage of an attack.

Pattern Differentiation

The patterns presented here are those we have observed in our clinic. You will see that they appear to be somewhat different from those that are usually provided. In the past we have always discussed the patterns for acute asthma as:

- heat
- cold
- Kidney deficiency

These are the patterns presented in Chinese textbooks describing the herbal treatment of children. Until now, we have followed these texts slavishly, assuming that if the Chinese say so, then it must be so. However, over the years it has gradually dawned on us that things are different for Western children, especially when you treat with acupuncture rather than herbs. There are many reasons for this, which are mainly to do with lifestyle and the free use of inhalers in Western children. In any event, the patterns, as we find them, are better described instead as:

- spasm
- phlegm
- heat

Spasm. This is the most common pattern. The whole chest and bronchi go into spasm, and the child has great difficulty breathing. It seems to be just as much effort to breath in as to breath out. This attack is typically seen in an allergic reaction, either to such things as cats, dogs, horses, or house mites, or else to foods. It is also seen in children who are confirmed asthmatics and who catch a cold, which then triggers an asthma attack. The main distinguishing feature is that the child just cannot breathe, although there does not seem to be anything else especially wrong.

Phlegm. This pattern is also common, although slightly less so. It has many similarities with the previous pattern, for the Lungs certainly go into spasm, but the difference is that there is lots of phlegm. It is the phlegm blocking the air passages which stops the child from breathing.

Heat.[1] Once again, there are similarities to the spasm pattern, for here too the chest may have seized up. The difference is that there is obviously an infection, probably bacterial (from the biomedical perspective), or an attack of wind which has transformed into phlegm-heat (from the traditional Chinese medical perspective). The distinguishing features are signs of heat, such as red face, hot forehead, red tongue, yellow coating, yellow nasal discharge.

Treatment

As noted in the introduction to this chapter, it is our belief that acupuncture is the best therapy for an asthma attack because of the simplicity of treatment. All three patterns above likely involve spasms, and there is an excellent point for relieving them:

ding chuan (M-BW-1)

Method: use two needles—one for each side—as you will probably want to retain them in place. Use 5mm needles for toddlers, but for five- or six-year-olds, you may need to use a longer and thicker needle, perhaps 15mm, 30 gauge needles. The needling method is to obtain qi and then give quite strong (but gentle) and continuous stimulation to the point. Do half a minute on one side, then half a minute on the other side. Return again to the first side. Continue for three to five minutes. (This is a very long time. Use a watch, for in an acute situation, half a minute seems like an eternity.) After three to five minutes there should be significant improvement in the breathing. It is then appropriate to use additional points based on the particular pattern.

Spasm-wheezing

P-6 *(nei guan)*	Opens the chest, calms the spirit
Liv-3 *(tai chong)*	Relaxes spasms
B-13 *(fei shu)*	Tonifies the Lungs

Method: strong dispersing method is used for all three patterns

Phlegm

With this pattern, you will instinctively want to clear the bronchi. Use the following points:

---

1. The important thing to realize is that while the hot-type asthma is hot, the phlegm and spasm types are not hot. Previously, they would have been called cold-type asthma. However, they do not have to be positively cold; there must simply be an absence of heat.

	CV-22 *(tian tu)*	Opens the bronchi
	CV-17 *(shan zhong)*	Opens the chest
	P-6 *(nei guan)*	Opens the chest
Heat	L-10 *(yu ji)*	Clears heat from the Lungs
	L-5 *(chi ze)*	Cools the Lungs

Prognosis: the effectiveness of the treatment depends very much on the underlying strength of the child. Continue to stimulate the points until the attack is relieved. If it is not, then you will have to resort to a combination of Chinese and Western medicine. After the initial treatment, you may need to see the child every six hours in a very severe case, but more likely once a day. This is even true for the heat pattern, which corresponds to bacterial infection in conventional medicine, and would usually be treated with antibiotics.

Other points

There are many other points which can be used. Those listed above are the points which seem to work for us. But there are others which are also known to work, such as G-21 *(jian jing)* and L-1 *(zhong fu)*, which we avoid during acute attack because of the danger of causing pneumothorax.

Emotional Factors

The big emotional factor is *fear* followed by *panic.* These two emotions certainly aggravate the situation and are part of the vicious circle which keeps asthma going. You can specifically treat the panic with remedies such as the Bach Rescue Remedy, but the main thing is to remain calm yourself. Just by touching the child and remaining calm and purposeful in your treatment, you will help to allay the fear and calm the panic, and this will help greatly. Another possibility is the submission reaction, which was touched on in the treatment of acute cough in Chapter 16.

CHRONIC ASTHMA IN CHILDREN UNDER FIVE

In this section we discuss the patterns seen in the very young (up to about five years), which are very different from those seen in older children or adults. This is because of the problems which they face in their lives, which are mainly about eating enough food and keeping warm. As they get older, the patterns change as the baby (whose main concern is breathing and eating) evolves into a toddler and then into a school child, with homework, friends and enemies, and computer games. Obviously, the patterns do not change on the fourth or fifth birthday; the change is gradual over the years, hence the time span can vary. You must assess each child individually and decide whether you think the child's condition is that of a younger or older child.

If a child under the age of five has asthma, two factors *must* be present:

1. phlegm, a characteristic of excess
2. Lung weakness, a characteristic of deficiency

In addition, the child almost always has a lingering pathogenic factor.

Other factors may play a role, but you can rely on the presence of these three things. This is actually quite useful. In children under the age of three and in those over the age of seven, the patterns are often simple, but in between those ages it is common to find mixed patterns. By remembering that these three factors are nearly always present, it gives you something to work with.

Patterns

Phlegm	• by itself • with accumulation disorder
Lung and Spleen qi deficiency	• normal • hyperactive
Lingering pathogenic factor	• hot • cold

═══

Remember: in all asthma, there is some aspect of Lung dysfunction.

═══

Note

Allergic asthma usually has at its base a lingering pathogenic factor which can be either hot or cold in nature. The cold type gives rise to allergies against such things as molds and penicillin, while the hot type gives rise to allergies against things like animals and house dust.

Case History

A few years ago while on holiday, we watched a child develop asthma. She was six years old, very thin and pale, and ate like a mouse. She would only eat ham and Italian cookies, and, of course, ice cream. This was certainly not due to a lack of variety in the hotel: where we stayed the proprietor would have cooked her anything! She also had bundles and bundles of energy. She went to the beach, ate ice cream, stayed up for dinner, and would go for a walk, a coffee, and a brandy afterwards in the local cafe. (The child did not actually have coffee and brandy. She was happy with ice cream.) She would then be up again at 7 A.M., bouncing around the hotel.

This child had a nasty cough, which had persisted for some weeks. Nothing much had been able to clear it, including antibiotics and herbal cough mixes. We offered an acupuncture treatment, but the howls and the wails were truly awful. It was quickly decided that it would be to no avail. So we sat back and watched, helplessly.

The cough was tight and harsh (she had a lingering pathogenic factor), but being in the sea air (the hotel overlooked the Mediterranean), the phlegm gradually began to loosen and she was able to cough some of it up. This made the cough worse, but to our minds, better out than in. However, to the father, not surprisingly, things were getting much worse. He could not bear to see his child suffering, so he decided that he would have to give her some ventolin. The results were rapid; she immediately recovered after a bad coughing fit and began to want things again—swimming, ice cream, and attention. Although she was given no more ventolin that day, she did receive it the next day and the next. As the days went on, she became wheezy more frequently, more hyperactive, and more . . . asthmatic.

Etiology

The main contributory factors are set forth earlier in this chapter. But the most common way to develop asthma is through the repeated treatment of acute coughs with antibiotics.

Pathogenesis

In children under the age of five with asthma there is always both Lung weakness and phlegm. There is often a lingering pathogenic factor, and sometimes accumulation disorder as well. All of these pathologies may combine to give rise to asthma.

Phlegm plus accumulation disorder

The accumulated food in the interior impairs the circulation of qi. The phlegm which is produced accumulates in the Lungs and leads to asthma.

Lung and Spleen qi deficiency	Weakness of the Lungs means that the qi is not governed properly. The weak Spleen leads to the formation of phlegm. These two factors give rise to asthma.
Lingering pathogenic factor	The pathogenesis is the same for both the cold and hot types. The presence of thick phlegm in the system retards the circulation of qi and obstructs the function of the Lungs, leading to asthma.

Signs & Symptoms

Pulse and tongue: note the frequent absence of pulse and tongue signs in the following pattern descriptions. This is because we have not found them to be reliable indicators in children under the age of five.

Phlegm	• gray facial color • cough with lots of phlegm • unable to breathe because of the excess of phlegm • nasal discharge • bubbly sputum *Pulse:* slippery
Phlegm plus accumulation disorder	All of the above, plus: • strong child • loud voice • red cheeks • irregular, green, smelly stools *Pulse:* slippery
Lung and Spleen qi deficiency (normal)	• child is weak, small, possibly undersized • possibly nasal discharge • small voice • easily out of breath • white or gray face • poor appetite or choosy about food • easily gets ill and difficulty in recovering
Lung and Spleen qi deficiency (hyperactive)	All of the preceding pattern, except: • lots of energy • often the parents are exhausted • manipulative
Lingering pathogenic factor (cold)	• reasonably strong child • very few visible signs of phlegm • gray face • vacant eyes • history of repeated attacks—treated with antibiotics • history of immunizations

• glands swollen
• worse in cold, damp weather
• often allergic to molds and/or penicillin, which can bring on attacks
• occasional abdominal aches with no obvious cause

Finger vein: if present it is blue

Lingering pathogenic factor (hot)

• reasonably strong child
• very few visible signs of phlegm
• white forehead, red cheeks or lips
• eyes vacant
• prone to fevers
• worse in hot weather
• often allergic to animals, which can bring on attacks

Treatment

The most important thing to remember in the treatment of asthma in children under five is that there is nearly always present, concurrently, a mixture of some phlegm, some Lung deficiency, and a lingering pathogenic factor. Of these, the phlegm or the Lung deficiency will be most obvious. Treat these first. *Do not begin by treating the lingering pathogenic factor.* Once you see a reduction in the phlegm or an increase in Lung qi, then you may proceed to treat the lingering pathogenic factor.

Main points[2]

L-5 *(chi ze)*
L-7 *(lie que)*
L-9 *(tai yuan)*
CV-12 *(zhong wan)*
CV-22 *(tian tu)*

Provided the child is not too full of phlegm, add:

S-40 *(feng long)*

═══════

**Remember to always use a Lung point.
You are treating a Lung disorder.**

═══════

Phlegm

The main points above will do, but *use S-40 (feng long) with care.* It is probably better to start with CV-22 *(tian tu)* for the first two or three treatments so as not to disturb too much phlegm and provoke an asthma attack.

---

2. Some people use *ding chuan* (M-BW-1) in the treatment of chronic asthma. We prefer to use it in treating acute attacks.

Prognosis: if phlegm is the main factor and the child is comparatively strong, you may be able to cure the asthma in fifteen treatments. Usually, however, this pattern has an underlying lingering pathogenic factor, and this may take another fifteen to thirty treatments to clear.

---

*If the child is drowning in phlegm,
do not start with S-40 (feng long).
Use CV-22 (tian tu) until much of the
phlegm has been resolved. Otherwise,
you may make things a lot worse.*

Phlegm plus accumulation disorder

Use the main points plus *si feng* (M-UE-9). A word of warning about using *si feng* (M-UE-9). Its use can release a large amount of heat and phlegm into the system. If the child is very phlegmy, you may make things worse by using this point. Start by using CV-22 *(tian tu)* and CV-12 *(zhong wan)* until much of the phlegm has been cleared, then proceed to *si feng* (M-UE-9) if necessary. You should already have advised the parents about the child's diet, so the accumulation may have cleared itself.

Prognosis: if the condition is a result of just accumulation disorder and phlegm, then it may take as little as five treatments. However, this is very rare, and you will usually have to clear a lingering pathogenic factor and strengthen the Lungs and the Spleen as well, which will take another ten to thirty treatments.

Advice: in the pure phlegm-type case, you will get a gradual expulsion of phlegm. If it is too violent, the child will have an asthma attack. This should be explained to parents beforehand so that they don't worry if phlegm starts coming out of all the orifices. If accumulation disorder is also present, the standard warning about the discharge of foul-smelling stools and irritability should be given. In addition, dietary advice is important (see end of this chapter).

---

*Si feng (M-UE-9) can release a lot of heat and phlegm,
so use it with care. If in doubt, use CV-22 (tian tu)
until the heat and phlegm are reduced.*

Lung and Spleen qi deficiency

Acupuncture treatment for both normal and hyperactive Lung and Spleen qi deficiency is similar, but the parental advice is different.

Treatment principle: tonify the Lungs and Spleen

Use the main points, plus:

Sp-6 *(san yin jiao)*
S-36 *(zu san li)*

Prognosis: progress is sure but slow. Depending on the strength of the child, fifteen to fifty treatments will be necessary. Treating twice a week may speed things up, but these children just need time to get their qi back to normal levels. As the qi strengthens, the child may start to expel the phlegm that is in the Lungs. Treat this using points listed above for the phlegm pattern.

Advice: explain to parents that progress will be sure but slow, and that the child just needs time to recover its qi. The child must rest and take light exercise every day. The diet should be warming to the Spleen (no ice cream, no fruit juice) and should follow the general guidelines for all children with asthma set out later in this chapter. If the child is hyperactive, it is a good idea to give advice about setting boundaries, if this is feasible.

Lingering pathogenic factor (cold)

Do not begin treating this until you have cleared up the phlegm and tonified most of the deficiency. Otherwise, you will make matters worse. Use the main points, plus:

bai lao (M-HN-30)
B-13 *(fei shu)*
B-20 *(pi shu)*
B-18 *(gan shu)*

Method: tonifying method at B-13 *(fei shu)*, dispersing or moving method at the other points. Moxibustion may also be used at CV-12 *(zhong wan)*, B-18 *(gan shu)*, and B-20 *(pi shu)*.

Lingering pathogenic factor (hot)

Use the same point prescription as the previous pattern. Surprisingly, you may still be able to use moxibustion at CV-12 *(zhong wan)* and the governing *(shū)* points on the back, if there is not too much heat.

If there is a lot of heat, use the main points with a dispersing method, especially L-5 *(chi ze)* and L-7 *(lie que)*. In addition, add Liv-2 *(xing jian)* and L-10 *(yu ji)*.

Advice: the diet should not include any phlegm-producing foods. Warn the parents that phlegm will start to come out and things may get temporarily worse. If you tell them before it happens, they are less likely to get upset!

What to Expect from Treatment

When you start treating a child with asthma the results will probably not be very dramatic. Gradually, the phlegm will diminish, the accumulation disorder will resolve, and the qi will strengthen.

Once you have achieved this much, you may proceed to treat the lingering pathogenic factor. After a few treatments the phlegm will start to loosen up and the child will begin to show such symptoms as cough, runny nose, or runny stools as the phlegm comes out. When the phlegm is loose, treat as if it were a phlegm condition. (This is similar to the approach used in treating chronic cough, described in Chapter 15.) Once the obvious phlegm has been resolved, then go back to treating the lingering pathogenic factor.

Once more, step-by-step:

1. Treat the phlegm or the Lung qi deficiency.
2. Treat the lingering pathogenic factor.
3. When the phlegm has loosened up, return to treating the phlegm.
4. When the visible phlegm is no longer present, return to treating the lingering pathogenic factor.
5. Continue in this way until the child has recovered.

Summary

Using acupuncture to treat asthma in children under five is very rewarding. It is also comparatively quick, taking only weeks instead of months or years, as is often the case with adults. The reasons for this are that the child is still comparatively strong, the disease will not have weakened the *zàng fǔ* organs too much, and the use of anti-asthmatic drugs will (hopefully) have been very limited. It therefore takes less time to strengthen the Lungs and cure the asthma. Even if there is a lingering pathogenic factor, acupuncture can still effect a cure in a matter of months, if the treatments are regular and the advice is followed.

It is awful to watch anyone gasping for breath, but somehow, to see a young baby or child under five wheezing and terrified as he or she fights for air is heart-rending. To prevent this from happening is one of the marvels of acupuncture.

CHRONIC ASTHMA IN OLDER CHILDREN

We will now turn our attention to treating chronic asthma in older children. It is fair to say that many of the children that we have seen with asthma have had the disease for many years before they come to us. They are often on a cocktail of drugs and have been weakened by the disease. The Kidneys gradually become more and more involved in the pathology of the asthma, and, consequently, it is more difficult to cure.

As with younger children, the older ones also suffer from a combination of patterns. You must decide which one is the most important, treat it, and then go on to treat the next and the next. You can, of course, treat more than one pattern at any one time with acupuncture. However, we feel that it is better to attack one aspect—putting all your energy into regulating one disharmony—before tackling the next.

Lingering Pathogenic Factor

In younger children with asthma there is very often a lingering pathogenic factor. As previously explained, once the child has crossed the seven- and fourteen-year transitions this problem becomes more serious. The majority of children that we see have a lingering pathogenic factor at the root of their asthma, which is deeply imbedded. In addition, the child is either deficient in energy, which must first be tonified, or there is some significant excess, such as Liver qi stagnation or much phlegm, which must first be dispersed. Consequently, it is only later on in the course of treatment that you can begin to expel the lingering pathogenic factor.

The main patterns are:

• Lung deficiency and weakness
• Lung and Spleen qi deficiency
• Lingering pathogenic factor
• Lung and Kidney deficiency and weakness
• Liver qi retarded (spasm type)

Both Lung and Spleen deficiency, and Lung and Kidney deficiency and weakness, can manifest as a hyperactive pattern as well, just as in chronic cough (see Chapter 15).

Etiology

The six patterns seen in younger children can evolve into the more adult patterns.

Phlegm. this pattern generally evolves into the Spleen qi deficiency or Lung qi deficiency type of asthma, or a combination of the two.

Accumulation disorder. Long-term accumulation disorder can lead to deficiency, and so the child may go on to develop the Spleen qi deficiency type of asthma. Alternatively, if the child remains strong, then the accumulation of food prevents the smooth flow of Liver qi, and the child's illness will evolve into the Liver qi retarded type of asthma.

Lingering pathogenic factor (cold and hot). These remain the same as the patterns seen in younger children. However, as explained earlier, these children will usually present with one or the other of the patterns, because by this time the lingering pathogenic factor has penetrated to a much deeper level.

Lung and Spleen qi deficiency. The normal type of Lung and Spleen qi deficiency gives way to the same pattern in older children. The hyperactive type gives rise to the Kidney deficient type, Spleen and Lung deficient type, or the Liver qi retarded type of asthma.

Lung deficiency and weakness. This condition usually arises from either

• severe Lung illness such as chronic cough, whooping cough, or pneumonia; or
• deep sadness

Lung and Spleen qi deficiency. The causes of this are many, and have all been discussed many times before in this book.

Lingering pathogenic factor. The most common causes include:

• a Lung illness that has never been cleared properly. This is usually a severe cough that has been treated with antibiotics.
• immunization for something like pertussis, which is especially harmful to the Lungs. Any immunization, however, can give rise to asthma because of the amount of thick phlegm it generates in the system, which in turn obstructs the Lungs. This is nearly always a deficiency type of lingering pathogenic factor, and so there will also be signs of Spleen qi deficiency.

Lung and Kidney deficiency and weakness. This pattern can stem from:

- congenital weakness from birth
- severe illness
- high, often prolonged fever
- overstimulation
- overwork at school
- too much pressure from parents
- use of steroid drugs
- long-term use of bronchodilators

Liver qi retarded. The main cause of this pattern is emotional stress at home or at school. It is often compounded by a severe lingering pathogenic factor that has also become an emotional problem. For further discussion of this subject, see Chapter 43.

Pathogenesis

The Lungs govern the qi and respiration and control the descending action of the qi. When the Lungs are weak, these functions are impaired. The qi then fails to circulate properly, and the regularity of breathing is interrupted, resulting in asthma.

The Spleen governs transformation and transportation. Weakness of the Spleen impairs these functions, resulting in the accumulation of dampness and phlegm. The Spleen makes phlegm, and the Lungs store phlegm. Dampness and phlegm prevent the smooth flow of qi in the body and obstruct the functioning of the Lungs, resulting in asthma. In addition, the Spleen relates to the earth element. When the earth is weak, it fails to nourish the metal (Lungs) element, further weakening the Lung energy.

The Kidneys govern the reception of qi. When they are weak, the qi is not brought downward but accumulates above in the upper burner, preventing one from breathing in. In addition, the Kidneys relate to the water element and are thus fundamental to the body; they are the 'root of life'. When the Kidneys fail to function properly, all the other *zàng* and *fŭ* organs will be affected.

The Liver governs the free flow of qi. When Liver function is impaired, the overall qi of the body readily stagnates, which in turn leads to stagnation of qi in the Lungs.

Signs & Symptoms

Lung deficiency and weakness

- pale, white face
- runny nose
- easily becomes out of breath
- catarrh is rather thin and sometimes frothy
- small voice

Tongue: pale, no coating
Pulse: thin, small

Lung and Spleen qi deficiency

- swollen abdomen
- loose stools, almost diarrhea
- poor appetite
- may produce gurgling sounds from the abdomen
- limbs weak, lethargic
- chronic catarrhal cough, which is productive
- possibly thick white catarrh coming from the nose; it may also be thin
- sometimes the face is rather yellow

Tongue: often coated
Pulse: weak

Lung and Spleen qi deficiency (hyperactive)

Symptoms as above, but the child appears full of energy, stays up late, and is rather manipulative.

Lingering pathogenic factor

Symptoms are identical to those of Lung and Spleen qi deficiency, plus:

- chronic cough which is harsh and nonproductive
- glands in neck swollen
- sudden drops in energy
- occasional unexplained abdominal aches and pains

Pulse: slippery, possibly weak

Lung and Kidney deficiency and weakness

- hunched shoulders
- underdeveloped
- weak bone structure
- thin
- lacking in vigor and will power
- listless
- veins may appear on the temples
- dark rings under the eyes

Tongue: no special indication
Pulse: rather small

Lung and Kidney deficiency and weakness (hyperactive)

Symptoms as above, but the child appears full of energy, stays up late, and is rather manipulative.

Liver qi retarded (spasm type)

- attacks brought on or aggravated by external stress or high emotion
- often the stress is between the parents, or in the family environment
- face is usually rather pale, with a greenish tinge
- possibly green around the mouth
- lips possibly red
- often has dark pools around the eyes

Tongue: often red, especially at the tip; purple body
Pulse: wiry

Note: if the child has had asthma for a long time, the tongue may have a granular coating

Treatment

Main points

As with the treatment of asthma in children under the age of five, certain points can be used regardless of the particular pattern. These include:

L-5 *(chi ze)*
L-7 *(lie que)*
L-9 *(tai yuan)*
B-13 *(fei shu)*

Lung deficiency and weakness

Use the main points with a tonifying technique.

Prognosis: usually good, with the number of treatments depending on the extent of the child's deficiency. The child should gradually improve over a period of fifteen to fifty treatments.

Lung and Spleen qi deficiency

Use the main points, plus:

S-36 *(zu san li)*
Sp-6 *(san yin jiao)*
B-20 *(pi shu)*
CV-12 *(zhong wan)*

Method: you can do moxibustion at CV-12 *(zhong wan).* You may also wish to add S-40 *(feng long)* or P-6 *(nei guan).* Use tonifying technique at all the points. However, S-40 *(feng long)* may cause phlegm to rise, aggravating the situation. Therefore, use it together with CV-22 *(tian tu).*

Prognosis: depending on how long the condition has persisted, it may take from ten to fifty treatments. In the hyperactive pattern the treatment is the same, but the prognosis is more variable. The child may well manipulate itself out of treatment.

Lingering pathogenic factor

Use the main points, plus:

B-18 *(gan shu)*
B-20 *(pi shu)*

Method: moving technique. Add *bai lao* (M-HN-30) when you feel that there is enough energy to move the phlegm in the channels.

Prognosis: expect slow progress, that is, thirty to fifty treatments. The results may be quicker if you use herbs as well as acupuncture.

===

Only attempt to clear a lingering pathogenic factor after the other deficiencies or excesses have been resolved.

===

Lung and Kidney deficiency and weakness

Acupuncture is not always the treatment of choice for this pattern. You may have to start with moxibustion at B-23 *(shen shu)*. If it is simply a question of weakness, then this will be enough. It is very rare to see this condition by itself without the added presence of Lung or Spleen deficiency. You will, therefore, usually need to treat the Spleen as well. Accordingly, use the main points plus:

S-36 *(zu san li)*
Sp-6 *(san yin jiao)*
B-20 *(pi shu)*
B-23 *(shen shu)*

Prognosis: this pattern responds well to acupuncture but will return if there is deep-seated weakness. The hyperactive pattern has a similar prognosis to that of the hyperactive Lung and Spleen qi deficiency pattern.

Liver qi retarded (spasm type)

Use the main points, plus:

Liv-3 *(tai chong)*
Liv-13 *(zhang men)*
P-6 *(nei guan)*

Prognosis: the response varies. If the stress continues or if the child becomes very introverted, treatment may serve only to maintain the status quo. If the stress passes, then ten to twenty treatments may restore the child's health.

Problems Encountered in the Treatment of Asthma

Removal from drugs

Perhaps one of the most disturbing things about the treatment of asthma in Western medicine is the addictive nature of the drugs that are used. The child will soon notice, either consciously or unconsciously, that it feels good after a puff of a steroid or bronchodilator. Even worse is that once the effects wear off, the child feels lousy. It does not take much imagination to realize that the child will prefer to feel good as opposed to feeling awful, so they take another dose. The cycle repeats itself again and again until the child is addicted. This effect is compounded by the fact that the drugs actually weaken the Lungs further and so increase the need for a boost.

Taking a child off these drugs must be done *slowly*. Do not attempt to reduce the dose until there is a great improvement in the child's breathing, that is, you have tonified the Lungs and resolved a lot of the phlegm. Then—and only then—reduce the dose of the drug they are on by a small amount. Leave them on that dose for a few weeks until you see that they have yet again improved. At that point, you can reduce the dose further. It is at the time of reducing the drug dose that you may see another attack. If you talk to the parents about this and explain that you know what you are doing, then you will, hopefully, retain their confidence.

Gradually, in small steps, the child will require less and less of the inhalant. When the child is well on the way to recovery, it will need the drug very little, if at all.

Problems with the parents

The main problem that we face is in trying to stave off disillusionment in the parents. There are many ways that this happens.

• Because the Lung qi is weak, the child will be susceptible to coughs and colds. When these occur, they can readily precipitate an asthma attack and the child can end up in hospital. When this happens, the parents will despair. All the time and energy (not to mention the money) spent in getting to your clinic seems to be in vain. The best way around this is to brief the parents well before you begin treating. Explain that progress is slow. Tell them there will be setbacks, and tell them when you most expect them, that is, during changes in the seasons, when the child is upset, when the child is near cats, and so forth. This helps them see that you actually know what is going on with their child.

• The treatment can seem very slow, long, and drawn out. It is often hard for the parents to see any improvement in their child, even after twenty or more treatments. You may detect a change in the pulse, color, and so on, but they may not. It is well worth every now and again going over things, pointing out the improvements *before* you get to the stage where you are defending yourself!

- Some parents find it hard to stop giving milk to their children. Provide alternatives that are easy to do. If they have a problem over calcium, explain that it is available elsewhere and give sources, or explain that many people in the world never touch milk and are still healthy. Many Africans, for example, grow into very big, beautiful people, yet they do not drink milk as children.

- The child starts to fight back. A child that has been a nice, docile, asthmatic wimp will often start to demand more attention as it gets better. Most parents are delighted by this as they can see their child becoming better, but some cannot cope. It is at this point that they stop coming.

- If, during the course of treatment, parents have to give antibiotics, they may feel very guilty. They are usually all too aware of our feelings toward antibiotics, and they feel as if they have let you down in some way, sometimes to such an extent that they stop coming. To prevent this, it is worth explaining to parents that there will be setbacks in the course of treatment and that it may be necessary to administer antibiotics. If possible, try to get them to see you first, as you can usually allay the need for the antibiotics. However, if this is not possible, then antibiotics may be given. Should this happen, acupuncture is very good at overcoming their side effects. In particular, you should point out that one course of antibiotics is unlikely to put things back to square one if the child has been coming for some time.

Problems with the children

- Manipulation of the parents by the child is a common problem. Many children take this to extremes by using their illness to extract anything they want from their parents, as in, "I'll get asthma if you do not give me a train!" It may be unsaid, but the message is definitely there. When this most valuable tool is about to be taken away from the child, it can rebel and cause real problems at home—to such an extent that parents decide to stop bringing the child.

- The main problem is that children do not want to come off the drugs that they are on. We have talked about the effects that the anti-asthmatic drugs have on children, that is, they become addicted as the drugs give them a real kick. As we progress and the child is able to reduce the amount of drug it takes, the child will often rebel. Schemes are dreamt up to persuade parents to stop treatment, the child's howls and wails increase during treatment, and life becomes harder for you, the parents, and the child! It is at this time that treatment can be stopped. The child will become difficult at home and make life hard for the parents. It is worth talking to the parents alone if you feel that this is happening. Many are ignorant of the fact that these drugs are addictive, and most are horrified by the idea.

• The other problem is confined to children who have the hyperactive Spleen qi deficiency pattern. These children are manipulative anyway, but when it comes to taking them off their drugs, they become devious as well. They will very often succeed in persuading their already exhausted parents to stop the treatment, and there is very little one can do!

Asthma and the Emotions

Increasingly, we are seeing an emotional component in the pathogenesis of asthma. We have emphasized that younger children under the age of seven do not generally suffer from Liver qi stagnation associated with constrained emotions. We like to think that children express their emotions and so prevent the Liver qi from stagnating. This is not always the case, however, and we are seeing more and more children who are being brought up unable to express themselves. This has much to do with the environment—inner cities with nowhere to play, poor housing conditions that are overcrowded with tense emotional family situations, and so on. Even in children as young as three, emotional factors can now be a part of the overall picture.

Traditionally, we would expect to see an emotional component in children older than seven years of age. This would coincide with going to a junior or preparatory school in England, with all the attendant pressures of the educational system. There would also be competition with other children to do well, and very often (in England) pressure from parents for the child to be an "achiever."

Younger and younger children are now put into the educational system for various reasons. As a consequence, these pressures start at an earlier age, and so these emotional components come into play earlier and earlier in the lives of children.

Asthma Drugs

Steroids and the Kidneys

The use of steroids to control asthma is commonplace. The side effects are numerous and well-documented in Western medical literature.

From a traditional Chinese medical point of view, the effect of steroids is to draw on Kidney energy. The initial effect is to give the whole system a huge boost—the Lungs can function well, as they suddenly have bundles of qi to draw in breath, and the whole system 'buzzes'—all at the expense of the Kidneys. This explains many of their side effects, for if steroids are used for a long time, the bones become brittle, the skin becomes dry and thin, and so forth.

Bronchodilators

Bronchodilators stimulate the Lungs. They give an immediate boost to the Lungs, enabling them to function properly and thereby preventing an asthma attack. However, in doing so, they deplete the yin of the Lungs, and when the Lung yin is depleted, it will inevitably draw on Kidney yin, thereby depleting yin in general. The time scale for this is usually many years, depending on how frequently bronchodilators are used.

General Advice

Although acupuncture is very helpful in the treatment of asthma, it is also necessary for the child to follow a strict diet, and probably make significant changes in lifestyle, if there is to be a complete cure. Without these changes, acupuncture can only slowly, if at all, effect changes. More likely, it will be palliative, simply preventing the condition from getting much worse.

The reason for this is found in the dual nature of the disease: it has elements of both deficiency and excess. It is deficient in that all children with asthma must have some Lung weakness. It is excessive in that there must be phlegm. To combat the weakness, the child must have a sensible lifestyle with rest, good diet, regular meals, and early nights. To combat the phlegm, the diet must contain no phlegm-producing foods. Although acupuncture is good at dealing with these two problems, if the patient will not cut down on cappuccinos and cheesecake or on parties, they will not get better.

Similarly, you will come across the parent who has already cut out dairy for some time, and it has made little difference. Try to persuade them to cut it out again. It seems that the *combination* of acupuncture, diet, and lifestyle changes, when made together, is very effective.

Changes in diet

- no dairy products
- no peanuts
- no oranges
- regular meals
- no ice-cold food or drink

Changes in lifestyle

Obviously, the changes in lifestyle that you will suggest will vary from child to child. It will depend on the strength of the child and on the cause of the asthma. Generally, one must encourage a child with asthma to rest. Television should be kept to a minimum, and exercise should be encouraged, preferably outside in the fresh air.

=====

Get enough sleep. No more than half an hour of television a day.

=====

Case History

It is very important to have agreement between husband and wife, and it is not always necessary to give the right advice, as this story about diet shows. I (JPS) had been treating this 3½ year-old boy for asthma for some time. He had a lot of phlegm, and although the results were good to begin with, they had become rather slow. So I started probing around to see what was going on at home. Was he still taking any cow's milk? "Well, yes, actually," the mother said, somewhat sheepishly. "It will slow the treatment down, you know," I said in a gentle voice, which I hoped concealed my true feelings of rage.

And so it went, for a couple more weeks, each time a gentle inquiry, each time a sheepish reply, and each time a gentle reproof.

"So what's the problem over stopping?" I eventually asked.

"Well, every time I am out (which is quite a lot), my husband will insist on giving him milk—cold milk at that, straight from the fridge. He doesn't believe that diet makes any difference. He thinks that since *he* likes milk, he doesn't see why his son shouldn't have it, too. I've tried to persuade him, but he is a bit obstinate."

So there it was: family discord, lousy diet.

"Well, keep trying to persuade him," I said. I didn't want a family row blamed on me.

And so it went. The next week the same, and the week after that, still the same "Keep trying to persuade him," resulting each time in a rather sheepish look.

But then the next time: what a display! She came in looking radiant, with fire blazing from her eyes. "You were absolutely wrong. It was stupid advice you gave 'em. Thank goodness I've realized."

"Er . . . yes? The milk . . ."

"Never mind the milk. You may be right about that, but certainly not over persuasion. I'm fed up with my husband not listening, so I've been to my solicitor who says he'll take my husband to court if he gives my darling boy so much as a drop of milk!"

Summary

Asthma in children over the age of five, and certainly over the age of seven, is a complicated disease. There are many factors involved—physical weakness, emotional problems, drug addiction, to mention but a few. Acupuncture is very effective at helping, but it is a long process. However, if you can persevere and treat regularly, and if the child and the parents are willing to cooperate, then you will succeed.

Asthma is a terrifying illness. It is so common now that we have almost lost the fear of it: many children use inhalers and can even be quite proud of the fact. But asthma kills, and kills in a horrific way: suffocation. To know that you have both the tools and the know-how to save many children's lives should fill you with great enthusiasm.

NOTE

• For case histories involving asthma, see Cases 3, 4, 5, 6, and 7 in Chapter 47.

❖

19 ❖ Immunizations and Their Side Effects

INTRODUCTION

The question of whether or not to have a child immunized is very difficult to answer. There are undoubtedly risks associated with immunizations, and there are also risks and suffering if a child contracts a disease. Before the event, it is impossible to say if the child will suffer side effects from the immunization, or if it will get the disease badly. The question of immunization thus comes down to balancing two unquantifiable evils. Since it is the child who may suffer it is no wonder that passions run high.

In this section we do not intend to embark upon a discussion of the pros and cons of immunization. The subject is complex, and it is so difficult to disentangle truth from prejudice, both in the scientific press and in broadsheets produced by alternative practitioners, that we feel it is best to refer you to some literature at the end of this chapter so that you can make up your own mind. We suggest that you read the sections on the treatment of childhood diseases before deciding. It is important that if you advise a parent against immunizing their child, you must either be able to give the treatment yourself, or be sure the child will be able to get treatment for the disease should the need arise.

You must also take account of the local conditions. The dangers associated with diseases like measles are very small in Europe and the United States. Estimates put the mortality at one to three per 100,000 cases. This is very different from Third World countries where measles can account for twenty-five percent of all infant mortality. In these countries, even a slight reduction in the severity of the disease has a large effect in saving lives. The same is not true in countries where living conditions are not so harsh.

━━

If you advise a parent against immunizing a child, you must either be able to give the child treatment yourself, or be sure the child will be able to get treatment for the disease should the need arise.

━━

The majority of children who visit your clinic will have had, or will be preparing to have, immunizations. Therefore, what we will outline in this chapter is (1) how to strengthen a child *before* an immunization (so that it does not have a violent reaction); and (2) how to treat the child *after* an immunization to avoid the subacute symptoms which tend to last for a long time. But first we will discuss the principle underlying immunizations, and some common side effects.

Principle Underlying Immunizations

The idea behind immunizations is to give the child a mild version of an illness. For example, in the case of whooping cough (pertussis), dead cells of *Bordetella pertussis* are injected. The immune system recognizes the dead cells and develops antibodies against them, which are also effective against live cells. In the case of polio, the virus is first attenuated by being given to monkeys. The virus which has adapted to monkeys is then less harmful to humans.

Thus, when you immunize a baby you actually give it a disease. Hopefully, the disease is a mild one which the child will get over quickly. But you *are* giving it a disease. It is this fact which explains the reactions. They are just what you would expect if a child suddenly caught an infection. This can be seen in the sudden symptoms which appear in the day or two after immunization and also in the longer term effects.

Errors in This Theory

Unfortunately, there are several factors which the orthodox theory does not take into account. First, the immune system is not merely a system for generating antibodies. There is a series of complex reactions which occur for the body to overcome diseases. Antibody response is simply one part of this series. Second, beneficial bacteria are an important part of our defense against disease. It has been shown that the bacteria on the skin and in the gut are mainly beneficial and that the bacteria themselves play an active part in overcoming other bacteria and viruses. Therefore, building up the population of beneficial bacteria is just as important as building up antibodies.

The third factor that is ignored is that by strengthening one part of the immune system, you may weaken another. It does seem that immunizations do have some effect in protecting the body against disease, but by focusing merely on one or two feared diseases, it often happens that the way is left open for other diseases. These diseases (like the common cold) would normally pose no danger, but when the immune system has been altered, they can become dangerous.

There is a fourth factor which we as alternative practitioners notice, namely, that diseases can often be beneficial. It is for this reason, above all, that we are strongly opposed to the use of any immunization.

Common Reactions to Immunization

There are three types of reactions to immunization: immediate, short term, and long term.[1]

Immediate reactions

These are fortunately rare and are due to an allergic reaction in the child. The child may go into acute toxic shock and require emergency medical attention.

Short-term reactions

These occur within the first few weeks post-immunization and are very common. The reactions are typical of a child combating a pathogenic factor which has been injected. Typically, they include the following symptoms:[2]

- **swollen lump at site of injection**
- **fever, restlessness, crying**
- **crying at night (excess) or excessive sleepiness (deficiency)**
- **diarrhea: stools green or of variable color, often with bad smell or lumps of phlegm**
- **poor appetite**
- seizures: convulsions, epilepsy, infantile spasms
- brain inflammation
- loss of muscle control (paralysis), often one-sided
- aching joints

1. The information provided here is based on the literature set forth in the bibliography at the end of this chapter.

2. The description of the pathogenesis of these symptoms is based on traditional Chinese medicine. The more common symptoms are in bold type.

- thrombocytopaenic purpura, hemolytic anemia
- diabetes and hypoglycemia
- cot death (sudden infant death syndrome)

PATHOGENESIS

Swollen lump at site of injection. This is a local reaction to the toxins.

Fever, restlessness, crying. These occur because the protective qi is fighting the pathogenic factor introduced during the immunization.

Crying at night (excess) or excessive sleepiness (deficiency). Again, these are due to the effort involved in fighting a pathogenic factor.

Diarrhea with stools that are green or variable in color, often with bad smell or lumps of phlegm. This occurs if the child had accumulation disorder before being immunized, which is aggravated by the pathogenic factor.

Poor appetite. This is due to the qi being injured.

Seizures, convulsions, epilepsy, infantile spasms. Attributable to the large quantities of heat and phlegm arising from the immunization.

Brain inflammation. This is symptomatic of heat in the Pericardium channel and is due to the pathogenic factor entering deep into the terminal yin level.

Loss of muscle control (paralysis), often one-sided. This is due to the pathogenic factor entering the channels and is a common sequelae to heat invading the Pericardium.

Aching joints. This is due to the pathogenic factor entering the channels.

Thrombocytopenic purpura, hemolytic anemia. Caused by a hot pathogenic factor that reaches the blood level, giving rise to heat in the blood.

Diabetes and hypoglycemia. Attributable to a hot pathogenic factor consuming the yin.

Cot death (sudden infant death syndrome). This is due to a deep invasion of the pathogenic factor, which usually occurs during sleep, when the qi is weak.

Long-term reactions

These are the most common types of reaction that you will see in the clinic. The longer term reactions belong to the category of lingering pathogenic factors, whose symptoms were described in Chapter 3. By way of reminder, there are three patterns—qi deficiency, phlegm, and thick phlegm—which underlie the specific reactions described below.

Specific Reactions to Certain Immunizations

In addition to the symptoms listed above, one sees symptoms relating to the actual immunization received. The pattern that emerges is usually a faint image of the disease that the immunization is designed to prevent.

Diphtheria-Pertussis-Tetanus (DPT) immunization

- **chronic cough**
- **chronic nasal discharge**
- **chronic or recurrent otitis media**
- **recurrent fever or earache (about once a month)**
- **vomiting phlegm**
- collapse and/or shock (may recur about once a month)

PATHOGENESIS

Cough. The cough that the child gets after the DPT immunization sounds a bit like whooping cough. The child does not actually 'whoop', but there is a cough with rather thick phlegm which is very difficult for the child to bring up. This often causes a croupy cough.

Hot patterns. One of the oddest long-term effects of DPT is the monthly recurrence of hot patterns. The heat can emerge in many different ways. For example, one child may have a fever monthly, while another child may get otitis media monthly. Yet another child who suffers from chronic cough or asthma may find that there are sudden monthly asthma attacks.

Vomiting. Vomiting phlegm is a symptom of whooping cough and also of the immunization.

Asthma. Recent research has shown that children who have received whole cell pertussis immunization are five times more likely to suffer from asthma.

Degree of protection. The immunization does give some protection, but not complete protection.

Polio immunization

- **thick, gray catarrh, which builds up over the month after immunization**
- **gray nasal discharge**
- **chronic catarrhal cough**
- **swollen glands**
- accumulation disorder
- abdominal pain

- cold-type insomnia
- paralysis
- brain damage

PATHOGENESIS

Phlegm. The unusual feature of the polio immunization is the *time* that the phlegm takes to build up and the *quality* of the phlegm. Very often there are few side effects from the immunization during the first week or two, especially if the child is healthy. The effects often only appear during the third, fourth, or even fifth week after the immunization. This is so long after the immunization that parents (and often the practitioner too!) do not relate the cause and effect.

The phlegm that gradually appears during the month after immunization is thick and gray-white in color. Once seen it is never forgotten, for it has a quality which is different from normal phlegm. It also has the unpleasant quality of being difficult to get rid of. It takes a lot more treatments to clear from the system than you would expect.

For relatively healthy children this phlegm is not a real problem; it gives rise to nasal discharge and a cough, which goes on for several months. However, for children who already have a respiratory problem, it is really serious. The phlegm in the lungs is the ideal breeding ground for bacteria, and these children quickly get bronchitis. Normally, the bronchitis is treated with antibiotics; but then, because of the difficulty in clearing the phlegm, the bronchitis soon returns. The child is then on a downward spiral of one respiratory infection followed by another, which leads toward asthma.

Degree of protection. Recent follow-up work on polio immunization suggests that the immunization does provide some, but not complete, immunity. The drawback is that those few children who do get polio after being immunized are more likely to become paralyzed, with the result that there is very little change in the overall number of children who suffer paralysis.

Measles-Mumps-Rubella (MMR) immunization

- **skin rash (intermittent, red)**
- **cough, nasal discharge, with yellow phlegm**
- **swollen glands**
- **hot-type insomnia with dreams**
- restless, cannot sit still
- clingy

Longer lasting side effects. The side effects of this immunization are less dramatic but longer lasting. The dominating symptom is insomnia and restlessness. Children who were calm and peaceful before become difficult to handle, and often their sleep pattern is disturbed for a long time after. But it is unusual to have the same devastating effects on the respiratory system that one sees with DPT or polio immunizations. On the other hand, the effects are much longer lasting and are much more difficult to eliminate. In Chapter 20 we provide considerably more detail about measles and its relation to poisons in the system. Recent research in England has shown that some children develop autism soon after the measles immunization, and also that there is a higher probability of developing Crohn's disease in teenagers.

Degree of protection. The immunization provides significant protection in the short term. Those few children who do get measles only do so mildly. However, it has been acknowledged that the effect wears off after five to ten years. Now the most common age for measles to occur is during the teenage years when the disease is much more severe. This disturbing observation led to an additional mass immunization of teenagers in the United Kingdom in 1994!

Another problem that had not been anticipated is that a child born to a mother who has not had measles does not receive any immunity at all. It is expected that such a child would be very vulnerable to an attack.

Contraindications to Immunization

From the conventional medical point of view, much depends on the individual, but in general, immunizations are contraindicated when:

• the child has had convulsions (fits)
• there is a family history of epilepsy
• the child has a weak immune system and suffers from recurrent coughs and colds
• the child has already had the disease
• there is hyperactivity

If one is immunized in these cases there may be a very violent reaction, possibly with convulsions, development of epilepsy, paralysis on one side of the body, or brain damage. In the United Kingdom, doctors are very enthusiastic about immunizations and very rarely check to see if a child has any of these contraindications. It is important to note that if the child is allergic to eggs, a specially prepared vaccine may be necessary, since many ordinary vaccines are made using egg protein. Other questions to ask include the following:

• is there much heat in the body, indicated by restlessness, great activity, insomnia, and bad behavior?
• does the child twitch? If so, this is an indication that he or she might get convulsions from an immunization.
• is the child teething? If so, wait until this has passed.

TREATMENT OF LONG-TERM REACTIONS

The basis of treatment is determined by the pattern from which the child is suffering. The first two patterns are straightforward; in fact, you don't need to know anything about lingering pathogenic factors, you just have to be able to recognize the patterns of qi deficiency and phlegm. The third pattern, thick phlegm, is often much more difficult to treat and may require many treatments.

Qi deficiency

L-9 *(tai yuan)*	Tonifies Lung qi
S-36 *(zu san li)*	Tonifies overall qi
Sp-6 *(san yin jiao)*	Tonifies Spleen qi

Method: reinforcing method

Prognosis: depending on the strength of the child, it will require between three and ten treatments. You may find that during the course of treatment this pattern evolves into the phlegm pattern.

Phlegm

L-7 *(lie que)*	Clears phlegm from the Lungs
S-40 *(feng long)*	Clears overall phlegm

Prognosis: as with all phlegm disorders, you may get a reaction, with much discharge of phlegm. For most immunizations, depending on the strength of the child, it will take about five to ten treatments. However, a child who has developed very thick gray phlegm after being immunized with the polio vaccine responds only very slowly to acupuncture.

Note

As we have seen, immunization with the polio vaccine seems to produce a particularly nasty form of phlegm, which appears about three weeks after the immunization. This does not respond particularly well to acupuncture, and it is frequently necessary to use the homeopathic treatment set out below.

Thick phlegm

This one is difficult to treat, especially if the symptoms are not very pronounced, since the nature of a lingering pathogenic factor is to be hidden and out of the way. What this means in clinical practice is that there are no special symptoms. This is especially true of immunizations, which seem to go to a deeper level; the symptoms are harder to see and to eliminate. Use such points as:

bai lao (M-HN-30)	Softens thick phlegm
B-18 *(gan shu)*	Strengthens Liver and Spleen, softens thick phlegm, and clears heat
B-20 *(pi shu)*	Strengthens the Spleen and softens thick phlegm

Accumulation disorder

This is a secondary pattern caused by the immunization, but often appears as a reaction. The treatment is straightforward:

si feng (M-UE-9)	Clears accumulation

But be careful! *Do not use this point at the first treatment if there is a lot of heat or a history of convulsions.* The heat may be aggravated, and, especially after immunizations, there is a risk of convulsions.

According to symptoms

The treatments listed above are for the overall condition of the child and apply when the symptoms are not too violent. But there are times when the symptom is really much more important than the overall condition. For example, if a child is vomiting a lot, it will not be able to hold food down, and it is this symptom that actually threatens the child's health.

Cough

Treating cough is simple: use almost any point on the Lung channel and also the governing *(shū)* point of the Lungs. The following points are all useful:

L-5 *(chi ze)*
L-7 *(lie que)*
L-9 *(tai yuan)*
B-13 *(fei shu)*

The treatment of cough is discussed in more detail in Chapters 15 and 16.

Vomiting

The treatment of vomiting is discussed in Chapter 11.

In general, use:
P-6 *(nei guan)*

Otitis Media

The treatment of otitis media is discussed in Chapter 25. Acute otitis media responds wonderfully to acupuncture. Often, just needling

TB-5 *(wai guan)*
is enough. Another point of local use is:

TB-17 *(yi feng)*

Overall results

With acupuncture, one can make a huge difference to the health of a child who has been badly affected by immunizations. In half to three-quarters of all cases, the child can be cured completely. However, there is a minority of cases where the cure somehow is not quite complete. You have great success during the first six to eight treatments, and then you seem to reach a plateau. Whatever you do, the child does not seem to be able to shake off that last bit. If you find this happening it is time to change therapy, and the treatment of choice in this situation is homeopathy. The homeopathic remedies which are based on the actual disease itself are often the key to getting rid of the last effects of immunization. Helpful remedies are set out below.

Administering homeopathic remedies

Wherever possible, find a qualified homeopathic practitioner and discuss your treatment with him or her. This can be a delicate situation, for of course no practitioner wants to be told what treatment to give!

The following remedies are recommended:

- whooping cough: Pertussin 30
- polio: Polio 30
- measles: Morbillinum 30

We strongly advise against administering these remedies if you do not have any experience with homeopathy. However, you may find yourself in a situation where you feel you must treat and there is just no possibility of referral to a homeopathic practitioner. In these circumstances we advise that you observe the following rules.

- Always treat with acupuncture first. *Never start with these remedies*, for if you do, you can provoke a very strong reaction.
- Only give the remedies when you have reached the third stage of treatment—the stage of thick phlegm—when there is enough qi for the homeopathic remedy to work.

• Give the remedy once, and wait for a reaction. It is very rare that you will need to give a second dose, but if you do, wait at least a month before doing so.

PREPARATION FOR IMMUNIZATION

There are always dangers in any medical intervention, and the dangers of immunization are quite significant. It does not require a lot of imagination to realize that a strong and healthy child is much less likely to suffer a bad reaction than a weak and sickly one. It follows, then, that if the parents do decide to have their child immunized, it is helpful to give the child acupuncture treatments *before* the immunization to ensure that it is as strong and healthy as possible.

Approach to the Treatments

What to treat

If the child is brought to you with significant symptoms such as catarrh, diarrhea, or screaming at night, then the treatment is relatively straightforward: simply treat the child until the symptoms have disappeared. What is much more likely is that the child will be brought to you without any special symptoms. You then have to decide:

• whether to give any treatment
• what treatment to give

It may sound rather daunting, but it is not all that difficult. There are three major imbalances to look out for which may be present in the child without giving rise to any significant symptoms. These should be treated before getting immunized. They are:

• accumulation disorder
• Spleen qi deficiency
• phlegm

These are the same patterns that are fully discussed in Chapter 15 on chronic cough.

Treatment

The principles of treatment are also set out in Chapter 15. To summarize, they include clearing the accumulation, tonifying the Spleen, or resolving phlegm.

Number of treatments

What is not so clear at this stage is the number of treatments you will need to give to the child. In fact, even in the clinic, it is never quite clear. What we suggest here is therefore just a guide.

Accumulation disorder. Typically, three treatments will be sufficient. Changes to look for include less phlegm and cheeks that are not so red.

Spleen qi deficiency. One to five treatments will be required. Changes to look for include improved appetite and facial color.

Phlegm. One to five treatments will be required. Look for a reduction in phlegm.

OUR PERSONAL FEELINGS ABOUT IMMUNIZATIONS

We do have our own feelings about immunizations, which we would like to share with you. You may well disagree with them; many people do. There is no right or wrong in this case, but we would like to tell you what we feel and our reasons for feeling that way. Please do not accept what we say as *right*. This is such a sensitive area, we would urge you to do some background reading and to make up your own mind.

On the whole, we are against immunizations. The short-term side effects can be treated effectively with acupuncture and are therefore not to be feared. However, we feel that the long-term side effects can be seriously detrimental to the health of the child and remain with the child for life, causing problems that can surface many years later.

We also feel that there are diseases such as measles that are positively beneficial for the child to have, since they clear poisons from the body that otherwise remain in the system.

We do not want to get into the situation of frightening parents away from immunizations. We are very careful in what we say and how we say it—trying to point out objectively how the particular child is likely to react to an immunization.

Certainly, not all children suffer ill effects from immunizations. Many cope very well; but some do not. We feel that we have to point this out to the parents of those children whom we feel *would* suffer as a result of immunization.

To Immunize or Not?

Many of the parents of the children we treat are rabid anti-vaccinationists, but there are also many pro-vaccinationists. When you meet one or other extreme, life is simple: there is no indecision. Anything you say will not make the slightest difference. The problems arise either when the parents are waverers, or when the parents are anti-vaccinationists while the rest of the family—grandparents, uncles, and aunts—are pro-vaccinationists. The parents are then in a difficult position, and so are you. Whatever advice you give, you are bound to incur somebody's wrath!

What we try to do in these circumstances is to point out to the parents the pressures that will be brought to bear if they do not have their child vaccinated: the full force of the medical establishment, well-meaning health visitors, as well as the family. The parents have to know what support you can give them against this fearful onslaught before making their decision.

The final choice is with the parents, and we always make this clear. If they decide to have the immunizations, we support them and will treat the child for side effects as needed.

If the child is going to be immunized, we suggest the child come in for a few treatments prior to the immunization to strengthen the qi and regulate the system. In this way, the child will cope much better. We also suggest that the child come for a few treatments afterward to clear up any side effects.

Similarly, we support parents if they decide not to have their child immunized, and we offer support if the child gets one of the childhood illnesses. It is very important that you offer this service if you advise against immunization. We do feel that you must work out some strategy for coping when the child does get the disease.

Immunizations: Which to Give?

Immunizations are routinely given to all babies unless there are strong contraindications (e.g., a history of convulsions or epilepsy in the family), because, according to Western medicine, there is no disadvantage to giving immunizations, only positive benefits. In the wider view of Chinese medicine, however, this simple view is rejected. Not only is there a significant risk that a disorder related to a lingering pathogenic factor will develop in the weeks following immunization, but in the case of the eruptive diseases of measles, mumps, and chicken pox, there is an actual disadvantage to being immunized—it prevents the expression of inherited toxins. A full discussion of this difficult problem is beyond the scope of this book and involves questions of herd immunity, eradication of disease, and individual freedom. We confine ourselves here to a brief discussion of the medical considerations.

As we have seen above, there is no such thing as immunization without risk; all of them carry some risk of brain damage and death which, within the error of statistical measurement, is comparable to the risk from the disease itself. Moreover, if anything, they carry a higher risk of sequelae in the form of a lingering pathogenic factor. Our own conclusions with respect to which immunizations should be given, and which should be avoided, are summarized below.

Measles

Avoid getting this immunization. According to the statistics, the reason for immunizing is that there is significant risk of brain damage from measles. In fact, the children most at risk are those who have a history of febrile convulsions, and these children are equally at risk of brain damage from the measles and the immunization. The risk of brain damage in healthy children is slight. Furthermore, measles is a disease which provides an opportunity for inherited toxins to come out. *Note:* this advice applies only to children in developed countries where measles has lost most of its severity. In Third World countries measles is still a major cause of infant mortality.

Pertussis (whooping cough)

This is still a dangerous disease, and even when there is no risk of brain damage, there remains a significant risk of injury to the Lungs, which can cause trouble much later in life. However, pertussis responds well to acupuncture (see Chapter 22). Thus, if acupuncture is available, immunization is unnecessary, but if acupuncture is not available and the child is sickly, then the decision is not so straightforward. A study in Germany showed that if a child was well looked after at home for the full three months needed to recuperate from whooping cough, there would be no ill effects. However, there are now very few families where the mother is willing and able to look after a sick child for so long a time. For most mothers, immunization of the child means that they can continue working. As a pediatrician, one does not have the same point of view as a parent!

Polio

Although the crippling effects of polio are far from beneficial, there is now strong evidence to show that most children contract polio but are unaffected by it. They simply develop a high fever. Those children who become paralyzed already have some kind of defect in the spinal cord. But we believe that these children are the very ones who are at risk from the vaccination.

Questions to Ask Yourself

- Can you treat it?
- What happens if you are on holiday or attending a course on acupuncture?

RECOMMENDED READING

James, W., *Immunization: The Reality Behind the Myth.* Westport, CT: Bergin and Garvey, Inc., 1988.

Chaitow, L., *Vaccinations and Immunizations-Dangers, Delusions and Alternatives.* Essex, England: C. W. Daniel Co., Saffron Walden, 1987.

Hume, E. D., *Pasteur Exposed.* Collingwood, Australia: Bookreal, W. A., 1989.

Neustaedter, R., *The Immunization Decision: A Guide for Parents.* Berkeley, CA: North Atlantic Books, 1990.

Coulter, H. L., & Fisher, B. L., *D.P.T.—A Shot in the Dark.* New York, NY: Avery Publishing Group, 1987.

Coulter, H. L., *Vaccination, Social Violence and Criminality.* Berkeley, CA: North Atlantic Books, 1990.

Moskowitz, R., *The Case Against Immunizations.* Northampton, England: The Society of Homeopaths, 1984.

U.K. Department of Health, *Immunization Against Infectious Disease.* London, England: HMSO Publications, 1990.

Miller, N. Z., *Vaccines: Are They Really Safe and Effective?* Santa Fe, NM: New Atlantean Press, 1992.

Miller, N. Z., *Immunization, Theory versus Reality.* Santa Fe, NM: New Atlantean Press, 1996.

O'Mara, P., ed., *Vaccination, the Issue of our Times.* Santa Fe, NM: Mothering Magazine, 1997.

❖

20 ❖ Measles

INTRODUCTION

Measles (also known as morbilli or rubeola) used to be regarded as one of the four scourges or epidemics to which children were most susceptible, and in the past, many children died from it. Fortunately, the disease is now usually much less severe in the developed world (and in China), and it is rare to see a serious attack. However, the risk of measles encephalitis, which does occur occasionally, is the principal motivation for giving children the measles vaccine.

The information in this chapter provides the basis for treating an uncomplicated attack of measles with acupuncture alone. More severe attacks may involve such complications as pneumonia, violent diarrhea, delirium, loss of consciousness, or collapse of the yang. The treatment of these complications usually requires more than just acupuncture. In the case of qi deficiency and collapse of the yang, the rash may not be fully expressed during the second stage (when it is supposed to emerge). Instead of heat signs, the patient shows signs of collapse with a white face and a rapid, feeble pulse. This is a dangerous condition for which the treatment principle is to tonify the qi; however, the use of acupuncture alone is usually not enough.

ETIOLOGY & PATHOGENESIS

Western view

Measles is a childhood illness which is simply due to an 'attack' by a virus. It can occur at any time, the most common being between the ages of one and three, with the incidence gradually decreasing as the age increases. An

263

attack of measles usually confers immunity for the remainder of life, but a tiny number of children do get measles twice or even three times. The later in life a person gets measles, the more dangerous it is; this is especially the case after puberty. Because of the partial success of the immunization (which wears off in five to ten years), the teenage years are now the most common time for measles to occur.

Chinese view

Measles is now considered to be due to both internal and external factors. This was not always the cause, however, and as late as the middle of the Song dynasty (960-1279), measles was attributed primarily to the internal factor of 'womb toxin'. The following passage written by Qian Yi in an early 12th-century work entitled *Craft of Medicinal Treatment for Childhood Disease Patterns (Xiao er yao zheng zhi jue)* reflects this view: "Babies are in the womb for ten months; the fluids, the five yin organs, and the blood become dirty; after birth, this toxin* must come out." Thus, the distinctive rash was regarded as poison, which was already present in the body, emerging on the skin. Later writers attributed measles to a combination of this factor and the action of an excessive disease. A work from the late Ming dynasty (1368-1644), *Records of Utmost Benevolence (Ren duan lu)*, notes that "Measles is from womb toxin combined with a seasonal change." When we reach the Qing dynasty (1644-1911), the causes of measles were understood to be seasonal change, the influence of plague qi *(lì qì)*, or even an external pathogenic factor. This is reflected in a writing of that era, *Survey of Measles (Ma zhen hui tong)*: "Measles is from womb toxin, change of season, warm weather, and infection."

Pathogenesis

The pathogenesis of measles is summarized in a passage from the *Complete Life-Saving Book of Measles (Ma ke huo ren quan shu)*, written in 1748: "The toxin influences the Spleen, the heat pours into the Heart, the organs are attacked, and the Lungs may also be affected." Elsewhere in the same work it is observed: "Initially it rises up into the yang; afterwards it settles into the yin." This is now interpreted to mean that the toxin enters through the nose and mouth and affects the Lung and Spleen channels. It attacks the protective qi of the Lungs, causing fever, cough, and watery eyes, and invades the Spleen,

---

*The poisons that appear on a physical level have a parallel on other levels, where they correspond to something equally poisonous—selfishness and greed. Measles is, in fact, a really important transition where the self-centeredness of the child is left behind, opening the way to more generous behavior.

causing dullness of mind, poor appetite, tired body, puffy eyelids, and eruption of the skin in little spots.

The Heart governs the blood, and if the measles toxin settles in the Heart, the normal qi and pathogenic factor struggle. The pathogenic factor then moves to the exterior, erupting in a bright-red rash accompanied by a weary spirit and desire for sleep. If the pathogenic factor causes constraint in the Liver channel, it 'rises smoking up to the eyes', leading to red, copiously watering eyes and an aversion to bright light. Measles is a yang toxin which transforms into heat and fire, and readily injures the yin and fluids. It is therefore common to see yin deficiency following an attack of measles.

If the child's body is weak and the normal qi is insufficient, the pathogenic toxin will flourish and rush inside, where it impairs and obstructs the Lungs. The regulation of qi circulation and breathing is thereby disrupted, the Lung qi is blocked, and there are symptoms of high fever without relief, cough, gasping for breath, alar flaring, and gurgling noise from the throat. If the measles toxin flourishes and blazes, 'steaming and smoking', into the Pericardium, and invades and injures the Liver, there are symptoms of wind stirring with twitching, high fever, incoherent speech, and even loss of consciousness. If the measles toxin moves downward, its heat will affect the Large Intestine by disrupting the transformation and transportation of food, causing diarrhea.

Symptoms Through Normal Course of the Disease

General

In the first or prodromal stage there is fever, but the patient is often calm and is neither irritable nor restless. There may be a severe cough, but neither alar flaring nor labored breathing. Three or four days after the fever starts a bright red rash will appear, usually at first behind the ears or on the neck, then on the head and face, chest and ribs, abdomen, limbs, palms, and soles.

Stage one

BEFORE THE RASH APPEARS

- the incubation period is about ten days, and there is a fever of three to four days before the rash appears, the fever increasing daily
- cough, mild at first
- eyes watery and red, photophobia
- eyelids puffy and swollen
- spirit tired, mental dullness
- possibly vomiting and diarrhea

- throat painful
- in extreme cases of high fever, possibly fear and nervousness
- characteristic grayish-white spots in the mouth with red borders (known as Koplik's spots)

Tongue coating: thin and white, or thin and yellow
Pulse: floating, rapid
Finger vein: purple

Treatment principle: gently cool, vent the rash, and release the exterior

Stage two

RASH APPEARS

- high fever which does not abate
- thirst with desire to drink
- severe cough
- spirit weary
- patient is floppy
- eyes very gummed up
- irritable and restless
- possibly prefers to sleep
- possibly has jerking and twitching movements, or convulsions
- a raised maculopapular rash then appears, starting first behind the ear, then spreading to the neck, face, head, chest, back, and limbs. The rash is bright red in color and may exude a watery fluid. Later the rash spreads and joins into larger areas, the color becoming darker.

Tongue body: red
Tongue coating: yellow
Pulse: overflowing, rapid
Finger vein: purple

If the patient had the measles immunization or was recently injected with gamma globulin, the fever and cough will be rather mild, the spots widely scattered and uneven, and the color of the rash will be pale red. The hands and feet may even be without rash.

Treatment principle: clear the heat, resolve the toxicity, and vent the rash

Stage three

RECOVERY STAGE

The most violent stage of the illness usually lasts between three and six days, after which the temperature starts to come down, and the rash changes color from a vivid red to a duller, slightly purple-red. Over the next few days to a week the rash fades completely, usually leaving no trace.

During this week the child is often confused and rather distant in behavior. The following changes are observed:

• the rash gradually diminishes; the skin becomes flaky with scales dropping off, and returns to normal color underneath within seven to ten days
• high fever diminishes
• spirit recovers
• digestion and appetite improve daily
• cough diminishes

Tongue coating: red, little sputum in mouth, little coating on tongue
Pulse: fine and soft, or fine and rapid
Finger vein: pale red

Treatment principle: enrich the yin and strengthen the qi, resolve the toxicity, and expel the remaining pathogenic factor

Complications

Complications may occur in severe cases. They can be understood from either a traditional Chinese medicine point of view, where the illness is regarded as a combination of external pathogenic wind and the expulsion of poisons, or a Western medical point of view, where the illness is seen as an invasion by a virus, with possible secondary bacterial infections.

Bronchopneumonia

From the traditional Chinese medical perspective, the pathogenic wind invades the Lungs, where it transforms into phlegm-heat and gives rise to a characteristic harsh, painful cough and rapid, slippery pulse. From a Western medical perspective, the phlegm that accumulates in the bronchi is an ideal breeding ground for bacteria, and the most common complication is bronchopneumonia, where a secondary infection invades the bronchi. The bronchi become inflamed, and there is a severe pain in the chest, often with shallow breathing or even asthma. This is a serious condition, and help should be sought immediately.

Encephalitis

The common reason for this complication is simply weakness, but in the past (and, perhaps, sometimes now), it arises because the rash did not come out. This has always been recognized as a serious disorder, and one of the indications for a number of herbs used in treating measles is 'to bring out the rash'. From a traditional Chinese medical perspective, the pathogenic factor transforms into heat and invades the Pericardium channel and the governing vessel. Symptoms of invasion of the Pericardium are extreme heat, delirium, loss of consciousness, and a rapid, thready pulse. The invasion of the governing vessel is manifest in the arching of the back (called 'the wheel of torture'). This is a very serious condition, and help should be sought immediately. From a Western medical perspective, the child will be delirious or even in a coma as a result of inflammation of the brain, brought about by the toxins 'caused' by the virus.

Diarrhea

From a traditional Chinese medical perspective, the excess heat-poison invades the Spleen, disturbing its function and giving rise to damp-heat diarrhea. This is serious in babies, who can easily become dehydrated. It is less serious in older children. From a Western medical perspective, one school of thought is that the poison which appears on the skin as a rash goes down to the intestines. This inflames the lining of the intestines and disturbs their function, giving rise to diarrhea. Another school of thought is that the diarrhea is due to secondary infection.

Sequelae

Tidal fever

Because the measles toxin is a warm pathogenic factor, it injures yin and damages qi such that they become insufficient, resulting in the following symptoms:

• fluctuating tidal fever
• irregular bowel movements
• emaciation
• cough without strength
• night sweats or spontaneous sweating
• dry skin
• stomach is full and packed
• possibly abdominal distention

Tongue: red with little coating
Pulse: fine, rapid
Finger vein: thin

Treatment principle: enrich the yin and clear the heat

Diarrhea

This occurs because the poisons affect the Intestines as well as the skin. Symptoms include:

• body is intermittently hot
• stools are in glutinous pieces, containing pus and blood
• abdominal pain
• diarrhea comes quickly and the child feels heavy

afterwards; diarrhea may occur five to ten times a day
• dull expression, tired spirit

Tongue coating: thick or greasy and yellow
Pulse: slippery, rapid
Finger vein: purple, broad

Treatment principle: clear the heat and resolve the toxicity, transform the dampness, and stop the diarrhea

Night terrors

This occurs because the heat poison is not expelled completely, often as a result of inadequate nursing, irregular feedings, improper foods, or unregulated feedings. The result is either insufficiency of blood and fluids, or an attack on the yin, either of which can lead to insufficiency of Liver yin. Symptoms include:

• unable to close eyes, which become dry for lack of nourishment
• night terrors
• possibly nebulae or cloudy film over eyes

Tongue: tip is red, little coating
Pulse: fine and rapid, or fine and soft
Finger vein: thin

Treatment principle: enrich the yin and brighten the eyes

Residual skin lesions

This is due to uncleared toxin remaining at the blood level, and pathogenic wind returning and lodging at the level of the skin. Symptoms include:

• skin has itchy patches, ulcers, boils, and rashes
• irritability
• poor appetite
• night terrors (in extreme cases)

Tongue coating: thin, yellow
Pulse: floating, slightly rapid

Treatment principle: nourish the yin and support the blood, expel the wind, and stop the itching

Impaired vision

The poison affects the optic nerve, giving rise to sensitivity to light and photophobia. In severe cases, and if the child is not kept in a darkened room, the optic nerve can be damaged and the whole of the eye has reduced energy and function.

Deafness

The wind and heat-poison may invade the ears, causing otitis media and, ultimately, severe damage to the ear. Very occasionally there is deafness as a result of middle ear infection from secondary invasion of bacilli.

Summary

First stage

- wind-cold
- wind-heat

Second stage

- full heat
- complications may include: (1) the rash does not come out; (2) phlegm-heat in the Lungs, causing bronchitis; (3) heat invades the Pericardium, causing delirium and coma: and (4) heat-poison invades the Spleen, causing damp-heat diarrhea

Third stage (recovery)

- qi deficiency
- yin deficiency

TREATMENT

Conventional Treatment

The only treatment available in orthodox medicine is prophylactic antibiotics to prevent the occurrence of bronchopneumonia and secondary bacterial otitis media.

Traditional Chinese Medicine

Acupuncture can be of great help. It is particularly effective in bringing down the fever. It is perhaps a bit less effective in resolving poisons (compared to herbs), but there is much less trouble in administration. In our experience, Western children hate taking Chinese herbs at the best of times, but even more so when they are ill. They may also dislike acupuncture, but it is easier to overcome their resistance.

Stage one

BEFORE THE RASH APPEARS

LI-4 *(he gu)*
TB-5 *(wai guan)* } Vents the rash and releases the exterior
L-7 *(lie que)*

Method: dispersing technique

According to symptom

Weak qi:
S-36 *(zu san li)* with tonifying technique

Painful eyes:
P-7 *(da ling)* with even method

High fever:
GV-14 *(da zhui)*, LI-11 *(qu chi)* with strong dispersing technique

Prognosis: treatment at this stage is beneficial and will help reduce the severity of the next stage. If there is a lot of poison to come out, the disease will inevitably progress to the next stage.

Stage two	**RASH APPEARS**

GV-14 *(da zhui)*
LI-11 *(qu chi)* — } Clears the heat and resolves the toxicity
LI-4 *(he gu)*

Liv-3 *(tai chong)* — Resolves poison
GV-10 *(ling tai)* — Resolves poison

Method: strong dispersing technique

According to symptom	Irritability: P-8 *(lao gong)*, P-3 *(qu ze)*

Convulsions:
shi xuan (M-UE-1)

Method: P-8 *(lao gong)* is needled; P-3 *(qu ze)* and *shi xuan* (M-UE-1) are pricked with the triangular needle to let a few drops of blood. P-3 *(qu ze)* is also indicated when the rash is very severe.

Prognosis: variable. For some children, one treatment may be sufficient at this stage. The child breaks into a sweat, falls asleep, and is cured within four hours. Severe cases may require more treatment. In fact, for some children the fever can go on for several days without any sign of abating, even with twice-daily treatment. The effect of acupuncture is to ensure that the fever does not rise too high and that there are no complications.

Stage three	**RASH FADES**

S-36 *(zu san li)* — Supplements the qi
Sp-6 *(san yin jiao)* — Enriches the yin
LI-11 *(qu chi)* — Reduces the rash

Method: tonifying technique

Prognosis: depends on the severity of the attack and the constitution of the patient. One treatment may be enough, or up to ten treatments in severe cases.

Complications

Bronchopneumonia (phlegm-heat invades the Lungs)	L-5 *(chi ze)* L-10 *(yu ji)* — } Clears heat in the Lungs L-1 *(zhong fu)*

	CV-17 *(shan zhong)*	Opens the chest and relieves pain in the chest

Method: even technique

Delirium or coma (heat invades the Pericardium)	*jǐng* (well) points GV-26 *(ren zhong)*	Restores consciousness

Method: bleed the well points, and use strong stimulation at GV-26 *(ren zhong)*

Note: if the delirium is due to failure of the rash to come out, another therapy should be considered, as acupuncture will not be especially effective. For example, homeopathic Aconite or homeopathic Pulsatilla may be considered as alternatives. There are also herbs in both the Chinese and Western pharmacopoeas.

Diarrhea	S-25 *(tian shu)*	Stops diarrhea
	S-44 *(nei ting)*	Clears heat in the Intestines

Method: even technique

Sequelae

Tidal fever	K-3 *(tai xi)*	
	CV-4 *(guan yuan)*	Tonifies the yin
	H-6 *(yin xi)*	

Method: tonifying technique

Diarrhea	S-25 *(tian shu)*	Stops the diarrhea
	S-36 (zu *san li)*	Strengthens the Spleen qi
	Sp-6 *(san yin jiao)*	Clears the damp-heat
	S-44 *(nei ting)*	Both points clear heat from
	LI-11 *(qu chi)*	the Stomach and Intestines

Method: even technique

Night terrors	H-9 *(shao chong)*	Clears the heat from the Heart
	P-9 *(zhong chong)*	and stops the terrors
	K-3 *(tai xi)*	
	Liv-3 *(tai chong)*	Resolves residual poisons

Method: even technique

Prognosis: this is fairly easy to cure, usually requiring only three to six treatments

Nebulae	Use even technique at G-20 *(feng chi)* and S-2 *(si bai)*. In addition, consider an eye wash with an appropriate herbal decoction.

Residual skin lesions	LI-11 *(qu chi)*

LI-11 *(qu chi)*
Sp-10 *(xue hai)* } Clears the heat from the skin
B-40 *(wei zhong)* and invigorates the blood

B-18 *(gan shu)*   Resolves phlegm and clears poisons

H-7 *(shen men)*   Invigorates the blood

Impaired vision

This must be treated as soon as possible. It is the retina, which is basically a network of nerves, that gets damaged. Like any nerve problem, it responds best if treated within three months of the injury. Use such points as:

B-1 *(jing ming)*
qiu hou (M-HN-8)
G-20 *(feng chi)*
Liv-3 *(tai chong)*

Method: B-1 *(jing ming)* and *qiu hou* (M-HN-8) must be needled to a depth of one to two units so that the sensation is felt at the back of the eye. Even technique is used at G-20 *(feng chi)* and Liv-3 *(tai chong)*.

Deafness

The deafness here is usually a result of nerve damage. Again, you have to use deep needling to be effective. Use such points as:

G-2 *(ting hui)*
TB-5 *(wai guan)*

Method: needle G-2 *(ting hui)* to a depth of one to two units, and obtain a sensation going up the arm when needling TB-5 *(wai guan)*. We have no direct experience in treating this, but the customary treatment for nerve deafness involves daily treatment with a rather painful technique. Unfortunately, this is a treatment that few Western children can tolerate.

Management

As soon as measles is confirmed, the child should be put to bed in a *darkened room*. The child may show no signs of the eyes being affected, but this measure should be taken to prevent permanent eye damage. Encourage parents to spend as much time as they can with the child to comfort it in times of distress. There is no doubt that careful nursing plays an important part in recovery from measles. Keep the child calm, reading it stories rather than allowing it to watch television or play computer games, which can put a strain on the eyes and the brain. Other helpful measures are described in *Natural Medicine for Children*.

Recovery

As the temperature starts to go down, the appetite will gradually return. Very simple foods, in very small quantities, should be given at first. Porridge or baby food is helpful as a first food. As the appetite returns and the digestion strengthens, a more varied diet can be given, and in cases of great weakness, beef broth can be very helpful.

Recuperation

A child who has had measles is in a wonderland for a week or more after the fever has gone down. Quite commonly, the child will wander around with a dazed and wondrous look in its eyes. The child looks like someone who has emerged from a very deep sleep, or has been through a mystical experience. When you consider the changes that have taken place, this is not surprising. What is not always realized is how tender the child is during this important time: all the defenses are down. If the child receives strong or violent impressions, they may have a lasting effect. For this reason, it can be helpful for a child to spend some time recovering in a quiet place in the country, if this is at all possible.

Treatment

For Western children, the extreme conditions described above under 'sequelae' are rare, so treatment is generally unnecessary. On the whole, it is better to let the child get better on its own. However, there are times when the child is extremely weak and has all the signs of qi deficiency. In such cases, a tonic treatment is necessary. Acupuncture can be helpful, but a simple herbal tonic is better.

AVOIDING THE COMPLICATIONS OF MEASLES

Any child is at risk from measles, even if the child has been immunized. But those who have not been immunized are more at risk, and the parents should be informed about how to avoid any complications when their child gets the illness.

General Advice

The main thrust of advice is to keep the child healthy and, in particular, to prevent the buildup of poisons in the system. This has several dietary implications.

- Avoid oranges, including orange juice. A child should not have more than one orange (or its equivalent in juice) a week. The poisons in oranges contribute to the measles poison.
- Avoid meat, especially red meat, as well as seafood, such as crabs and shell fish. A child's digestion is not as strong as an adult's, and it is difficult for children to digest meat completely without generating poisons. In our opinion, children should eat a predominantly vegetarian diet up to the age of seven, except in special circumstances such as recuperation after illness.
- Artificial colorings and flavorings should be kept out of children's foods altogether.

Treatment

As a practitioner, you can strengthen a child so that if it does get measles it will not develop complications. This is worth doing at any time, and especially if there is an epidemic. It is never too late to start treatment.

Avoiding bronchopneumonia

The obvious extra thing to look out for is phlegm. Make sure that the child does not have symptoms of phlegm build-up, or get frequent coughs and colds. Dietary advice includes avoiding dairy products.

Avoiding encephalitis

It has been ascertained that any attack of measles affects the brain, and that the poisons released have a disrupting effect on brain activity. In the normal progress of the disease, this poison gives rise to the temporary dulling of consciousness, which passes as the poison levels subside. When the poison levels become too severe and the temperature of the brain becomes too high, the resulting inflammation of the brain can lead to permanent damage. However, this will only occur if the brain is already too active and overstimulated. So if a child already has a 'hot head', then it is much more likely to suffer from encephalitis and its complications. All of this points the way for reducing this risk, namely, to ensure that the brain is as cool as possible. This means bringing up the child in as calm and peaceful a manner as is practical. In particular, we advise against stimulation by:

- exposure to television
- early learning methods
- introducing the child to too many exciting activities

On the positive side, do encourage the child's imagination by reading to it, encourage painting, outside play, and simple daydreaming.

Avoiding diarrhea

Once again, the main advice is dietary. Ensure that the child has regular meals, and in younger children, ensure that steps are taken to prevent the build-up of the accumulation disorder.

IMMUNIZATION

Among conventional medical practitioners, the case for and against immunization is argued on both sides with great passion. Those arguing for immunization point to the discomforts, the dangers of complication, and even the risk of death from measles. Those arguing against immunization point to the reduction in severity of measles in recent years, the dangers of immunization, and even the risk of death from the immunization itself. Each side can produce statistics to prove their case. On account of the large samples needed to give accurate results, it has been found to be nearly impossible to obtain a sample that is free from bias.

What the statistics *do* tell us, is that there is a risk from measles of brain damage and even death. However, there is also a risk from immunization of brain damage or death, and the risk is similar, that is, about twenty per million. So it is not completely safe to have the measles, nor is it safe to have the immunization. There is no completely safe course, and in deciding whether or not to have the immunization, other factors have to be taken into account.

Personally, we are vehemently opposed to the measles immunization. We feel that if the measles poison remains in the system, it is likely to cause a multitude of nasty diseases later in life. We also feel that the wave of selfishness that seems to have engulfed the developed world can only be made worse by the immunization, as the measles poison is associated with a very self-centered attitude.

What Can Be Done for the Immunized Child?

A child who reaches puberty without contracting measles is unlikely to get them, but there are other opportunities and ways for the poison to come out. A common way is for a low-grade rash to appear at puberty and stay for a year or more. A distinctive feature is that the rash is more pronounced at times when the child is healthier and more energetic, typically at the end of the summer holidays. If the child can be supported (both medically and psychologically) during this time, the transition (which is so full of risk at a young age) can be more gentle, with the pain and the danger spread over a longer period. Another way the poison can come out is in the form of glandular fever (mononucleosis), when the child is in its teens. This is discussed at greater length in Chapters 43 and 44.

❖

21 ❖ Mumps

INTRODUCTION

Mumps (epidemic parotitis) is one of the diseases that all children are expected to get. It usually passes without any complications, often with only a mild swelling of the glands. Mumps generally affects one side at a time, such that after the swelling has gone down on one side, it is common for the other side to swell up. In common with all glandular problems, the speed with which the condition changes is relatively slow, and the results of acupuncture are accordingly not as dramatic as in measles and febrile convulsions. For severe attacks, however, acupuncture treatment can be of great help in reducing the severity of the pain and other symptoms, and in shortening the course of the disease. Complications can be avoided, and when they do arise from neglect, they can be quickly treated. Also, in some children, an attack of mumps can make them feel tired and depressed for quite a long time (six to eight weeks during the illness, plus another six to eight weeks thereafter). Acupuncture treatment is very effective in restoring energy and cheering the child up.

ETIOLOGY & PATHOGENESIS

The root cause of mumps is very similar to that of measles, that is, another aspect of heat poison which is present at birth and needs to come out. The difference between measles and mumps is partly one of degree—measles is much worse than mumps—and partly due to the poison being in a different system. From the point of view of traditional Chinese medicine, the poison of measles is deep in the interior, in the *zàng fǔ* organs, while that of

277

mumps is more exterior, in the channels. One can see a parallel in conventional medicine where measles is likely to 'attack' the brain and spinal cord, while mumps only 'attacks' the glandular system.

Beneficial aspects

Just as measles rids the system of a really nasty poison, mumps rids the body of a slightly less nasty poison. It has the effect of clearing out the channels, especially the Liver channel. If a child does not get mumps (either because of lack of exposure to the active disease or because of immunization), it will be more prone to glandular fever at a later age. Alternatively, if the child does get mumps later, it is likely to affect the Liver channel, causing orchitis (swelling and inflammation of the testicles) or ovaritis (swelling and inflammation of the ovaries).

Chinese view

Mumps is attributed to the rising up of a wind-damp-heat infection (known as a warm toxin). The disease enters via the mouth and nose, accumulates in the leg lesser yang Gallbladder channel, where it obstructs the circulation of qi and blood, and collects in the area of the jaw. The parotid gland becomes enlarged and painful.

The leg lesser yang channel has an exterior-interior relationship with the leg terminal yin Liver channel, which passes to the genitals. If the pathogenic toxin enters this channel, the complication of orchitis arises. If the damp toxin steams upward, it can reach the nutritive level and enter the Pericardium (also a terminal yin channel), giving rise to convulsions and loss of consciousness.

PATTERNS & SYMPTOMS

Warm toxin at the superficial level

Symptoms characteristic of this pattern include:

• parotid gland is swollen and painful; the border of the swelling is not distinct
• swelling may appear on one or both sides
• chewing is difficult

Tongue coating: thin, white, or yellow
Pulse: floating, rapid (sometimes deep and slippery)

Treatment principle: dispel the wind and clear the heat, disperse the knots, and reduce the swelling

Heat toxin accumulating and collecting

This condition is rarely seen in the West. Symptoms include:

• high fever
• headache

- irritability
- thirst
- no appetite or even vomiting
- fatigued and dispirited
- parotid gland is enormously swollen, with scorching heat and pain
- throat is red and swollen
- difficulty chewing and swallowing
- dry stools or constipation
- urine yellow and scanty

Tongue coating: yellow, thin, slippery
Pulse: slippery, rapid

Treatment principle: clear the heat and resolve the toxicity, soften the hardness, and disperse the swelling

TREATMENT

Main points	TB-17 *(yi feng)*	Local point
	S-6 *(jia che)*	Local point
	LI-4 *(he gu)*	Distal point to move the qi in the face and jaw
Secondary points	TB-5 *(wai guan)*	Clears the pathogenic wind
	G-20 *(feng chi)*	Clears the pathogenic wind

Method: in principle, a dispersing technique should be used, but in practice an even technique is enough

According to Symptom

Fever	Add GV-14 *(da zhui)* and LI-11 *(qu chi)*
Orchitis	Add Sp-10 *(xue hai)*, Liv-2 *(xing jian)*, and G-43 *(xia xi)*
Pain	Add L-11 *(shao shang)* and LI-1 *(shang yang)*

Method: strong dispersing technique is used at all the points. Needles may be retained for twenty minutes, with stimulation given every five minutes.

According to Pattern

Warm toxin at the superficial level

The points listed above should be sufficient. If there is no fever, moxibustion on ginger may be applied to the swelling.

Prognosis: each treatment should bring a noticeable improvement, but several treatments may be necessary

Heat toxin accumulating and collecting

Use the main points listed above, plus the following:

TB-2 *(ye men)*	Clears the heat and disperses obstruction in the channel
CV-24 *(cheng jiang)*	Circulates the fluids and relieves thirst

In addition, the center of the swollen gland may be needled to a depth of 2.5 units, or the swollen gland may be pricked at its upper, middle, and lower parts. After pricking with a triangular needle, cupping should be applied to withdraw the toxin which is mixed with the blood. Another effective folk technique is simply to use a wick made of string or from the herb Medulla Junci Effusi *(deng xin cao)* which has been dipped in sesame oil. The wick is lit and the tip is quickly extinguished at a point one unit above the upper tip of the ear.

Prognosis: treat once daily; several treatments will be required to achieve a cure

Complications

If an adult gets mumps, there is high risk of orchitis or ovaritis. This is extremely uncomfortable and worrying for men (less so for women, for once), as they fear for their manhood. In fact, it is very rare for either impotence or sterility to follow even a bad attack of orchitis. The following two points can be used in treating this disorder:

Sp-10 *(xue hai)*
Liv-2 *(xing jian)*

We do not know how effective these points are for we have never treated orchitis. However, traditional Chinese medical textbooks are virtually unanimous in recommending their use.

❖

22 ❖ Pertussis

INTRODUCTION

Pertussis ('whooping cough') is still a dangerous disease for children, and, unlike measles and scarlet fever, it has not lost any of its severity. There are epidemics of pertussis every three to four years in the United Kingdom, which the health authorities try to eliminate by means of immunization. These efforts are not wholly successful because the vaccine has yet to be perfected, and with the whole-cell vaccine, there is significant risk of severe brain damage and even death. This makes parents somewhat reluctant to subject their children to this treatment. (The new serum vaccine developed in Japan is considerably safer.)

In Chinese medicine pertussis is attributed to an external pathogenic factor, but it is thought that it can only progress to a serious illness if the digestive system is already somewhat blocked. The pathogenic factor injures the Spleen qi, leading to accumulation disorder and giving rise to the characteristic ropy sputum. Our opinion, however, differs somewhat from the Chinese view. It seems to us that whooping cough is a disease where thick phlegm, which was there already, is eliminated from the body. In this respect, it is somewhat similar to measles, although with measles it is the heat poison which is eliminated. It is not something that is mentioned in the Chinese medical literature (perhaps it does not occur in China), but one can speak of 'womb phlegm', that is, phlegm that occurred as a result of the nine months in the womb when the body fluids could not flow freely. Pertussis, then, can be viewed more as a therapeutic transition because it throws out this phlegm.

Pertussis is really only a danger to children under three years of age. At this tender age, their digestive systems and lungs are fragile and can easily be injured by the release of large amounts of thick phlegm. Acupuncture, however, is especially good at treating pertussis. With regular treatment there is no need for the child to suffer any ill effects from pertussis, and because of the release of 'womb phlegm', the child will genuinely benefit from getting the illness.

For many people, the idea that whooping cough might be good for the child is plain nonsense. This is especially true for older people, who can point to someone they knew who died from whooping cough in the years before the Great War. At that time whooping cough really was dangerous, and many children did die from it or suffered permanent damage to their Lungs. But this is no longer the case, and most children now do benefit from whooping cough. The main benefit is to be seen in the appetite: children who have had whooping cough invariably have very good appetites and rarely show any sign of allergies. From the Western point of view this correlation is unintelligible, but it is straightforward enough in traditional Chinese medicine: if phlegm has been cleared out of the system, then of course the Spleen will function better.

In the absence of any treatment, pertussis can persist for about three months, hence its Chinese name, 'hundred-day cough' *(bǎi rì ké)*. The continued coughing over this period of time causes great distress to the child (and its family) and can severely injure the Lungs. Many cases of asthma that appear at a later age can be traced to an attack of pertussis that injured the Lungs when the person was very young. Even mild cases can leave one with a bad, dry cough which can persist for a lifetime. Such risks surely explain the desire to immunize one's children. However, if acupuncture is used, none of these sequelae need occur, for the disease can be treated before it has had time to injure the Lungs.

In Western medicine pertussis is attributed to a bacterial infection by *Bordetella pertussis.* In recent years, however, some viruses have evolved which present symptoms that are very close to pertussis. There are slight differences in the nature of the cough and of the sputum, but to the casual eye the two types of cough look identical. Pertussis immunization is not effective against the latter type of cough. Acupuncture is helpful, although the results are less effective and may require up to two or three times as many treatments.

Concerning the differentiation of patterns, the disease is divided into two stages, followed by a recovery stage. In each of these stages there are two types, one hot and one cold. The hot pattern used to be more common, but now the cold pattern predominates. In addition, we now see a deficiency pattern (occurring in weak children) which is not mentioned in the Chinese texts. From a Western perspective, the hot type is attributed to an opportunistic bacterial infection in addition to the pertussis. This infection is usually treated with antibiotics.

ETIOLOGY & PATHOGENESIS

Etiology

According to traditional Chinese medical textbooks this disease is caused by an attack of epidemic pathogenic wind. If the child's body is weak and phlegm has accumulated, the pathogenic factor can take hold, giving rise to the second stage with the characteristic convulsive cough.

Pathogenesis

First stage

The epidemic wind pathogenic factor enters via the mouth and nose and battles with the protective qi of the Lungs. At this stage it presents as an exterior pattern of either wind-cold or wind-heat. If the child is healthy the disease will gradually go away without advancing to the second stage. However, if phlegm or accumulation disorder is already present, or if the child is weak, it will progress to the second stage.

Second stage

If the pathogenic wind blocks and obstructs, this can transform into heat, which consumes the body fluids. As a result, the phlegm will thicken and obstruct the bronchi, interfering with the free passage of air in the Lungs. The Lung qi thereupon rises up in rebellion with convulsive cough and vomiting of mucus and fluid. The regulation of the qi mechanism is disrupted by the convulsive cough, and the circulation of blood in turn is impaired. This is evidenced in such symptoms as purple face and ears, veins on the neck standing out, and spontaneous sweating. In extreme cases there may be urinary incontinence.

If the convulsive cough is severe or if the coughing continues for a long time, the heat may injure the Lungs and affect the Lung connecting channels. This can lead to coughing blood or nosebleeds. Because the organs in children under two years of age are weak, the spirit diminishes as the baby gives up fighting, leading to collapse of the

Lungs. Phlegm-heat then rises to the sensory orifices, with such symptoms as twitching, delirium, and loss of consciousness.

Third stage | Most children in the West come through the second stage to the third stage. The child shows exhaustion of either qi or yin.

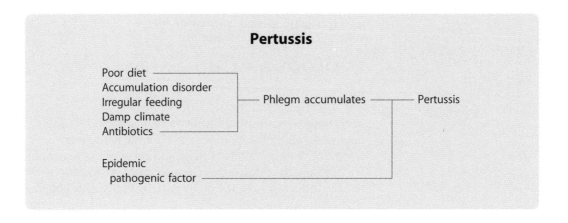

PATTERNS & SYMPTOMS

First Stage (10-20 days)

- cough begins with exterior pattern symptoms, but quickly leads to wheezing and coughing with bubbly, frothy sputum
- often, there is copious nasal discharge

Tongue coating: thin, white
Pulse: floating, with strength

Treatment principle: cause the Lung qi to descend and transform the phlegm

Second Stage (40-60 days)

General | • much convulsive coughing, followed by characteristic croup; better in the daytime, worse at night
- abdominal pain
- much mucus in the Lungs
- convulsive cough is relieved by vomiting

Phlegm-cold binds up the Lungs | • sputum is more liquid
- clear nasal discharge

Tongue coating: white, greasy
Pulse: floating, tight

Treatment principle: warm and disperse the Lung qi, stop the cough, and transform the phlegm

Phlegm-heat injures the Lungs

- sputum is sticky, thick, difficult to bring up
- sputum may be flecked with blood
- epistaxis
- mouth dry, thirst with desire to drink

Tongue coating: yellow, dry
Pulse: slippery, rapid

Note

This pattern corresponds to the Western complication of opportunistic infection. The idea is that a quite different bacterium starts to proliferate in the Lungs. It is able to do this because of the poor health of the Lungs and the large amount of phlegm contained in them.

Treatment principle: clear the heat and disperse the Lung qi, stop the cough, and transform the phlegm

Lung and Spleen qi deficiency

This pattern is seen in the West but not in China. Characteristic symptoms include:

- pale looking, even white
- very thin
- history of poor appetite
- lethargic
- possibly fits of coughing, but not as violent as in strong children (although they can still be alarming to watch)

Tongue: pale, wet
Pulse: weak or soft

Treatment principle: tonify the Lungs and nourish the Spleen

Complications (rare in the West)

If the disease continues untreated for a long time, the following symptoms are commonly seen:

- pathogenic factor attacks the yin; typical yin deficiency
- pathogenic factor attacks the Lung passages giving rise to asthma
- violent vomiting
- stifling sensation and fullness in the chest, painful ribs
- vomiting blood
- periorbital edema
- constipation
- poor appetite, swollen abdomen
- delirium

Third Stage: Recovery (20-30 days)

General

- cough is reduced and barely paroxysmal
- vomiting is reduced

Lung and Spleen qi deficiency

- body is weak and deficient
- cough and voice weak, without strength
- small amount of watery sputum
- shortness of breath
- tired and without strength
- cold hands and feet
- spontaneous sweating
- poor appetite, choosy about food
- distended abdomen
- watery stools
- copious, pale urine

Tongue coating: thin, white
Pulse: deep, forceless
Finger vein: pale, thin

Treatment principle: tonify the Lungs and nourish the Spleen

Yin deficiency (rare in the West)

- dry cough without strength
- hot soles and palms
- restlessness, wakes up at night
- irritability
- night sweats
- red cheeks
- lips dry

Tongue coating: thin, yellow
Pulse: rapid, forceless
Finger vein: thin, purple

Treatment principle: nourish the yin and moisten the Lungs

TREATMENT

First Stage

L-7 *(lie que)*	Both points direct the Lung qi
LI-4 *(he gu)*	downward, transform the phlegm, and clear the wind
G-20 *(feng chi)*	Clears the wind

In weak children it may be beneficial to tonify the qi with S-36 *(zu san li)*. If the back is tender to palpation or the Lungs are weak, add B-12 *(feng men)*. For wind-cold, add L-9 *(tai yuan)*, and for wind-heat, add L-5 *(chi ze)* and L-11 *(shao shang)*. If there is any sign of accumulation disorder, this should be treated with points such as *si feng* (M-UE-9) to prevent the disease from progressing to the second stage.

Method: L-7 *(lie que)*, LI-4 *(he gu)*, and G-20 *(feng chi)* are needled. B-12 *(feng men)* may be needled or cupped. L-9 *(tai yuan)* is needled for wind-cold. Use moxibustion (or moxibustion on garlic) at B-12 *(feng men)* or other tender back points. For wind-heat, L-5 *(chi ze)* is needled and L-11 *(shao shang)* is pricked with the triangular needle to withdraw a few drops of blood.

Prognosis: this depends very much on the patient's overall health. In a reasonably healthy child, one or two treatments should be sufficient to prevent the cough from progressing to the second stage.

Second Stage

Main points

si feng (M-UE-9)

This point may be combined with P-6 *(nei guan)* and LI-4 *(he gu)*, with L-7 *(lie que)*, or with L-9 *(tai yuan)*.

Method: according to *all* the Chinese texts, *si feng* (M-UE-9) is pricked with the triangular needle to withdraw a few drops of yellow fluid, but in our experience the fluid is red!

According to symptoms

Much sputum:
add S-40 *(feng long)*

Difficulty in breathing:
add CV-22 *(tian tu)* and CV-17 *(shan zhong)*

Phlegm-cold binds the Lungs

In addition to the main points, use the following:

B-13 *(fei shu)*	Strengthens the Lungs and directs the Lung qi downward
CV-12 *(zhong wan)*	Transforms the phlegm
CV-17 *(shan zhong)*	Transforms the phlegm

Method: moxibustion may be used, especially moxibustion on garlic

Phlegm-heat injures the Lungs

In addition to the main points, also use L-11 *(shao shang)* to clear the phlegm-heat.

Method: use a triangular needle to withdraw a few drops of blood

Prognosis: in both phlegm-cold and phlegm-heat, the prognosis depends on the overall health of the patient and how much time elapsed between the onset of the illness and the treatment. In a reasonably healthy patient treated within a week or so of onset, one or two treatments should be enough to loosen the phlegm, with three or four additional treatments to consolidate the effect.* In weaker patients, or if the disease is not treated until a month or so after onset, more treatments may be required. *Treatment should then be given at least twice a week for the next month or two, to avoid relapse between treatments.* This may sound like a long time, and it is. It simply takes time to get rid of the thick phlegm which has been in the system since birth.

If the 'pertussis' is not in fact due to the pertussis organism, a more frequent treatment plan is required. It is often necessary to treat such patients every day for about two weeks, followed by two or three weeks of twice-a-week treatment.

Lung and Spleen qi deficiency

The main thrust of treatment is to tonify the child. To begin with, use a tonifying technique with moxibustion at points such as the following:

L-9 *(tai yuan)*
L-5 *(chi ze)*
S-36 *(zu san li)*

Then, after a few treatments, use a tonifying technique with moxibustion at these points:

B-13 *(fei shu)*
B-20 *(pi shu)*
L-9 *(tai yuan)*

Prognosis: if it is at all possible, treat three times a week; once a week will not be enough. Results are quite variable and depend a lot on the child. If it is simple deficiency, it may take quite a number of treatments to bring the energy up. If the child is hyperactive Spleen qi deficient, the child may become very depressed after the treatments and strongly resist coming again.

---

*Loosening the phlegm throughout the body will give rise to a productive cough. In some patients, the resultant loose cough can be quite severe. In fact, it may seem to be worse than the pertussis; with further treatment, however, it soon passes.

Complications	Yin deficiency: add B-38 *(gao huang shu)*, K-3 *(tai xi)*, and B-23 *(shen shu)*

Asthma:
add CV-22 *(tian tu)* and *ding chuan* (M-BW-1)

Vomiting:
add P-6 *(nei guan)* and S-36 *(zu san li)*

Stifling sensation and fullness in the chest, painful ribs:
add G-34 *(yang ling quan)* and S-40 *(feng long)*

Vomiting blood:
add P-6 *(nei guan)*, S-36 *(zu san li)*, S-34 *(liang qiu)*, and S-21 *(liang men)*

Periorbital edema:
add Sp-4 *(gong sun)*

Constipation:
add L-5 *(chi ze)*

Poor appetite, swollen abdomen:
add Sp-6 *(san yin jiao)*

Delirium:
bleed *shi xuan* (M-UE-1) and needle GV-14 *(da zhui)*, LI-11 *(qu chi)*, and LI-4 *(he gu)*

Third Stage

Lung and Spleen	S-36 *(zu san li)*	Tonifies Spleen qi
qi deficiency	CV-12 *(zhong wan)*	Tonifies Spleen qi
	L-9 *(tai yuan)*	Tonifies Lung qi
	B-13 *(fei shu)*	Tonifies Lung qi

Method: tonifying method; indirect moxibustion, or moxibustion on ginger, may be used at B-13 *(fei shu)* and CV-12 *(zhong wan)*

Prognosis: this depends largely on the severity of the attack and the constitution of the patient. It can range from one to ten treatments.

Yin deficiency	L-9 *(tai yuan)*	Tonifies Lung qi
	B-38 *(gao huang shu)*	Tonifies the yin of the whole body
	B-23 *(shen shu)*	Tonifies Kidney yin
	K-3 *(tai xi)*	Tonifies Kidney yin

Method: tonifying method; no moxibustion

Prognosis: one to three treatments are usually enough to clear the heat. The condition may then transform into the qi-deficiency type.

PREVENTIVE MEDICINE

Homeopathic 'immunization'

There is a lot of mystique surrounding homeopathic immunization against whooping cough. However, within the perspective of traditional Chinese medicine we can see how it works.

The treatment consists, first of all, of treating the child for any major imbalances, and then giving it a single dose of Pertussin 30, a nosode prepared from a child with whooping cough. This treatment is repeated every spring and autumn during the first three years of life. What this nosode seems to do is to activate the system in a way that is similar to a real attack, so that the child throws out a lot of phlegm. The effects are much milder than real whooping cough, so its administration does not threaten the health of the child; nor does it completely rid the body of all the thick phlegm that should be expelled. However, enough phlegm is expelled for the child to be able to cope with *Bordetella* when it comes along. The child does not really have genuine immunity against *Bordetella*, so it does 'catch' it. However, the illness remains one of *wind at the superficial level,* and does not go any deeper. The child may have a harsh cough for a week or two, but after that, the cough goes away.

So, to look at the effects in terms of symptoms, the treatment is effective. To look at it literally in terms of genuine immunization against *Bordetella*, it is not effective!

Acupuncture 'immunization'

What can we as acupuncturists do to prevent a bad attack of whooping cough? The answer is: a lot. We can follow exactly the same principles as the homeopath. First of all, we treat any obvious imbalances. The old saying "Tonify in deficiency and disperse in excess" is useful here.

It is true that we do not have quite the same specific remedies as the homeopath, and if it were easy to take a child to a homeopathic practitioner, I would do so. But we can do a lot for the child who does not have access to homeopathy.

LOOKING AFTER THE CHILD

A study carried out by anthroposophical doctors in Germany has shown that children who are well nursed during whooping cough suffer no ill effects. Those who do suffer long-term injury are those who are not properly looked after. This is the case even without any treatment! This point has to be labored, because home conditions have changed so much during this century. In the past it was much more common for the father to go out to work and for the mother to stay at home. Whatever we may think of gender inequality, this situation meant that if a child was ill, mother was always around to look after the child. This is no longer the case, for it is common for both parents to go out to work or for the mother to be a single parent. This means that special provisions must be made for looking after a child that is ill.

The consequence is that, if it is at all possible for a child to go to school, then off it goes. Many children are sent to school who quite definitely should be resting at home. This dilemma is particularly acute in whooping cough. Once the illness has reached the whooping stage, according to conventional medicine, the child is no longer infectious. Moreover, the child may have its worst coughing fits during the night, so the child can be sent to school without causing too much disruption in the classroom. However, when a child has whooping cough, it really should be kept at home and only taken for short walks, enough to get some fresh air into the Lungs. For many parents the temptation to go back to work and send the child to school (or creche) at this stage is irresistible. This is a pity.

NOTES

- While the patient has pertussis, all phlegm-producing foods should be avoided.

- The main meal should be given early in the day so that most of the food can be absorbed before the evening and nighttime attacks, which often lead to vomiting.

- The spasmodic cough at night can be alleviated by giving the child a thyme bath. Make an infusion of one teaspoon of thyme to one pint of water. When this has cooled, strain it into the baby's bath.

- The panic which accompanies an episode of spasmodic coughing can be alleviated by using Bach Rescue Remedy. Put a few drops of this remedy in a glass of water beside the bed. When the child awakes in a coughing fit, give it a sip or two to allay the panic which it will feel when it cannot breathe.

- For a case history involving pertussis, see Case 8 in Chapter 47.

❖

23 ❖ Tonsillitis

INTRODUCTION

Tonsillitis is one of the most common of chronic childhood complaints, so much so that in the recent past it was standard procedure to remove children's tonsils regardless of whether they had problems. This surgery is rarely, if ever, necessary for patients who are prepared to undergo acupuncture treatment, for acupuncture is dramatically successful in treating acute tonsillitis and can effect a cure in most chronic cases as well.

From a Western medical point of view, tonsillitis is caused by either a bacterial or viral infection. From the traditional Chinese medical point of view, it can be caused by external factors, but it is recognized that internal factors also play an important role. Among the common causes of both acute and chronic tonsillitis are those discussed below.

Epidemic

These are most common at the beginning of spring and autumn, when the weather changes suddenly and there is often wind as well. Under these conditions, an external pathogenic factor can invade the throat, giving rise to acute tonsillitis.

Dysfunction of the Lungs and Stomach

The throat is known as the 'gateway' of both the Lungs and the Stomach. Therefore, problems associated with the Lungs, such as inflammation of the chest, ears, and nose, can give rise to acute or chronic tonsillitis. Similarly, if there is much heat and phlegm in the Stomach, this too can rise up to the throat and cause acute or chronic tonsillitis.

292

Environment	The tonsils filter airborne poisons: tobacco fumes and chemical fumes (e.g., paint and cavity wall insulation). These poisons can predispose a child to tonsillitis as they cause dampness and heat to accumulate in the body and obstruct the channels of the throat.
Repeated infections	If a child suffers repeated acute attacks of tonsillitis, this will gradually weaken the qi in the throat and may lead to chronic tonsillitis. This is especially so if these acute attacks are not treated well, which is to say, if antibiotics are routinely prescribed.
Immunizations	Certain immunizations—pertussis being the most common—have the effect of giving rise to chronic tonsillitis.
Emotions	Problems of the throat are often linked to the emotions, most commonly, bottled-up anger.
While treating otitis media	It is not uncommon for tonsillitis to appear when you are treating chronic otitis media. The lingering pathogenic factor which was in the ears moves downward. This is not a bad reaction, but it may need to be treated. It certainly needs to be explained to the parents!

Tonsillitis and the Emotions

Perhaps one of the most glaring differences between conventional Western medicine and traditional Chinese medicine is that, according to the former, virtually all acute diseases are caused by *external* factors, for example, a bacteria or virus. Obviously, this is true in some cases, but what the Chinese noticed a long time ago is that this need not be the case: acute illness may come from an internal problem. Tonsillitis is a good example. The Western medical diagnosis is that it must be a bacterial or viral infection. The Chinese say that this can happen (an external pathogenic factor), but it may also be due to internal heat from diet or emotional frustration.

This is borne out by looking at the common pattern that tonsillitis follows: it is rarely seen in children under the age of two, and becomes common in two- to three-year olds. At this time, the most important factors that have changed in the child's life are trying to communicate effectively and properly, and wanting to do things but not quite accomplishing them. There is another peak around the age of six to seven years when children become more self-conscious and self-reflective about their emotions.

Although it is rare for tonsillitis to be only emotionally based, emotions are very often an important factor. Usually, the child also has a lingering pathogenic factor or an inappropriate diet.

ETIOLOGY & PATHOGENESIS

There are two patterns for acute tonsillitis and two for chronic tonsillitis.

Acute Tonsillitis

Wind-heat

This type of tonsillitis can arise as a complication from another illness in the body, most commonly from an infection in the upper respiratory tract, ears, or nose. For example, cough, rhinitis, or otitis media can all give rise to tonsillitis as the pathogenic factor passes from the Lungs, ears, or nose to the throat.

An external attack of pathogenic wind-heat, or wind-cold that transforms into wind-heat, can lead directly to an acute attack of tonsillitis. This is the type seen when there is an epidemic.

The Lungs govern the exterior and are affected by all exterior patterns. The throat is known as the 'gateway' of the Lungs; if wind-heat invades the Lungs, it can accumulate in the throat and condense the body fluids, which then become phlegm. Phlegm and heat obstruct the qi in the channels, which causes them to become enlarged, painful, and bright red.

Lung and Stomach heat

Actually, this is two conditions, each with a different etiology and therefore with a different treatment. The first is a progression of a wind-heat disorder to the yang brightness *(yáng míng)* fever stage. The second is caused by an acute attack of chronic tonsillitis which is brought on by something overheating the Stomach, for example, spicy, greasy foods.

Yang ming fever. This is a progression of the previous pattern of wind-heat. The pathogenic factor moves inside and turns into the yang ming fever stage.

Heat in the Stomach. This is caused by internal factors that result in Stomach heat. The most common are:

• accumulation disorder in younger children
• hot, spicy, greasy food in older children

The throat is also the gateway to the Stomach. If pathogenic heat accumulates in the Stomach, it will readily rise up to the throat and, as described above, condense the body fluids to form phlegm, which obstructs the qi in the channels, and thus give rise to tonsillitis.

Chronic Tonsillitis

Lingering pathogenic factor

This is called 'stone moth' *(shí é)* in traditional Chinese medicine because it feels like a stone in the throat and looks like the wings of a moth or butterfly. This is the most common pattern for chronic tonsillitis in children. There are two main causes of this type of tonsillitis:

- repeated attacks of acute tonsillitis, especially if treated with antibiotics
- immunizations, especially the pertussis vaccine, can give rise to a lingering pathogenic factor in the throat

These are aggravated by such things as pollution, chemicals, or tobacco smoke. This lingering pathogenic factor can occur in children of either the excess or deficient type (see Chapter 3), and this differentiation will influence the treatment.

The pathogenic factor that originally invades the throat—be it external or from an immunization—is never completely cleared from the throat and remains lodged there, obstructing the flow of qi and blood in the channels. This can lead to phlegm accumulating in the tonsils, causing them to swell, and to stagnation and heat, making them red and inflamed. Since the qi does not circulate well in the throat area, the risk of an external pathogenic attack is increased, leading to an acute infection on top of the chronic condition.

Yin deficiency

This is called 'milk moth' *(rǔ é)* because there is often a milky film over the tonsils. Although this pattern is the one with characteristic purulent spots, in fact both chronic patterns can be purulent. The genuine yin deficiency pattern is rarely seen in Western children for there is little cause for them to become truly exhausted. When it is seen, it tends to be caused by a prolonged or severe febrile disease, but this is usually treated with antibiotics. It can occur in a mild form, with intermittent sore throats, from about the age of seven upward, especially in children who have ambitious parents. Alternatively, it can be seen in children who are Kidney deficient and are continually overstimulated by television, overexcitement, and so on, which leads to exhaustion and yin deficiency. The fire from deficiency rises up to the throat, causing burning and soreness.

Tonsillitis

Acute: Wind-heat —— Invades throat ┐
             Otitis media — Spreads to throat ┘├— Tonsillitis

             Yang brightness fever ┐
             Otitis media ————————┘├— Heat in Stomach and Lungs rises up — Tonsillitis

Chronic: Lingering pathogenic factor in throat —— Tonsillitis never cleared
             Yin deficiency — Fire blazes up to throat — Tonsillitis

PATTERNS & SYMPTOMS

Acute Tonsillitis

Wind-heat

- sudden attack, with symptoms of the pathogenic factor at the superficial level
- fever with chills
- throat pain with difficulty in swallowing
- tonsils red and swollen
- face red
- headache, aches all over the body

Tongue body: red
Tongue coating: thin, yellow
Pulse: floating, rapid

Treatment principle: disperse the wind and clear the heat, reduce the swelling, and benefit the throat

Lung and Stomach heat

Both patterns will have certain symptoms in common:

- copious perspiration
- constipation
- thirst with preference for cold drinks
- tonsils extremely red or swollen with yellow or white spots
- yellow or red urine

Tongue body: red
Tongue coating: yellow
Pulse: rapid, overflowing

There are also individual signs and symptoms for each pattern.

YANG MING FEVER

- pathogenic factor moves inside, which leads to the 'big four' (big fever which becomes very high at times, big

thirst with preference for cold drinks, big sweating, and big pulse which is rapid and overflowing)
- abdomen may feel full and bloated
- constipation may be severe

Treatment principle: clear the heat and bring down the fire from the throat, disperse the knots, and move the bowels

HEAT IN THE STOMACH

- large appetite
- whining and miserable
- possibly a full or burning sensation in the stomach

Treatment principle: clear the heat and bring down the fire; if necessary, move the retained food

Chronic Tonsillitis

Lingering pathogenic factor ('stone moth')

STRONG (EXCESS-TYPE) CHILD WITH LINGERING PATHOGENIC FACTOR

- child is generally strong
- tonsils swollen enormously and brightly colored
- sore pain in throat, or throat is swollen and uncomfortable
- dry, hard cough
- snoring sound from nose
- lymph glands in neck are enlarged
- colds quickly develop into tonsillitis

Tongue body: maybe red or pale
Pulse: slippery

Note: the lingering pathogenic factor may be either hot or cold. If it is hot, there will be signs of heat, such as a red tongue and red face, while if it is cold, the tongue and face will be pale. In addition to the above signs, the child may show signs of phlegm: there may be a productive cough, and there will be visible signs of phlegm.

Treatment principle: harmonize the qi and blood, disperse the phlegm, and expel the lingering pathogenic factor

SPLEEN QI DEFICIENCY PLUS A LINGERING PATHOGENIC FACTOR

- child weak, floppy, and lethargic
- prone to recurrent infections
- cough is usually weak
- glands swollen in neck
- muscle tone flabby
- poor appetite, picky over food
- pale, dribbling

Tongue body: pale
Pulse: weak

Note: these children may also have visible signs of phlegm, for example, runny nose or productive cough.

Treatment principle: tonify the qi, disperse the phlegm, and expel the lingering pathogenic factor

Yin deficiency

- throat is swollen, red, painful, and dry
- tonsils appear to be covered with a dry paste and some pus
- symptoms are worse in the early morning or when overexcited
- possibly bright red phlegm

Tongue: dry, red
Pulse: fine and rapid

Treatment principle: enrich the yin, bring down the fire, and benefit the throat

TREATMENT

Acute Tonsillitis

Main points

LI-4 *(he gu)*	Clears the wind-heat and benefits the throat
S-44 *(nei ting)*	Benefits the throat and clears the Stomach heat

These points are usually enough to stop the pain and start the healing process. The pain should start to subside during the treatment. If it does not, or if the tonsillitis is very severe, the following points will be helpful.

L-11 *(shao shang)*	Clears the pain and swelling in the throat
CV-22 *(tian tu)*	Benefits the throat
SI-17 *(tian rong)*	Local point for tonsils
TB-17 *(yi feng)*	Local point for tonsils

Method: strong dispersing method; if the pain and swelling in the throat is very severe, bleed L-11 *(shao shang)* with a triangular needle

According to symptoms

Headache and other wind symptoms:
G-20 *(feng chi)*

Fever:
LI-11 *(qu chi)*

Delirium:
P-9 *(zhang chong)*

In severe cases which do not respond to treatment, or where there is danger of the throat becoming blocked, prick the tonsils themselves with a triangular needle.

Special treatments

1. Prick the engorged vein on the back of the ear.
2. 'Without heat' moxibustion: apply a paste of crushed garlic at LI-4 *(he gu)* for one to two hours to cause irritation of the skin. The paste must not be left in place too long, as severe blistering can occur.

According to pattern

WIND-HEAT

The main points listed above are adequate.

Prognosis: one treatment is usually enough to relieve the pain, but more may be required to reduce the swelling. In young children, LI-4 *(he gu)* alone is sufficient, while in older children it may be combined with L-7 *(lie que)*.

YANG MING FEVER

GV-14 *(da zhui)*
LI-11 *(qu chi)* } Clears heat and releases the exterior
LI-4 *(he gu)*

The main points listed above may also be used. In severe cases a purgative such as a preparation of Senna *(Cassia angustifolia)* should be administered.

Prognosis: one treatment is usually sufficient to stop the pain; further treatments may be required to clear the yang brightness fever

HEAT IN THE STOMACH

Use the main points, but especially S-44 *(nei ting)* and LI-4 *(he gu)*.

Chronic Tonsillitis

Main points

LI-4 *(he gu)*	Benefits the throat
S-44 *(nei ting)*	Benefits the throat and clears the Stomach heat

In chronic tonsillitis there have often been so many attacks that the qi in the throat is very weak. We often find that it is necessary to add some local points to the prescription for the first few treatments—even though children hate points on the throat. Consider such points as:

CV-22 *(tian tu)*	Benefits the throat
SI-17 *(tian rong)*	Local point for tonsils
TB-17 *(yi feng)*	Local point for tonsils

Lingering pathogenic factor

IN STRONG CHILD

In addition to the main points, the points below are helpful in expelling lingering pathogenic factors that block the channels.

bai lao (M-HN-30)	Clears lingering pathogenic factors from the channels; used for all glandular congestion problems
B-13 *(fei shu)*	Tonifies Lung qi, resolves knotted phlegm
B-18 *(gan shu)*	Benefits the Liver function of maintaining the free flow of qi, tonifies the Spleen
B-20 *(pi shu)*	Tonifies the Spleen, transforms the phlegm

Method: use a dispersing technique. If the lingering pathogenic factor is cold in nature, you may use moxibustion; if it is hot in nature, you may add such points as:

LI-4 *(he gu)*
S-44 *(nei ting)*
Liv-2 *(xing jian)*

Prognosis: in cases of recent origin, three to five treatments may be enough; in long-standing cases, twenty to forty treatments may be required. The patient may have a discharge of catarrh and develop a cough after the treatments as the thick phlegm is resolved. If phlegm begins to appear, use S-40 *(feng long)*.

WITH SPLEEN QI DEFICIENCY

Use the following points to tonify the qi, plus one or two local points to bring qi to the throat:

S-36 *(zu san li)*
Sp-6 *(san yin jiao)*
L-9 *(tai yuan)*
CV-12 *(zhong wan)*

Method: use a tonifying technique as well as moxibustion

Prognosis: depending on the extent of the deficiency, thirty to forty treatments may be needed. As the child becomes stronger, you must alter your point prescription and needle technique accordingly to expel the lingering pathogenic factor, as described in Chapter 3.

Yin deficiency

Using needles on a genuinely yin-deficient child is difficult, as the child is truly frightened by them. Start by using moxibustion at the points, and then progress to using needles. Use the following points:

L-7 *(lie que)*	Both points act on the throat and
K-6 *(zhao hai)*	tonify the yin of the body
B-13 *(fei shu)*	Tonifies the yin of the Lungs
B-38 *(gao huang shu)*	Tonifies the yin of the entire body
B-23 *(shen shu)*	Tonifies the yin of the Kidneys
K-3 *(tai xi)*	Tonifies the yin of the Kidneys
B-18 *(gan shu)*	Tonifies the yin of the Liver

Prognosis: in mild cases, five to ten treatments are needed; in severe cases, ten to twenty treatments

NOTES

• In chronic tonsillitis, pay attention to the diet, avoiding phlegm-producing and warming foods such as milk, cheese, lamb, spicy foods, and greasy foods.

• In yin deficiency disorders, it is important for the patient to rest. If there is insomnia, this should also be treated.

• The lingering pathogenic factor variety of tonsillitis is cured much more quickly if herbs are combined with acupuncture. One Western herb that should be considered is Poke root *(Phytolacca decandra)*.

• Tonsillitis is sometimes seen during the treatment of chronic otitis media. The otitis media should be treated as described in Chapter 25, and the parents should be reassured that this is a normal progression during treatment.

• For a case history involving tonsillitis, see Case 9 in Chapter 47.

❖

24 ❖ Conjunctivitis

INTRODUCTION

Conjunctivitis is not commonly seen in the clinic as a presenting complaint . However, it is found in children that are being treated for other problems, and in these cases it is well worth treating with acupuncture because the effects are very good. The severity of the problem varies from a mild itchy eye that is uncomfortable to both eyes being red and very sore. It ranges from a single attack to a chronic condition that has been around for months. In all these variations, acupuncture can be extremely helpful.

In an acute attack you can often reduce the itching and discomfort in the eye in just one treatment, and in most cases it rarely takes more than three. In children where the problem is more long-standing, you can nearly always help and usually cure the condition altogether in under twenty treatments, even in very complex cases.

It is therefore well worth treating and is very simple to treat. Even just adding a point such as G-20 *(feng chi)* to your prescription if the child has come in with some other complaint will help. It is also worthwhile because conjunctivitis is miserable to have, and you can stop a lot of the symptoms with acupuncture.

What Is Conjunctivitis?

Western medicine

Acute conjunctivitis is inflammation of the conjunctiva of the eye. In Western medical terms it is said to be caused by a virus, bacteria, or an allergic reaction. When the culprit is a virus, the symptoms are said to be milder. Chronic conjunctivitis is a chronic inflammation of the conjunctiva with exacerbation and remissions over months or years.

The causes are said to be the same as for acute conjunctivitis. The general symptoms include:

- bloodshot eye
- gritty, sore eye
- discharge of pus
- eyelids gummed together after sleep

The standard Western treatment depends on the cause:

- if bacterial, antibiotic eye drops are administered
- if allergy-based, a short course of topical corticosteroids and antibiotics are administered; tests, however, should be done in advance to rule out the presence of the herpes simplex virus
- if viral, then no treatment is usually given

Traditional Chinese medicine

By contrast, the view of traditional Chinese medicine is that both external and internal factors are important for both acute and chronic conditions. There are two patterns for acute conjunctivitis and two for chronic conjunctivitis. The patterns for acute conjunctivitis are:

- attack of wind-heat
- uprising of heat and dampness

The patterns for chronic conjunctivitis are:

- lingering pathogenic factor
- Liver and Gallbladder heat

We will first discuss acute conjunctivitis, and then chronic conjunctivitis.

ACUTE CONJUNCTIVITIS

Etiology & Pathogenesis

Wind-heat

This is a straightforward invasion of wind-heat attacking the eyes. The flow of qi and fluids is disrupted, leading to sore, dry, itchy eyes.

Uprising of heat and dampness

Heat and dampness from the interior rise up to the eye. In younger children, common causes include:

- accumulation disorder
- latent heat in springtime

In older children, sources include:

- spicy, greasy foods
- Liver qi constraint which combines with dampness

The dampness can come from the diet or from a lingering pathogenic factor. (A lingering pathogenic factor may be both damp and hot in nature and may alone cause an acute attack.) The heat and dampness enter the Liver channel and rise up to the eye, causing them to become sore, red, and painful.

As noted above, latent spring heat can cause conjunctivitis. Latent spring heat is discussed more fully in Chapter 14. The most common time to see this will be in the spring as the child begins to release the excess heat generated during the winter. Although it is quite 'normal' to release heat in the spring, it is still worth treating if it manifests as conjunctivitis.

Signs & Symptoms

Wind-Heat

If the heat predominates there will be more redness in the eye. If the wind predominates there will be more watery secretions.

• red, sore, itchy eyes
• possibly watery eyes
• sudden onset
• signs of an attack of wind-heat
• possibly fever
• possibly thirst

Tongue: thin coating, red tip
Pulse: floating, rapid

Latent heat

If the conjunctivitis is caused by latent heat there will be typical signs of wind-heat, plus:

• irritability
• restlessness
• general feeling of unease, that is, a feeling that the child is not quite all right

Uprising of heat and dampness

• signs of pus and dampness in the eye
• signs of dampness or phlegm in the other parts of the body
• possibly the classic signs of accumulation disorder
• possibly the classic signs of a lingering pathogenic factor (swollen glands, etc.)
• in older children the heat may come from constrained Liver qi

In practice it can be very hard to tell these three patterns apart as they often appear suddenly, and are all hot disorders which may contain signs of dampness. The best way to distinguish among them is through the pulse and tongue signs:

- a child suffering from an external attack will have a floating pulse and possibly a thin tongue coating
- a child with interior heat will have a red tongue, and the pulse will be full, rapid, and possibly wiry

Having said this, a young baby, or an older child for that matter, may well decide that you are not going to see its tongue today, and that there is absolutely no way that he or she will sit still for pulse taking. Luckily, it is not that important, for when it comes to treatment, they are all quite similar.

Treatment

Main points

In the treatment of all attacks of acute conjunctivitis you can use:

G-20 *(feng chi)*
LI-4 *(he gu)*

Another point which is frequently used is G-37 *(guang ming)*.

If there is obvious dampness and goo in the eye, add:

G-34 *(yang ling quan)*

Method: use a reducing method at all points

If you are clear about the cause, then add points according to the pattern.

Wind-heat

Treatment principle: clear the wind-heat, cool and nourish the eyes

L-7 *(lie que)*
TB-5 *(wai guan)*
tai yang (M-HN-9)

Prognosis: one treatment should be enough; occasionally, you may need to treat a second time. We have not treated many cases, but in those we have the reaction was what you would expect when treating wind-heat: the child sweated profusely for about two hours and was then completely better.

Uprising of heat and dampness

Treatment principle: clear the heat and dampness from the eyes

Use the main points. If there is emotional constraint, add:

Liv-3 *(tai chong)*
B-18 *(gan shu)*

If there is accumulation disorder, add:

si feng (M-UE-9)

If there is latent heat, add:

P-7 *(da ling)*
Liv-2 *(xing jian)*

The reaction to treatment is a bit variable. It rather depends on the underlying cause of the heat. If it is due to accumulation disorder, you know what to expect. If it is due to latent heat, then the child may become hot and sweaty for a day or two. If it is due to suppressed rage, expect the emotions to come out—sometimes quite violently.

Prognosis: depends on the cause, but one to three treatments should be enough to clear the eyes. Then you must go on to resolve any underlying problem, with dietary advice and so forth.

CHRONIC CONJUNCTIVITIS

Etiology & Pathogenesis

Lingering pathogenic factor

In some children the eye always seems to have something the matter with it: either there is a stye or it is sore and itchy. In addition, there may be episodes of acute conjunctivitis. The child is typically deficient in energy, with all the classic signs: poor appetite, weak, floppy. There may also be signs of phlegm, but not necessarily. Since this pattern has at its base a lingering pathogenic factor, the phlegm may be too thick to be seen. The thick phlegm in the channels blocks the circulation of qi to the eyes, giving rise to recurrent bouts of conjunctivitis and related problems.

It should be noted that although the child is deficient, the lingering pathogenic factor can be hot in nature. This is often seen after measles when the child has used its eyes too much, too soon, or inappropriately after the illness. The qi is further hindered in reaching the eyes, exacerbating the situation.

Liver and Gallbladder heat

The most common cause of this pattern in older children is constrained emotions or even anger. It is usually combined with a diet that is rich in greasy, hot, or spicy foods. The heat and dampness enter the Liver and Gallbladder channels and rise up to the eyes.

It should be noted that in both of the chronic patterns, the child is more prone to acute attacks because the qi in the eyes is already weak.

Signs & Symptoms

Lingering pathogenic factor

- eyes are often causing problems
- possibly visible signs of phlegm, for example, glue-like discharge from the eyes
- swollen glands
- child has no spirit and the eyes too lack spirit
- child is often weak and is prone to recurrent infections

Pulse: slippery or weak

Treatment principle: clear the lingering pathogenic factor

Liver and Gallbladder heat

- at times the eyes are red, swollen, and painful, while at other times they are fine
- red face
- possibly red scanty urine, especially when the eyes are bad
- often worse when the child is upset or angry

Tongue: red
Pulse: wiry

Treatment principle: clear Liver and Gallbladder heat

Treatment

Use points to bring qi to the eyes, such as:

G-20 *(feng chi)*
LI-4 *(he gu)*

Add additional points according to the individual condition.

Lingering pathogenic factor

S-36 *(zu san li)*
B-20 *(pi shu)*
B-18 *(gan shu)*

Method: even or moving technique; add moxibustion if the child is cold

If there is a hot lingering pathogenic factor, use:

Liv-3 *(tai chong)*
B-18 *(gan shu)*

Prognosis: variable, depending on the state of the child; ten to twenty-five treatments should be enough

Liver and Gallbladder heat

Use the main points, plus:

Liv-3 *(tai chong)*
G-37 *(guang ming)*
Liv-2 *(xing jian)*

Method: dispersing technique

Advice

- All the usual: rest, no dairy products, eat warming foods.

- If the condition follows an episode of measles, the child must rest the eyes.

- Try and explain what is going on to the parents, and hopefully, they will start allowing the child to express his or her emotions more freely.

- If needed, change the diet. In particular, avoid eggs and peanuts in all types of conjunctivitis.

SUMMARY

Although we do not see many cases of conjunctivitis, those we have seen and treated have produced impressive results. In an acute attack the eye is often better after only one treatment. Even in chronic cases you can do a lot of good in a relatively short space of time. As the treatment is so simple—just a couple of points—it is well worth the small effort, especially since conjunctivitis is such a miserable thing for a child to have.

NOTE

- For a case history involving conjunctivitis, see Case 25 in Chapter 47.

❖

25 ❖ Otitis Media

INTRODUCTION

Otitis media is very common in babies and children, although it does vary in both its severity and frequency. In some children it is just a mild discomfort, while in others it is very painful. It may happen only occasionally in an otherwise healthy child, or the attacks may be recurrent and frequent. In some children the pain in the ear may even be continuous with acute flare-ups.

Otitis media is regarded with fear by many people, as it is said that there are risks of serious complications, including, occasionally, the risk of deafness. However, there is a certain amount of paranoia here, for if the condition is left alone by both orthodox and alternative healthcare practitioners, ninety percent of ear infections will resolve themselves, leaving no damage behind. This is not to say you should not treat it. No one wants to see a child suffer if help can be given, and acupuncture is very successful at treating otitis media. In fact, in the acute stage, the effects of using acupuncture are just short of miraculous. In young babies and in simple cases it is possible to relieve the pain in one treatment and effect a cure in two or three treatments. In more complex cases (where there have been repeated attacks) it takes longer, but success is almost certain, provided your diagnosis is correct and the parents are prepared to follow your advice. Even in those cases where there is risk of complications—and, of course, there are some—giving acupuncture regularly and frequently reduces the risk. This is in contrast to Western medicine, which has little to offer in the way of a cure, especially if the cause is a viral infection.

In Western medicine, acute otitis media is always attributed to external attack by a virus or bacteria, while in Chinese medicine the internal and external factors are given equal weight. Internal factors are heat or cold,* possibly accompanied by dampness, which come from a variety of causes. The heat is most commonly attributable to accumulation disorder in younger children, and to emotional factors causing Liver qi constraint in older children. The cold usually comes from the diet, overuse of antibiotics, or a cold lingering pathogenic factor.

External factors are external wind, cold, or heat invading the ear. This is common after swimming, or accompanying another illness such as tonsillitis or an upper respiratory tract infection. (Wind-cold and wind-heat can pass down the Eustachian tube.)

Chronic otitis media is usually caused by a lingering pathogenic factor, which is easily established when frequent attacks of otitis are treated with antibiotics. Alternatively, the lingering pathogenic factor can be traced to an immunization, commonly the pertussis vaccine. Rarely, chronic otitis media is caused by yin deficiency.

PATTERN DIFFERENTIATION

The treatment of otitis media is, from the acupuncturist's point of view, quite straightforward, especially in the acute condition. This is because otitis media is regarded as a channel problem. Heat, cold, and/or dampness enter the channels of the ear—Triple Burner and Gallbladder—and obstruct the flow of qi in the ear. These pathogenic factors may stem from a *zàng fǔ* (organ) disharmony, and this will obviously need to be cleared eventually. However, to stop the pain, one need simply regulate the qi in the channels. Therefore, the choice of points is straightforward.

The diagnosis, however, is complicated by the fact that it is often hard to differentiate the patterns, since they can blend into each other. This is especially true in acute cases. For example, a young angry child is much more likely to suffer an external invasion of a pathogenic factor. Similarly, a child who is unwell is much more likely to be irritable. A child with accumulation disorder is predisposed to either an external pathogenic attack or Liver and Gallbladder damp-heat, both of which can

---

*The differentiation of patterns in this chapter is for Western children. Previously, it was thought that an ear infection had to be a hot disease. We are now seeing many children with cold symptoms.

cause otitis media and are often difficult to distinguish in the acute situation.

Fortunately for acupuncturists, an accurate diagnosis is not always necessary in order to relieve the symptoms and the pain. However, once the acute condition has passed, you should make an accurate diagnosis in order to effect a lasting cure and prevent the problem from returning.

In chronic otitis media differentiation is often straightforward, but the treatment can take a long time, depending on the severity of the condition. The child may suffer acute attacks during the course of treatment, causing minor setbacks if they are treated with antibiotics.

Listed below are the key points used in the differentiation of otitis media.

Acute vs. chronic

Chronic otitis media is defined here as a more or less permanent earache, or as earaches that return frequently. Acute otitis media is an actual inflammation of the ear, with the child usually in great pain.

Serous (nonsuppurative) vs. suppurative

The serous type often has little or no discharge from the ears or nose, and if there is a discharge, it is clear and watery. By contrast, the suppurative type always has a thick, yellow discharge, often foul-smelling. From a traditional Chinese medical point of view, the suppurative type is basically similar to the serous type, with the additional complication of a systemic build-up of phlegm-dampness.

External cause vs. internal cause

The external cause is wind-heat or wind-cold, with or without dampness obstructing the ear cavities. The internal cause stems from heat or damp-heat, either from the digestion or the Liver, which enters the channel and causes obstruction. In practice, many acute attacks have both an internal and an external factor. With this knowledge, the practitioner must decide on the proper course of treatment.

In diagnosing a child with acute or recurrent attacks, the area surrounding the ear should be palpated for tenderness and for swollen glands. The otoscope is useful in determining the severity of the condition and in assessing the progress of treatment.

Deficient or Excessive?

Acute otitis media is, by definition, a condition of excess by virtue of the fact that it is caused by a pathogenic factor: wind, cold, heat, or dampness. Therefore, a dispersing needle technique is used. However, it can occur in deficient- or excess-type children alike. It may be necessary to tonify the qi after an attack in deficient children to prevent it from recurring. Chronic otitis media is either a deficient disorder or a combination of excess and deficiency. Some tonification must therefore be done.

Hot or Cold?

Acute otitis media can manifest as a hot or a cold disorder. In the Chinese texts that we have consulted, it is defined as a hot, inflammatory condition. The hot condition arises from an invasion of wind-heat, or wind-cold which transforms into wind-heat. We have found, however, that this does not always fit in with our observations of Western children. Many children will present with a cold condition where the child has obvious ear pain but no heat signs at all. This occurs when the child has an underlying cold disorder, usually cold-phlegm (often from a cold lingering pathogenic factor). On top of this, there is an invasion of wind-cold. The cold enters the channels of the ear and causes pain. When you see otitis media with no signs of heat, moxibustion can be used with great effect.

It is fair to say that from an acupuncturist's point of view, it is less important to make the distinction between hot and cold. For example, TB-5 *(wai guan)* is used in the treatment of acute otitis media regardless of whether it is hot or cold in origin.

Chronic otitis media may also manifest as hot or cold, depending on whether the lingering pathogenic factor is hot or cold, and on the diet of the child.

We begin our discussion with acute otitis media, followed by chronic otitis media.

ACUTE OTITIS MEDIA

Patterns

• external attack of wind-heat or wind-cold
• Liver and Gallbladder heat

These patterns may combine with dampness into new patterns:

• external attack of wind-heat or wind-cold plus dampness
• Liver and Gallbladder damp-heat

Although the syndrome is called Liver and Gallbladder heat, it would probably be better to call it 'heat enters the Liver and Gallbladder channels' because this is a channel disorder. It can result from a dysfunction of the organ; if the organ is weak, then the channel will not be strong.

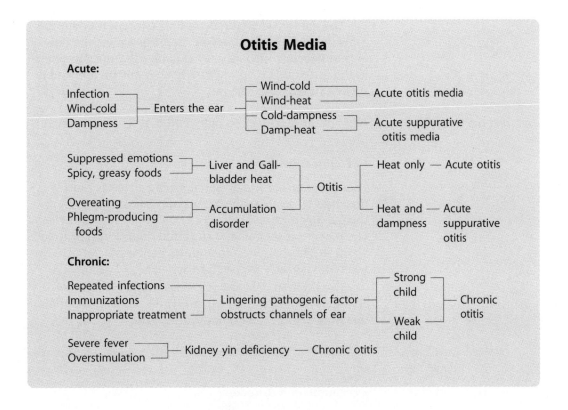

Otitis Media

Acute:

Infection
Wind-cold
Dampness
— Enters the ear —

Wind-cold
Wind-heat
— Acute otitis media

Cold-dampness
Damp-heat
— Acute suppurative
otitis media

Suppressed emotions
Spicy, greasy foods
— Liver and Gall-
bladder heat

Overeating
Phlegm-producing
foods
— Accumulation
disorder

— Otitis —

Heat only — Acute otitis

Heat and — Acute
dampness suppurative
otitis

Chronic:

Repeated infections
Immunizations
Inappropriate treatment
— Lingering pathogenic factor
obstructs channels of ear —

Strong
child

Weak
child
— Chronic
otitis

Severe fever
Overstimulation
— Kidney yin deficiency — Chronic otitis

Etiology & Pathogenesis

External invasion of wind-heat or wind-cold

Invasion of an external pathogenic factor can have many causes. The two most common are:

• getting cold after swimming or after washing the hair
• being in a cold wind

It is possible for the pathogenic factor to transfer from another place in the body—most commonly an upper respiratory tract infection—to the ear. In some children the external cold transforms into heat, while in others the cold remains cold. In both cases the external pathogenic factor blocks the circulation of qi and causes pain.

External invasion of wind-heat or wind-cold plus dampness

The common causes for an invasion of an external pathogenic factor are outlined above. The dampness usually comes from:

• diet: too many greasy, spicy foods, or too many dairy products
• antibiotics
• accumulation disorder in younger children

In theory, external damp-heat can invade the ear. While this rarely happens in the United Kingdom, it may in warmer and more humid climates.

The dampness accumulates in the interior. When the ear is invaded by a pathogenic factor, as above, the flow of qi is impaired, which causes the pain. Also, the dampness in the interior rises up to cause further obstruction and a sticky exudate from the ear.

Liver and Gallbladder heat

This condition is seen in older children. The heat comes from:

• Liver qi constraint

There is often some emotional problem that is causing the child to become upset. This may not be obvious; even the parents may be unaware of it! The problem, for example, may be at school, and the child does not want to talk about it. This pattern also appears in "pushy" families, where the child is expected to achieve.

The internal heat enters the Liver and Gallbladder channels and rises up to the ear. The heat obstructs the free flow of qi in the ear and causes pain.

Liver and Gallbladder damp-heat

In younger children, the source of the heat and dampness is:

• accumulation disorder

The cause is therefore an inappropriate diet, feeding schedule, and the like. The heat and dampness find their way to the Liver and Gallbladder channels, rising up to the ear and causing pain.

In older children, the heat is caused by:

• Liver qi constraint

The damp aspect most commonly comes from:

• diet
• antibiotics
• lingering pathogenic factor

It is common to see this type of otitis media as an acute flare-up in cases of chronic otitis media.

Internal dampness and heat enter the Liver and Gallbladder channels and rise up to the ear where they collect and form pus. Both the dampness and the heat obstruct the flow of qi in the ear and cause pain.

Signs & Symptoms

External invasion of wind-heat or wind-cold

The onset is sudden, usually with an easily recognized reason: getting cold after swimming, going out in the rain. The pain is often excruciating, and the child will be screaming in agony. There are other signs of an external attack, such as fever, aversion to cold, and sweating, depending on whether the condition is wind-heat or wind-cold in origin.

You can also see this condition while the child has another infection, commonly an upper respiratory tract infection, as the pathogenic factor can find its way into the ear. There are no special characteristics to distinguish children who suffer from an attack of this kind: it can happen to excess- or deficient-type children, happy or sad children.

- ear feels stuffed up
- pain in the ear
- some hearing loss
- possibly tinnitus
- headache
- aversion to cold or wind
- possibly upper respiratory tract infection
- nasal discharge

Depending on whether the condition is caused by heat or cold:

- fever (high or low)
- sweating, if due to wind-heat

Pulse: if wind-heat, floating, or floating and rapid; if wind-cold, tight, or tight and floating

Treatment principle: expel wind, release the exterior, and regulate the qi in the ear cavity

External invasion of wind-heat or wind-cold plus dampness

This pattern is the same as the one above with the added factor of dampness. The dampness is of internal origin. Hence, these children have *signs of dampness* prior to and during the attack, for example, runny nose or productive cough. The symptoms are thus the same as those above, plus:

- pus in the ear: sticky, milky, white, or yellowish
- usually signs of dampness and phlegm elsewhere in the body
- accumulation disorder in younger children

Tongue coating: thin
Pulse: floating and slippery, or tight

Treatment principle: expel the wind and release the exterior, resolve the dampness, and regulate the qi in the ear cavity

Liver and Gallbladder heat

This generally occurs in older children. The heat comes from Liver qi constraint, usually due to constrained emotions. These children are typically cross, bad-tempered, and irritable. It usually occurs more in excess-type children, but it can occur in the deficient-type as well, in which case they hide their irritability and are anxious to please. Symptoms include:

• inner ear distended and full
• possibly the ear drum is bleeding
• possibly some fluid in the ear
• often very painful
• diminished hearing
• headache with swollen feeling, pressure, dizziness, or burning sensation

Tongue body: red
Tongue coat: yellow
Pulse: wiry, rapid, or slippery

Treatment principle: clear heat from the Liver and Gallbladder channels and regulate the qi in the ear cavity

Liver and Gallbladder damp-heat

This occurs in both young and older children. In younger children the cause of both the heat and dampness tends to be accumulation disorder; hence, they will show all the typical signs of this disorder.

In older children there is some Liver qi constraint plus dampness in the system, usually attributable to the diet. Once again, the older children tend to be irritable and quick tempered. Often there are signs of dampness before the attack, such as a productive cough or catarrh. Symptoms include:

• yellow pus in ear
• signs of phlegm and dampness in the body
• inflammation that does not subside
• headache
• ear region is swollen and painful
• ear drum bleeding
• mastoid process is mildly painful
• possibly wind signs
• possibly vomiting and twitching

Tongue: greasy, yellow
Pulse: wiry, slippery

If there is accumulation disorder:

• smelly, vile stools
• red cheeks
• green nasal discharge

Treatment principle: clear heat from the Liver and Gallbladder channels, resolve dampness, clear heat and regulate qi in the ear cavity; if necessary, clear accumulation disorder

Treatment

The main points for the treatment of acute otitis media are on the *shao yang* channels of the hands and feet. The ear is encircled by the hand *shao yang* (Triple Burner) channel, and secondary channels pass through the ear from TB-17 *(yi feng)* and G-20 *(feng chi)*. You can, therefore, use:

TB-5 *(wai guan)*	Expels wind and regulates the channel
TB-17 *(yi feng)*	Expels wind and benefits the ear
G-41 *(zu lin qi)*	Regulates the Liver and Gallbladder
G-20 *(feng chi)*	Expels wind and regulates the Liver and Gallbladder
G-2 *(ting hui)*	Local point for otitis media

Method: TB-5 *(wai guan)* and G-41 *(zu lin qi)* are needled to a depth of 0.5 to 1 unit, and the sensation should travel upward along the limb and toward the head. For children under the age of three, these distal points usually suffice. They also cause less distress than the local points. The angle of insertion at G-20 *(feng chi)* is slightly lateral in order to direct the sensation to the ear. TB-17 *(yi feng)* is needled to a depth of 1 unit. G-2 *(ting hui)* may be needled to a depth of 1.5 units, but for conditions of excess it is usually sufficient to needle to a depth of 0.5 units. The sensation should radiate to the inner ear and is usually rather painful. This is because the qi of the ear is stuck, owing to the presence of the pathogenic factor. As you remove this obstruction, it causes temporary, but sharp, pain. We have found that, for most cases, needling the points on the infected side only is sufficient.

The following combination will bring quick relief:

TB-17 *(yi feng)*
LI-4 *(he gu)*

Use a moxibustion stick at TB-17 *(yi feng)* if there are no signs of heat.

If there are signs of heat, use:

GV-14 *(da zhui)*
LI-4 *(he gu)*
LI-11 *(qu chi)*

If there are signs of cold, use moxibustion around the ear if you can. We suggest you try:

CV-12 *(zhong wan)* with moxa

Prognosis: it is not uncommon for the pain to subside with-in minutes. In young children and babies, one treatment using distal points will usually be enough. The child will break into a sweat, fall asleep, and be cured. In older chil-dren, a series of three treatments during the same day may be necessary to reduce the pain.

External wind-heat or wind-cold invasion plus dampness

Use the same points as you would for the previous pattern, plus:

G-34 *(yang ling quan)*	Transforms dampness in the *shao yang* channel

If the dampness is chronic in nature, add:

S-40 *(feng long)*	Resolves dampness and phlegm
Sp-6 *(san yin jiao)*	Tonifies the Spleen, resolves dampness

Prognosis: one or two treatments are usually enough, although it may take more in stubborn cases

Liver and Gallbladder heat

The main points listed above are usually sufficient. Some sources substitute TB-3 *(zhong shu)* for TB-5 *(wai guan)* and G-40 *(qiu xu)* for G-41 *(zu lin qi)*. Other sources recommend using all four points.

Prognosis: this pattern is common among older children and may take three to five treatments to cure. If the pain is very strong, first treat two to three times a day, and then daily. If a deficient-type child comes to you with this pattern and the pulse is wiry—that is to say, a deficient child with an excess pulse—the prognosis is less favorable.

Liver and Gallbladder damp-heat

Use the main points until the pain subsides, and then add:

G-34 *(yang ling quan)*	Clears Liver and Gallbladder damp-heat, resolves dampness and phlegm
Liv-13 *(zhang men)*	Transforms dampness
Sp-9 *(yin ling quan)*	Resolves dampness

If there is accumulation disorder, add:

si feng (M-UE-9)	Clears accumulation disorder

Prognosis: while any pain that accompanies this problem is reduced quickly (usually after the first treatment), the main problem (pus) is usually rather slow to change. If the child is treated daily, there may be no appreciable reduction in the pus until after the third or fourth treatment. Eight to ten treatments are generally sufficient. For the first two or three treatments, combine a local point with a distal point.

This is very effective in bringing the qi to the ear.

If the child is clearly under emotional stress, the condition will most likely return. Acupuncture can still be of great help, as you can add points like Liv-3 *(tai chong)* to regulate the qi. Doing this can often give the child enough resolve to sort out the problems, or at least come to terms with them.

Other Remedies

There are other remedies that are useful to know about. They can be given to the parent to take home, or, if you are phoned in the middle of the night, they can be offered for temporary relief until the child can be seen.

- The patent herbal formula Cattle Gallstone Pill to Relieve Toxicity *(niu huang jie du pian)* should be considered in an acute attack. It has an almost immediate effect in calming the pain.

- The essential oils of lavender and chamomile can be put in a teaspoon of warm olive oil and gently poured in the ear. Use two to three drops of essential oil per teaspoon.

- Optrex (or any other proprietary eye lotion) is soothing if the ear is very hot and inflamed because it relieves inflammation in mucous membranes. Soak cotton wool in it and drip it into the ear. (Although these lotions are marketed primarily for eye problems, their function is to soothe inflamed mucous membranes, so they are good for the ear too.)

- If there is a cold disorder in the ear, use ginger compresses. You will know for certain if it is a cold disorder, for if so, the ginger will be very soothing.

- You can use a small slither of garlic—not too big or too small—taped over the ear. First, place some cotton wool over it, and leave it there for an hour or so. This is useful only for a wind-cold disorder.

Antibiotics and Acupuncture

Many of the children you see will either be on, or will have recently had, a course of antibiotics. Even if this is the case, it is still helpful to treat the child. Not only will the cure be that much quicker (antibiotics do not always help), but if antibiotics have been used in the treatment of otitis media, then acupuncture can be used to prevent the ensuing buildup of dampness.

CHRONIC OTITIS MEDIA

Chronic otitis media is defined here as more or less continuous earache, usually with discharge, with periods of acute flare-ups. From the Chinese medical point of view, chronic otitis media also includes recurrent ear infections, such as monthly infections. We also consider 'glue ear' (chronic secretory otitis media) under the heading of chronic otitis media.

Patterns

There are three patterns:

- lingering pathogenic factor with much phlegm (excess disorder)
- Spleen qi deficiency with an underlying lingering pathogenic factor (excess disorder with a basis of deficiency)
- Liver and Kidney yin deficiency (deficiency disorder)

The first two patterns are by far the most common; the third, yin deficiency, is hardly ever seen. The first two patterns can present as either predominantly cold or predominantly hot.

Etiology & Pathogenesis

Lingering pathogenic factor

This pattern is caused by:

- immunizations, especially the pertussis immunization
- treatment of acute otitis media with antibiotics

The original pathogenic factor—be it from an immunization or an acute attack of otitis media—is not completely cleared from the body. The presence of the lingering pathogenic factor produces much phlegm, which obstructs the flow of qi in the ear cavity, causing pain and discomfort. Since the qi is weak locally in the area of the ear, the ear is much more prone to acute flare-ups, either from external attacks or internal disharmony.

There are two disorders here, one hot and the other cold. They both can arise from the same factors; it depends on how the child reacts to the cause. For example, one child who has had the DPT immunization may get masses of thick and cold phlegm in the system: a cold lingering pathogenic factor. Usually, there is a chronic, underlying cold disorder as a result of a cold diet or repeated use of antibiotics. This child will tend to get the cold type of chronic otitis media.

Another child may have a tendency toward heat in the system, perhaps due to a history of accumulation disorder. In this case, the immunization will produce a tendency toward the hot type of otitis media.

These children are not especially deficient in energy; it's just that the whole system is clogged up with thick phlegm. It is possible for these children to throw off the lingering pathogenic factor themselves through one of the childhood illnesses. For example, during an attack of whooping cough the thick phlegm associated with the lingering pathogenic factor may be expelled from the body. However, most children are immunized against this disease, and they need the help of acupuncture, herbs, or homeopathy to expel any lingering pathogenic factor.

Spleen qi deficiency plus lingering pathogenic factor

The Spleen qi becomes depleted for the reasons explained in Chapter 3. In addition, here there is a lingering pathogenic factor. This is commonly caused by immunizations or the frequent use of antibiotics. The symptoms are worse when the child is:

• exhausted
• pushed too hard at school
• under emotional stress

As with the previously described pattern of lingering pathogenic factor, this disorder can present as either hot or cold, depending on the child, the diet, and the nature of the lingering pathogenic factor. The pathological process is the same as described above, except that there is the added problem of the qi being weak. This means that these children do not have sufficient qi to throw off the lingering pathogenic factor. In them, the phlegm is less a problem than the qi deficiency. Since the whole qi system is weak, the child is much more prone to invasion from external pathogenic factors, which usually attack the ear. In addition, recurrent coughs and colds are a feature of this type of otitis media.

Liver and Kidney yin deficiency

• high fever depleting the yin

The Liver and Kidney yin are deficient, which deprives the ear of the nourishment from the essence. With the introduction of antibiotics this is rarely seen nowadays, but it is becoming more common in older children who:

• work on computers
• watch video games and television all day

These activities seem to deplete the Kidney yin. Such children also tend to be slightly hyperactive. Hence, the

condition can get slowly worse as they do not allow themselves the rest that is essential to cure this condition.

Signs & Symptoms

In general, the symptoms are:

- tinnitus
- deafness
- middle ear is full and packed
- examination shows a distended eardrum

Lingering pathogenic factor

- main symptom may be hearing loss
- continuous feeling of pressure (a bursting, distended sensation) in the middle ear
- ear feels blocked, and, on examination, one or both eardrums may be bleeding or discharging fluid
- child may not complain of pain unless the ear is palpated
- possibly nosebleed
- possibly nose and throat inflammation
- swollen glands
- often has recurrent attacks of otitis media

Pulse: slippery

Treatment principle: resolve the phlegm, regulate the qi of the ear, and eliminate the lingering pathogenic factor

Spleen qi deficiency plus lingering pathogenic factor

- inner ear is swollen and bursting
- eardrum is gray or white in color
- often is lazy, has little strength, and is easily discouraged
- mouth and lips are pale
- limbs thin and weak
- poor appetite
- swollen glands

Tongue: pale
Pulse: weak

Treatment principle: tonify the qi and eliminate the lingering pathogenic factor; resolve phlegm as it appears

In cases of both lingering pathogenic factor and Spleen qi deficiency, the pattern may be either hot or cold in nature. If it is cold, you will then see:

- pale face
- cold-type abdominal pain

Pulse: tight and full

If it is hot, you will see:

• irritability and restlessness
• red face, or red cheeks

Pulse: rapid

Liver and Kidney yin deficiency

• dizziness
• sticky fluid on the eardrum
• possibly a sore back
• tends to be hyperactive in the evening
• may have history of febrile disease
• possibly watches a lot of television and/or video games
• possibly red cheeks

Tongue body: red
Pulse: fine, rapid

Treatment principle: tonify Liver and Kidney yin

Treatment

The treatment of chronic otitis media is aimed at regulating the qi of the channels around the ear. In order to do so successfully, you must resolve the lingering pathogenic factor. So, although some of the points may be the same as those used in treating acute otitis media, you must add others to treat the underlying condition.

Distal points are more commonly used than local points, except when the qi in the ear has been severely depleted. You must then use local points for one or two treatments to draw qi to the area.

Main points

TB-5 *(wai guan)*	Expels wind and regulates the channel
TB-17 *(yi feng)*	Expels wind and benefits the ear
G-41 *(zu lin qi)*	Regulates the Liver and Gallbladder
G-20 *(feng chi)*	Expels wind and regulates the Liver and Gallbladder
G-2 *(ting hui)*	Local point for otitis media

Lingering pathogenic factor

Use the main points, plus:

bai lao (M-HN-30)	Clears the lingering pathogenic factor (point located 2 units superior to GV-14 *(da zhui)* and 1 unit lateral to the spine)
B-18 *(gan shu)*	Regulates the Liver and Gallbladder, and moves the blood and qi

| B-20 *(pi shu)* | Regulates the Spleen, moves the blood and qi, and transforms the dampness |

Method: either needling or moxibustion may be used at these points. Local points are important if the qi in the ear is very weak, which occurs with a long-standing lingering pathogenic factor.

Prognosis: clearing the body completely of the pathogenic factor may take ten to twenty treatments (see discussion of lingering pathogenic factors in Chapter 3). After the first few treatments there are often signs of catarrh, such as cough and nasal discharge, as the thick, clogged phlegm that has accumulated in the channels begins to soften. This process can be considerably accelerated by the use of herbs such as poke root *(Phytolacca decandra)* and blue flag *(Iris versicolor)*, but there is no substitute for acupuncture in bringing the qi to the ears. To effect a complete cure, two or three months of weekly treatment are usually required, even if herbs and acupuncture are combined. More frequent treatment will not significantly hasten the cure, for it simply takes time for this kind of change to take place.

Spleen qi deficiency plus lingering pathogenic factor

Local points are often needed here in the beginning stages of treatment to bring the qi to the ears. Points to use include:

| TB-17 *(yi feng)* | Regulates qi in the ears |
| G-2 *(ting hui)* | Regulates qi in the ears |

In addition, add the following governing *(shu)* points on the back to tonify the qi so that the lingering pathogenic factor can be expelled:

| B-18 *(gan shu)* | Tonifies Liver and Spleen |
| B-20 *(pi shu)* | Tonifies Liver and Spleen |

Additional points that tonify the qi and resolve dampness include:

S-36 *(zu san li)*	Tonifies qi
Sp-6 *(san yin jiao)*	Tonifies qi and resolves dampness
CV-12 *(zhong wan)*	Tonifies the Spleen

Method: moxibustion is useful at the governing *(shū)* points and at CV-12 *(zhong wan)*

Prognosis: treat two to three times a week, if possible; if you cannot, then once a week will still produce good results, but obviously takes longer. Fifteen-plus treatments are usually required, depending on the strength of the child. As you treat, the child will get stronger and start to expel the phlegm associated with the lingering pathogenic factor. This is a good sign!

Liver and Kidney yin deficiency

Acupuncture is not really the treatment of choice here. You can do moxibustion at B-23 *(shen shu)* as well as massage along the Triple Burner channel in the direction of the ear.

Once the Kidney energy is stronger, you will be able to use needles. Use the main points, plus:

B-18 *(gan shu)*
B-23 *(shen shu)*
Liv-3 *(tai chong)*
K-3 *(tai xi)*
} Tonifies the Liver and Kidney yin

Prognosis: this condition is uncommon in children except after febrile diseases, when a few treatments will suffice provided that the child is eating normally. If the condition occurs without a history of febrile disease, it is essential to ascertain the cause of the deficient yin. If the child is addicted to computer games or some other form of stimulation, it may be difficult to cure.

NOTES

• Acute attacks of otitis media are often treated with antibiotics. If such treatments are given repeatedly, they can lead to a buildup of dampness. After an acute attack of otitis media has been treated successfully (with either acupuncture or antibiotics), it is a good idea to give further treatments to resolve the remaining dampness.

• In all cases of otitis media, the patient should avoid red meat and spicy, fried, or other warming foods. If dampness is present, the patient should also avoid eggs, cheese, milk, peanuts, and sugar.

• During the treatment of chronic otitis media, tonsillitis sometimes develops, as the toxins drain away from the ear into the throat. This is usually short-lived and is an indication that the treatment is working (see Chapter 23 for treatment of tonsillitis).

• If attacks of acute otitis seem to recur every month, one may suspect a lingering pathogenic factor from a pertussis immunization.

- The Western medical treatment for recurrent catarrhal otitis and hearing loss is to insert small tubes (grommets) in the ear. This can usually be avoided by timely acupuncture treatment, provided it begins three months before the date of the proposed surgery. Some recent research has shown that children with recurrent otitis media who undergo this operation are more likely to have hearing deficits later in life than those who do not undergo the operation.

- Otitis media is overdiagnosed. If a child is irritable and out of sorts, it is very likely to get this diagnosis.

- For case histories involving otitis media, see Cases 23 and 24 in Chapter 47.

❖

26 ❖ Hay Fever

INTRODUCTION

The material in this chapter is based on our experience and observations. It therefore reflects what we have seen in the clinic and the way that we view hay fever. It is by no means a definitive account!

What Do We Mean by Hay Fever?

In the long-distant past, hay fever was a real fever that people got when they were making hay or were near others who were doing so. Over the years the meaning has changed, so that now it has come to mean allergic rhinitis that occurs in late spring and early summer. At least, that is the way we understand it, and that is the problem we will be discussing. Typical symptoms include:

- nasal congestion and irritation, with discharge
- sneezing
- red and watery eyes

Often there is also:

- difficulty in concentrating
- discharge of thick mucus
- headache
- photophobia

The onset is seasonal and is usually identified with pollen of various sorts, some people being more upset by grass pollens and others more by flowers and trees. For some people the sheer joy of seeing an old-fashioned meadow full of flowers is replaced by the sheer misery of hay fever. For some the effect is so violent that they have to stay indoors for a few weeks. Others have adopted drastic solutions like wearing a sort of space suit when they are outside, with a perspex pollen-free dome around their head!

Conventional Approach

In conventional Western medicine, hay fever is seen as an allergic histamine response to foreign bodies which attack the lining of the nasal cavity. The emphasis in this theory is on the external attacking agent, identifying the pollen as an outside invading force.

There are two types of treatments: desensitization treatments and antihistamines. They both have drawbacks. The desensitizing treatment is quite variable in its results and can lead to anaphylactic shock; antihistamines make patients feel drowsy (see case history below). This, however, is all that is available, and many people would rather put up with the drowsiness than the intense irritation of hay fever.

Traditional Chinese Medical Approach

The emphasis in traditional Chinese medicine is on internal factors. Although the hay fever appears at a certain time of year, it is related more to the time of the year than to the pollen which happens to be around at that time. In fact, the time of onset—both the time of year and the age of the children who most likely develop hay fever—provide the key to its etiology and pathogenesis.

Time of year

The time of year when people develop hay fever, late spring to early summer, is characterized by a change in temperature from cold to hot. The hottest days have not yet been reached, and the average temperature is still increasing. In this book, we have encountered seasonal problems before in discussing spring fevers, which are often a manifestation of latent heat. Latent heat is more of a problem when there is a Liver imbalance, leading to difficulty in adapting to changes in the weather. The onset of hay fever is also a manifestation of some kind of latent heat, either simple seasonal latent heat or heat from a long-standing lingering pathogenic factor.

Time of life

Hay fever is rarely seen in children under seven years of age, and this is an important clue, for this is the age when the emotions develop and become controllable (see Chapter 43 for a discussion of stages of development). This is, therefore, the age when the stagnation of Liver qi first appears. Before this age there is little in the way of restraint of emotions, and so the incidence of hay fever is very small. In our clinic we have seen hay fever only once in a child under seven years of age, and that was a five-year-old child who already had nasal discharge. The discharge was made slightly worse when the pollen count was extremely high.

This relationship between hay fever and the Liver is confirmed by the Chinese medical texts, which mention damp-heat in the Liver and Gallbladder as one of the patterns. It is also confirmed by observing people with hay fever. Above all, one gets from them a feeling of irritation and frustration. Something, or some*one* (other than simply pollen), is obviously "getting up their nose"!

PATTERNS & SYMPTOMS

It must be understood that there is *always* some heat accumulating in the nose and that there is *always* some stagnation of Liver qi from repressed emotions. With that in mind, one can distinguish the following patterns:

- Liver yang rising
- lingering pathogenic factor
- Lung and Spleen qi deficiency (also hyperactive Spleen qi deficiency)

Each of these patterns may or may not be accompanied by phlegm-dampness (in this respect, it is similar to otitis media). Some adults also have the pattern of Lung and Kidney yin deficiency. This may also be a pattern for children, but we have not seen it in the clinic.

Apart from the general symptom of hay fever, one can distinguish the symptoms according to the patterns.

Liver yang rising

There are only two key symptoms here:

- frequently flies into a rage
- facial color may be red or white, but becomes purple when in a rage

Pulse: wiry

In an adult you would expect to see a purple tongue with a yellow coating, but you are unlikely to see this in a child. This pattern is often seen in redheads.

Lingering pathogenic factor

Again, there are really not many distinguishing features. The following will (nearly) always be seen:

- gray face

- swollen glands
- vacant look in eyes
- greasy skin
- may be rather aggressive
- sudden collapse of energy

Pulse: possibly slippery

Lung and Spleen qi deficiency

This is the familiar pattern of:

- white face
- droopy, cannot stand up straight
- probably poor appetite

Pulse: weak

TREATMENT

Main points

The following prescription is good for all types of hay fever. You may want to modify it for each patient, but it is a good starting point.

L-7 *(lie que)*	Tonifies the Lungs, clears phlegm, and opens the nose
LI-4 *(he gu)*	Benefits the nose and face
LI-20 *(ying xiang)*	Local point for nose and tonifies the Lungs

On the whole, children dislike being needled at LI-20 *(ying xiang)*. Some may put up with it, as being better than suffering from hay fever, but others will simply freak out. An alternative point (near the nose, rather than local) is:

GV-23 *(shang xing)*	Opens the nose

Additional points

There are two other points of special use:

G-39 *(xuan zhong)*	Benefits the nose and brings down Liver yang
Liv-3 *(tai chong)*	Regulates the Liver

These points are likely to be the main ones you will use during the hay fever season, when the main thrust of treatment is to relieve the symptoms. If you are treating before the season, then you will probably want to give more emphasis to the underlying patterns.

When to Treat

You can, of course, wait until the season starts and the child is streaming from the nose. Some families prefer to do it this way, especially if they are suspicious of alternative medicine in general and acupuncture in particular. Why treat for something that might not happen? they ask.

However, the best time to treat is during the month preceding the hay fever season. This is mid-springtime and is the ideal time to treat all Liver-related disorders. Often, two or three treatments at this time can make a huge difference in the severity of symptoms when the time comes. (If you are treating adults, you may need to start a bit earlier in the spring and give a few more treatments.)

Hay Fever and Influenza

As we saw at the beginning, one aspect of hay fever is latent heat, either in the form of an inadaptability to changes in the weather, or in the form of a lingering pathogenic factor. One of the surest ways of permanently clearing the problem is for the child to have a good fever in the spring and to get over it unassisted. In this way the suppressed heat can be burnt off, never to reappear. Sometimes this point of view can be explained to the parents, but more often than not we find that it is met with incredulity.

Does Acupuncture Cure It?

We are often asked if acupuncture can cure hay fever, and if so, what about the pollen, which every one knows is out there and is a serious problem for all mankind. The answer is yes, acupuncture can very often provide a complete cure. To be sure, the pollen will go on being there—hopefully, for millions of years—but acupuncture has the effect of reducing or eliminating the sensitivity of the body to the allergens.

❖

Case History: Liver Yang Rising

One does not normally think of Liver yang rising being a child's problem, but this child, a friend of the family, certainly had it. The first signs of it came when he was about six months old. At this time his rages were put down to 'colic'. Soon after, he started teething, a process which lasted for a year or two. During this time the rages were put down to 'teething'. Then at eighteen months they were put down to the 'terrible twos', and at about four years of age to 'preschool nerves'.

His tempers really were amazing, even from this young age. I think they probably were not helped by his mother, who felt quite helpless when he flew into a temper and did not know how to handle them. His rages at six or seven years were truly spectacular, according to his parents. He would shout and scream and kick and hit the floor. We did not actually ever see one, but more than once we came to the house and heard a sound like the kitchen scene in Alice in Wonderland: all scream-ing and shouting from both parents and children. Of course, the appearance of someone else took their mind off what they were doing, and so we never actually saw these rages.

But we did see them when the child was about nine of ten years old. They were spectacular. He normally had a pale face with bright ginger hair (always a dangerous combination). What happened was this:

-His mother criticized him.

-He replied.

-An argument developed.

-The argument escalated into all-out shouting.

-Then, suddenly, rage and fury enveloped him. His face went purple, his eyes bulged, and he held his breath in fury. He was paroxysmal with rage and quite unable to breathe. He stayed in this state for about thirty seconds, until he passed out and fell on the floor. This enabled him to relax and breathe, and he soon came back to consciousness.

When he came round like this he felt much better. He would quite calmly pick himself up and go off and do something constructive, as though nothing had happened (although the adults around needed a stiff drink to steady their nerves!)

The first onset of hay fever that he had was at about eight years of age. At first it was mild, but as the years progressed it became really very severe: he could not even go outside on fine dry days in the season.

He did come to me (JPS) for treatment, but he hated the needles and hated being treated by me, a friend of his parents. Moreover, I was unable to do anything about the special relationship that he had with his mother. For some reason which I could never fathom, they just set each other off. The slightest criticism by one would be taken the wrong way by the other, who would then reply with some acid and biting remark. Two or three full scale arguments a day were the norm during school holidays!

The problem of the arguments (and also of the hay fever symptoms) were reduced a bit when the mother took a "good parenting" course. But still, the incompatibility is there, and he still gets hay fever.

27 ❖ Insomnia and Night Terrors

INTRODUCTION

Insomnia and screaming at night is a very common problem. It is also one which frequently brings parents to the clinic, since the screams of their children wake them up and tire them out as well. Western medicine has some answers in the form of narcotics, but these are not suitable for all patterns of this disorder, and may cause the child to be dull-witted during the day.

We have found that acupuncture is extremely effective in treating insomnia and night terrors in children, more so than any other therapy we have encountered. We also consider it an important problem to treat because a child needs to sleep well in order to thrive. If the sleep is continually disturbed, then it is likely that the child will become weaker in some respect to the point where they may develop additional illnesses. Similarly, if the child is otherwise ill, then it is unlikely to get better without adequate sleep.

There are four basic patterns of insomnia and night terrors which will be discussed here.

Spleen cold (excess, or excess with underlying deficiency)

The common factor with all of these children is that they have cold digestion, that is, the Spleen is cold. This means that food is not easily digested and accumulates in the Intestines. There are many causes, but by far the most common is eating too many cold foods, especially bananas and cow's milk. Moreover, the diet need not necessarily be cold, it may just be inappropriate—too many rough foods, for example. If the digestion were alright or hot, then this sort of diet would lead to accumulation disorder, but because the Spleen is cold, it leads instead to a cold type of stagnation which causes the child to wake with colicky pain, clenching its fists and grinding its teeth. Other causes of a cold Spleen are taking cold medicines, or the use of anesthetics in childbirth. This is a disorder of excess in that there is cold from excess in the Intestines; it is thus frequently seen in excess-type children. However, it can also be seen in deficient-type children when they come down with cold from excess.

Obstructed heat in the Heart channel (interior heat from excess)

These children cannot sleep because there is heat from excess in the body. This causes them to be restless during sleep, and often to wake early as well. When they do wake up, they are wide awake. The heat can come from many sources, the most common of which are accumulation disorder from overfeeding, or feeding inappropriate foods, eating excessively heating foods (spicy, greasy), and a lingering pathogenic factor from immunization or illness, or from the mother during pregnancy. Treatment is similar in all cases, but the cause should be identified for there to be a lasting cure.

Fright (interior heat from excess)

Although children are easily frightened by events they see (and sometimes events that they alone see, such as lions on top of the wardrobe), their fright is usually discharged with a loud cry, which brings comfort from their parents. The fright that causes problems is of a type that is not, or cannot be, expressed. For example, a child may not appear to react at all to some frightening situation, such as a car accident; or a child in the womb is unable to express the fright that is transmitted to it when the mother herself suffers a shock. Exactly why this happens has no clear explanation; it is similar to unexpressed anger, which can also harm the physical body. This pattern, while usually a result of such a shock, can also be caused by constant overstimulation, for example, watching too much television or playing too many computer games, or living in a very tense and high-strung family. These children wake at night with nightmares, screaming and frightened.

Qi and blood deficiency (interior deficiency)

Although this pattern is referred to as blood deficiency in Chinese textbooks, it also includes Spleen qi deficiency and Heart qi deficiency. The blood deficiency is considered to be the most important aspect because restlessness of the spirit is attributed to a failure of the blood in nourishing the Heart. Another aspect of this pattern is that it involves the Liver, since the blood should return to that organ during sleep. Clinically, blood deficiency may be due to a prolonged illness, actual hemorrhage, or anemia. But it may also occur as an effect of deficient qi: even though there is no blood deficiency per se, not enough blood reaches the Heart to nourish the spirit. These children wake many times in the night. They will often drink a little and then fall asleep for a couple of hours before waking again.

ETIOLOGY & PATHOGENESIS

Spleen cold

The Spleen is the central yin organ. It is extremely yin, and has an affinity to warmth and an aversion to cold. In young children, cold can easily invade the middle burner; in addition, the Spleen qi is often weak. The night is a time of yin; since cold is a yin pathogenic factor, it readily overcomes the yang at night and causes obstruction. The cold obstruction gives rise to colicky pain, and the child awakes screaming.

Common causes include:

- much cold-energy food in the diet: bananas, yoghurt, ice cream
- use of anesthetics during childbirth, which depletes the qi of the baby, and is cooling to the Spleen
- use of 'cold' medicines, especially antibiotics

Obstructed heat in the Heart channel

Heat and fire in the body rise up and affect the Heart channel, causing insomnia. The heat can come from a variety of sources: diet, womb heat, immunizations, illness. The child usually does not wake crying, because it is the heat that causes the child to wake up. However, the heat affects the Heart and disturbs the spirit, so on waking, the child becomes easily frightened by the darkness of the room and will begin crying. Consequently, this pattern is helped by a night light: the child can wake, orient itself, and may then go back to sleep. Such children also tend to wake very early, around 5 A.M. They are wide awake and want to play, and will start to cry when no one else seems to be in a playful mood.

This pattern arises when the child becomes too hot, internally. Common causes include:

- accumulation disorder
- hot or greasy food in the diet
- lingering pathogenic factor that causes heat in the body; this may be the result of an immunization, for example, HIB or Pertussis, or it may be due to a hot illness that has never been cleared
- womb heat, which is to say, heat that is transmitted from the mother during pregnancy; it may be because the mother herself has a hot constitution, or because she ate heating foods during the pregnancy
- child has too little to drink

Fright

Children are easily frightened. Their Heart spirit is easily disturbed and becomes restless. The fright that we speak of here can be caused by something the child has imagined, or, more commonly, by a very real event like an accident, a traumatic experience, a sudden shock. When a child is frightened like this it "scatters" the five spirits *(shén)*. This is different from the fear that depletes the Kidney energy, which is more long term. The five spirits reside in the Heart and are related to the five elements. It is the Heart spirit in particular that is affected, hence the child will often have nightmares and wake up terrified in the middle of the night. However, you may also notice that such children are fearful (the water element is affected), they lack concentration (earth), and are tearful (metal). Fright is characteristically seen on the child's face as a blue hue between the eyes.

Other factors that shock the child, suddenly, and cause the five spirits to be scattered:

• mother experiences a shock while pregnant
• child sees something that frightens it; this is usually something quite awful; it is unlikely that this sleep pattern would become chronic after just being startled by a car starting, for example
• increasingly, overstimulation due to watching television and playing computer games; so-called "children's" television is often full of violence and frightening googly-eyed monsters, and some computer games are genuinely terrifying

Note: usually when a child has a fright, he or she will cry out and get immediate comfort from the parents. But sometimes the child does not react—it may be that it cannot: the accident may have happened to the mother while pregnant, or the event was so shocking that the child did not know how to react. In such cases there may be no mention of the incident by the parents.

Blood and qi deficiency

If the qi and the blood are deficient, the Heart will not be properly supported. The Heart spirit is then easily disturbed, and the child will wake up whimpering or crying. The child will wake often in the night because the qi and blood are weak, and the circulation of qi and blood normally slows down in the night anyway; thus, the child has to wake in order to get the qi moving again. For this reason, the child characteristically takes a small amount of food, and then goes back to sleep again with little trouble, only to wake up a couple hours later in order to move the qi and blood again. Another aspect of this condition is that the Liver is involved, as blood returns to the Liver at night.

This condition may arise from deficiency of both qi and blood, from deficiency of qi alone in failing to move the blood (which does not reach the Heart), and from deficiency of blood alone. It can therefore be caused by anything that depletes the qi or blood, including:

- long-term disease, anemia
- blood loss after an accident
- immunization
- difficult childbirth (e.g., long, or with the use of anesthetics)
- constitutional weakness
- deficiency of the mother during pregnancy: anemia, exhaustion, overwork

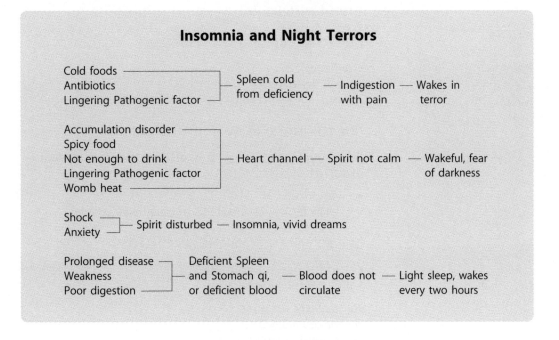

Insomnia and Night Terrors

Cold foods
Antibiotics
Lingering Pathogenic factor

— Spleen cold from deficiency — Indigestion with pain — Wakes in terror

Accumulation disorder
Spicy food
Not enough to drink
Lingering Pathogenic factor
Womb heat

— Heart channel — Spirit not calm — Wakeful, fear of darkness

Shock
Anxiety

— Spirit disturbed — Insomnia, vivid dreams

Prolonged disease
Weakness
Poor digestion

— Deficient Spleen and Stomach qi, or deficient blood — Blood does not circulate — Light sleep, wakes every two hours

PATTERNS & SYMPTOMS

Spleen cold

- wakes up because of pain, screaming
- goes to sleep easily, but wakes up terrified with colicky pain and arched back
- often wakes up crying
- pain may cause the child to sweat
- prefers to sleep lying face down
- clenched fists
- pale face
- cold limbs
- possibly poor appetite
- loose stools
- tongue and lips pale or white

Tongue coating: white
Pulse: deep, strong, and wiry or fine
Finger vein: dull red

Treatment principle: warm the Spleen and disperse the cold

Obstructed heat in the Heart channel

- prefers to sleep lying face up
- wakes in fear, but fear and crying is cured if there is a night light
- may have difficulty falling asleep, or may lie awake for several hours after midnight
- restless and irritable
- upon waking is wide awake, wanting to play
- urine possibly scanty and red
- possibly constipated
- face scarlet, lips red

DUE TO ACCUMULATION DISORDER

- red cheeks
- nasal discharge
- green, sour-smelling, or foul-smelling stools

DUE TO LINGERING PATHOGENIC HEAT

For example, after febrile convulsions, delirium, or immunizations:

- vivid dreams
- lives in fantasy world, talks to imaginary people

DUE TO WEAKNESS OF THE HEART ORGAN

- pain in chest on exertion
- blue complexion or lips

Tongue body: tip is red
Tongue coating: white
Pulse: rapid, forceful
Finger vein: dull purple (with lingering pathogenic heat)

Treatment principle: clear the heat and stop the terrors

Fright

- starts up in the middle of sleep
- wakes up frightened and is inconsolable
- at times has dread and fear, may fear going to sleep
- lips and face may be white or bluish
- often jumpy and nervous
- bluish color around eyes, or on bridge of nose
- cuddles close to mother (clinging)
- some history of fright and trauma

The pulse and tongue may show no signs, or the pulse may be wiry and rapid at night.

Treatment principle: control the fear and calm the spirit

Qi and blood deficiency

- pale face, listless
- often develops after an illness
- weak and feeble
- restless and irritable
- poor appetite
- can fall asleep, but wakes at regular intervals through the night, as frequently as every half hour

Tongue and lips: pale red or cherry red
Tongue body: tip is red
Tongue coating: little or no coating
Pulse: deficient, rapid

Treatment principle: nourish the Heart and calm the spirit

TREATMENT

Main point   H-7 *(shen men)* for all sleeping disorders

Spleen Cold

In addition to H-7 *(shen men),* use the points below.

For babies, add *si feng* (M-UE-9), and moxa at CV-12 *(zhong wan)* to tonify the Spleen qi and disperse the cold.

Method: textbooks recommend using a triangular needle at *si feng* (M-UE-9) to withdraw a few drops of clear yellow fluid. In practice, however, it is enough to simply needle the points.

For older children, the following groups of points are of service:

GROUP I

S-36 *(zu son li)*	Tonifies the Spleen qi
Sp-6 *(san yin jiao)*	Tonifies the Spleen qi
CV-12 *(zhong wan)*	Tonifies the Spleen qi and disperses the cold; use needling and indirect moxa, or only indirect moxa

GROUP II

Sp-4 *(gong sun)*	Regulates the qi in the abdomen
P-6 *(nei guan)*	and calms the spirit

Prognosis: usually one to three treatments are sufficient, but sometimes as many as ten treatments are required. Often the baby or child is quite irritable for up to twenty-four hours after treatment, and may have foul-smelling stools as the bad food is expelled. This may be accompanied by small red pimples on the cheeks, or sometimes on the body.

Advice: diet is important in the treatment of this pattern. Ensure that the child has no cold-energy foods, or the mother, if she is breast feeding.

Obstructed Heat in the Heart Channel

This pattern really encompasses three different patterns, each of which gives rise to heat in the Heart channel: accumulation disorder (food blockage giving rise to heat); lingering pathogenic heat from a febrile disease or immunization; and weakness of the Heart organ.

In addition to H-7 *(shen men)*, use the points set forth below.

Accumulation disorder

For babies, use *si feng* (M-UE-9) to clear the blockage from the Intestines.

For toddlers and children:

S-44 *(nei ting)*	Both points clear heat from the
LI-4 *(he gu)*	Stomach and Intestines
Liv-3 *(tai chong)*	Benefits digestion and clears heat
CV-12 *(zhong wan)*	Benefits digestion and clears heat

If the child is awake from 1 to 3 A.M., use B-18 *(gan shu)* and Liv-3 *(tai chong)*.

Prognosis: the symptoms are usually cleared in one to three treatments, with the same discharges described under the first pattern, but more violent. This pattern is often difficult to clear completely, and may recur at three to six month intervals if the child's digestion is weak, or if the child has a tendency to overeat. If the blockage is treated soon after each recurrence, the attacks will gradually diminish in severity as the child grows older.

Lingering pathogenic heat

The main point is P-8 *(lao gong)*, but many other points may be of service, especially H-7 *(shen men)*, SI-3 *(hou xi)*, and B-60 *(kun lun)*.

Prognosis: one to three treatments may be sufficient if the lingering pathogenic heat is of recent origin, but if the underlying febrile disease occurred long before, or if it is due to an immunization, then more treatments may be required.

Weakness of the Heart organ

The Heart should be strengthened, and the heat cleared, using such points as:

H-7 *(shen men)*	Calms the spirit and strengthens the Heart
P-6 *(nei guan)*	Both points tonify the Heart qi
B-15 *(xin shu)*	and regulate the Heart
K-3 *(tai xi)*	Indirectly clears heat from the Heart

Prognosis: the primary symptom of night terrors can usually be cured in six to eight treatments, but it may not be possible to cure organic heart lesions such as septal defects. In our experience, children with congenital heart defects usually have heat in the Heart, often accompanied by intense anger. It seems that these children have anger from before birth, and this disrupts the normal flow of qi in the chest.

Fright

The groups of points below are useful in calming the spirit.

GROUP I

P-6 *(nei guan)*
P-7 *(da ling)*
H-7 *(shen men)*

GROUP II

P-6 *(nei guan)*
B-15 *(xin shu)*
Sp-6 *(san yin jiao)*

Prognosis: one to three treatments are usually sufficient. The insomnia resulting from a shock can last many months, even years, if untreated. As a result of treatment, the heat is discharged through the Stomach and Intestines, and it is common to have symptoms such as diarrhea with sore anus, painful tongue and gums, nasal discharge, and irritability during the first few days following treatment.

Special treatment: search for small blisters in an area up to one inch on either side of the thoracic spine, and prick these with a triangular needle to withdraw a few drops of clear fluid. This fluid is thought to contain the toxin.

Qi and Blood Deficiency

This pattern encompasses Spleen and Stomach qi deficiency, as well as blood deficiency. The patient will appear to be weaker if suffering from the blood-deficient type.

S-36 *(zu san li)*	Both points tonify the Spleen and
CV-12 *(zhong wan)*	Stomach qi
CV-6 *(qi hai)*	Tonifies the qi of the entire body
Sp-6 *(san yin jiao)*	Tonifies the Spleen qi
GV-20 *(bai hui)*	Brings qi and blood to the head
H-6 *(yin xi)*	Regulates the circulation of blood and calms the spirit

Method: abdominal points should be treated with needles and indirect moxa, or indirect moxa alone. The tonifying method is used. When needling GV-20 *(bai hui)* on babies, take care to avoid the fontanel.

Prognosis: one to two treatments in mild cases, five to ten (or more) treatments if the child is really weak. In some cases the insomnia will appear to be cured after one treatment, but will recur a few days to a week later unless a full course of treatment is given.

NOTES

- There is a saying in Chinese medicine which is relevant to the first two patterns: "If the Stomach is not harmonized, then the mind will not be peaceful."

- The patterns presented in this chapter do appear quite frequently, but it is also common to have a mixture of patterns, as there may be more than one cause, for example, improper food as well as overstimulation. When such mixed patterns appear, the mother should be questioned carefully to identify the multiple causes.

- The child's pattern of sleep is often a reliable guide to the pathological pattern.

  Spleen cold from deficiency: crying before waking up, screaming the moment the child awakes

  Obstructed heat in the Heart channel: afraid of the dark, light sleep; no crying when child first awakes

  Fright: frightening dreams

  Qi and blood deficiency: wakes every hour or two at night; takes a little food or water and goes straight back to sleep

- For case histories involving insomnia and night terrors, see Cases 10, 21, and 22 in Chapter 47.

❖

28 ❖ Eczema in Infants and Young Children

INTRODUCTION

Eczema is one of the most common complaints that we see in the clinic. It is almost as if every child has had, at one time, some sort of itchy rash that has been described as eczema. It can range from a small area of the skin that itches, to the whole body itching, almost unbearably. In its worst form it can drive a child to distraction. The itching keeps it awake at night, and makes it miserable in the day. Children inevitably scratch the affected areas—sometimes so viciously that they tear at the skin, causing bleeding and making the skin red-raw.

For the acupuncturist the treatment of eczema is both easy and complicated. It is easy in that the theory is simple, and the choice of points needed is small. But it is complicated in that the results of treatment are variable, and it is often difficult to work out what is really going on and why. Some children respond very well, while others initially do well, then relapse or make no further improvement.

However, it is well worth treating because the possible relief that you can offer is incredible. In some cases the child will be totally cured, and in nearly all there will be some improvement in the symptoms. With regular treatment you can save a child from a life of misery: itching, scratching, sleepless nights, corticosteroid creams, oils, lotions, and scarred skin.

One of the problems in treating eczema is that the word itself is used to describe a wide variety of complaints. It can be temporary—an itchy rash starts after an illness, say, and passes— or it can be there virtually all the time; the child may even have been born with it. It can be confined to just a few areas—commonly the back of the legs, and in the creases of the arms—or it can spread to almost the entire body. As the condition becomes more serious the affected areas tend to spread, commonly to the wrists and ankles and down the legs and arms.

In its mildest form there may just be a roughening of the skin: instead of feeling soft and smooth, the skin feels like sandpaper. There are then varying degrees of severity as the skin becomes not just rough, but flaky as well, with a fine powder or small flakes coming off when the skin is rubbed.

The degree of discomfort varies as well. There may be no itching: it is just the concern of the parents that the condition *might* develop which provides the impetus for bringing the child for treatment. There may be a mild discomfort that comes and goes, and can be alleviated by various things such as moisturizers or proper diet. There may be almost continual itching and scratching through the day and night that drives the child to distraction and is not alleviated by anything except very powerful drugs, and then only temporarily.

Although this is a complete hodge podge of symptoms, the underlying cause of the condition in children tends to be straightforward. By asking simple questions about the diet, history of illness, quality of the rash, and so on, it is usually quite easy to make a diagnosis and to treat the underlying cause.

UNDERLYING FACTORS

The root cause of eczema is that the skin is not being properly nourished. It is said in Chinese medicine that the blood nourishes the skin; thus, for eczema to occur, there must be something preventing good circulation of blood—or preventing circulation of good blood—to the skin. In children, by far the most common reason for this is the accumulation of phlegm and dampness under the skin, which prevents blood from nourishing the skin. Other causes can be heat in the blood, or blood deficiency, or a combination of the two.

For eczema to occur, there must be something preventing good circulation of blood—or preventing circulation of good blood—to the skin.

General Etiology

There are three factors that tend to underlie eczema in children. When they combine, it leaves the way open for the eczema to take hold.

Heredity

It is well known that eczema (and asthma) runs in families. It is often found that children in these families have skin problems.

Lung dysfunction

That the Lungs govern the skin is one of the axioms of traditional Chinese medicine. If a child has any chronic problem of the Lungs, then the descending and dispersing of fluids becomes impaired, and fluids can accumulate in the skin. Over time these stagnant fluids transform into phlegm-dampness, and may be the cause of eczema.

The most common pattern of Lung disorder associated with eczema is that of a lingering pathogenic factor. The child may have had a Lung illness that was never completely cured, or an immunization that injured the Lungs. A lingering pathogenic factor may also be a cause of heat in the system, when the pathogenic factor is hot in nature. The heat aggravates the symptoms.

Spleen dysfunction

"The Spleen is the generator of phlegm; the Lungs are the container of phlegm" goes the saying. By far the most common cause of phlegm in children is a dysfunction of the Spleen. Either it is a little weak and there is difficulty in digesting foods, or the child may be eating food that the Spleen cannot cope with such as oranges, cow's milk, or cow's cheese, which directly injures the Spleen and allows for the formation of dampness, phlegm, or damp-heat. Once phlegm and dampness have formed they can accumulate under the skin where they obstruct the flow of qi and blood there, resulting in eczema.

The Spleen is also integral to the manufacture of blood. If the Spleen function is impaired it may lead to blood deficiency, which may in turn cause eczema.

In the majority of children there is a combination of all these predisposing factors: the family has a history of skin problems; the child has had all the regular immunizations and a few courses of antibiotics, giving rise to a lingering pathogenic factor in the Lungs; and the diet is often poor and hard on the Spleen, which leads to the formation of phlegm and dampness. Obviously, one cannot change the family history, but by strengthening the Lungs and Spleen, resolving the phlegm and dampness, and eliminating the lingering pathogenic factor, one can open the way to overcome any familial tendencies.

The importance of Spleen and Lung dysfunction cannot be overemphasized: one need only look at the common ages of onset of eczema in children to realize their importance. Eczema typically appears at four to six months—about the time the first solids are introduced—and the baby has to struggle a bit to digest food. At this time the Spleen is taxed, and it is easy for phlegm and dampness to be produced. Or it may appear earlier when the baby is first given bottle food (usually based on cow's milk), which is often too rich for the child, and contributes to the formation of phlegm.

Another common time for the disease to make an appearance is around the time of the first immunizations, or after a bad Lung disease, which has been treated with large doses of antibiotics. Both of these situations can give rise to lingering pathogenic factors, and thus impair the functioning of the Lungs.

Symptoms

Heat

Many cases of eczema are accompanied by symptoms associated with heat such as hot, itchy, red, and inflamed skin. There are two main reasons for this. First, the child may have systemic heat which obstructs the flow of qi and blood to the skin. This is commonly seen after an immunization which leaves a hot lingering pathogenic factor, such as after the measles immunization. Or the heat may come from the digestion and relate to diet. In young babies it is often due to accumulation disorder, in older children to damp-heat in the Stomach and Intestines. These children are typically hot and irritable, and sometimes even hyperactive. It should be said that it is very rare for the heat to enter the blood, and when it does, it is usually a rather severe condition. The main symptom of heat in the blood is purpura.

The other leading cause of the heat is local stagnation, as opposed to systemic heat in the blood. There is obstruction under the skin due to phlegm and dampness, which causes stagnation of qi, which in turn leads to heat. However, the child need not be hot inside; indeed, often the child actually has a cold, and possibly deficient digestion.

Dampness

Some cases of eczema present with an oozing, suppurative rash. This is due to the accumulation of dampness below the skin. It is frequently accompanied by a weak and deficient Spleen, or is associated with the consumption of too many cold, damp-forming foods, especially cow's milk, fruits, and ice-cold foods.

Dry, rough skin

Eczema that presents with dry or flaky skin is caused by there being more phlegm than dampness under the skin. The phlegm is often very thick and prevents blood from nourishing the skin. In addition, there may be heat in the child: the heat dries up the fluids, which are then unable to nourish the skin. Another cause of dry, rough skin is found in children with deficient blood, where the blood fails to moisten the skin.

Itching

This is the symptom that causes more distress to the child than any of the others. Itching can occur for many reasons in children. In acute disease like impetigo, it is often caused by wind. Occasionally, itching is caused by stagnant blood, but most often in children by stagnation of qi: its flow beneath the skin is impaired and so the skin itches. By scratching, the qi moves and the itching is relieved. This explains why the itching in many children gets worse at night: it is at that time that the qi and blood slow down and easily stagnate.

However, in order for the qi to stagnate under the skin, something must be preventing it from moving smoothly. The reason for this in children is most commonly the accumulation of phlegm and dampness under the skin. This helps explain why certain foods that cause phlegm and dampness—such as a small amount of cow's milk, or a few peanuts—can precipitate such a dramatic increase in the itching of a child with eczema, and why eliminating them from the child's diet can have such a beneficial effect.

In some children there are additional factors such as systemic heat, blood deficiency, or damp-heat, all of which may obstruct the flow of qi under the skin and thereby aggravate any stagnation and thus itching.

The other cause of itching in a child is rarely spoken about in textbooks, and is considered under the category of *yì bìng* diseases, which may be translated as "imbalance in the seven emotions." As previously explained, the flow of good quality blood is essential to nourishing the skin. If blood is deficienct or hot, the skin will not be nourished and eczema can result. However, even if the quality of the blood is good, if it is prevented from reaching the skin it will be deprived of nourishment and eczema will result. One way this can happen is if the Heart spirit is disturbed. The Heart is directly linked to the flow of blood. If its spirit is unsettled, the flow of blood is impaired, preventing it from nourishing the skin. This can cause itching, sometimes very severe.

This helps explain why in many children something as tenuous as an unpleasant thought (e.g., an acupuncture treatment) or an emotional upset can send the child into a paroxysm of scratching. It is especially true in children who have had some history of shock or trauma, where the Heart spirit is less firmly rooted, that a disturbance of the emotions can cause such a dramatic effect.

The role of the emotions in eczema is important and should be understood. Very often the emotional component is not obvious, but as one treats the child it is very common for the temperament and character of the child to alter. A docile child may become more assertive, an angry child more docile. The reason for this is that something has happened that causes the child to act out of character. Often a shock or tauma is easy to identify, but it can also be something more insidious, like the after effect of an immunization. These situations can profoundly affect a child, especially its spirit.

The importance of this for the acupuncturist is that it is often necessary to add *shén* (spirit) points—that is, points with *shén* in their name, like *shen men* (H-7)—to the prescription. By itself this will not cure the condition, but combined with treating the other underlying problems—phlegm, dampness, Spleen dysfunction, Lung dysfunction, lingering pathogenic factor—it can make the difference between curing or not curing the eczema.

ETIOLOGY & PATHOGENESIS

Underlying virtually all cases of eczema that we see in the clinic is a lingering pathogenic factor (LPF). The LPF is usually the result of an immunization or an illness treated inappropriately, and thus not cleared properly from the body. In eczema the LPF is usually in the Lungs or directly in the skin, for example, after an acute skin infection such as staphpylococcus is treated with topical or systemic antibiotics. However, the most important thing is to distinguish whether phlegm, heat, or deficiency is the dominant factor, and then treat it first before tackling the LPF. In some cases you may find that the LPF is itself the dominant factor, which means you must start there.

Here is a list of commonly seen patterns in children with eczema:

• phlegm and dampness accumulate in the system
• heat obstructs the flow of blood to the skin
• qi and blood deficiency
• lingering pathogenic factor

- accumulation disorder
- accumulation disorder with greed

Phlegm and dampness accumulate in the system

These children present with many signs of phlegm and dampness in the system. They often have constant congestion or even asthma, as the Lungs are full of phlegm. The most common sources of the phlegm and dampness are the diet, medicines, or the direct result of an LPF. The phlegm and dampness may be hot or cold in nature. The child may itself be hot due to the presence of a hot LPF, or it may eat many phlegm-forming, hot-energy foods, thus causing phlegm-heat in the system. Or the child may be more cold, eating cold-energy foods, or having taken many cold medicines such as antibiotics, resulting in cold-phlegm. The phlegm and dampness accumulate under the skin, preventing the flow of qi and blood there, which gives rise to eczema. The eczema will be more suppurative if there is more dampness than phlegm.

Heat obstructs the flow of blood to the skin

Children with this pattern tend to be hot and irritable. They may even be hyperactive. The heat is usually derived from immunizations, a hot diet, or from the mother as womb heat or womb poison. The heat disturbs the flow of blood to the skin, resulting in eczema. The eczema may be hot and inflamed, depending on the extent of the heat in the system.

Qi and blood deficiency

These children tend to be pale, weak, and are frequently ill. Often, they will suffer from insomnia, waking many times a night. The main causes are anemia in pregnancy, anesthetics during birth, and frequent illnesses, typically treated with antibiotics and immunizations. When the qi and blood are weak, the blood does not reach the skin to nourish it, resulting in eczema.

Lingering pathogenic factor

In these children the main factor is that of the LPF. There is little in the way of phlegm or heat or deficiency, just the thick phlegm that is so characteristic of this pattern. The skin in these children is often dry and flaky, and they frequently have dull, vacant eyes and exhibit sudden collapses of energy. The thick phlegm accumulates under the skin, obstructing the flow of qi and blood, and thereby causing eczema.

Combinations of Patterns

In some children, especially older ones, you will see a combination of the above patterns. Among the most common:

- phlegm or dampness and heat
- qi deficiency and a hot LPF
- qi and phlegm and/or dampness

Whether one treats all the presenting symptoms at once, or tackles one symptom at a time, depends on the particular child. One might, for example, first clear any heat and then go on to resolve the phlegm.

In addition, in younger children under the age of four you may see:

- accumulation disorder
- accumulation disorder with greed

These two patterns present when the child is given an inappropriate diet. They usually have an underlying LPF.

We have not listed any of the patterns of spirit disturbance because it is not helpful to treat this disorder until the underlying physical cause has been at least partly addressed.

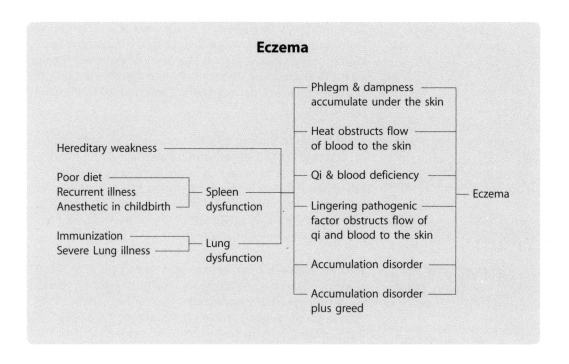

PATTERNS & SYMPTOMS

As most cases of eczema involve a lingering pathogenic factor underlying another pattern, they will generally share the following symptoms:

- swollen glands in the neck or groin
- history of repeated illness or of immunizations

- eyes lack vibrancy or spirit *(shén)*
- frequent collapses of energy

In any of the patterns for eczema the skin may appear to be red and hot. This is often due to local stagnation and repeated scratching, although the underlying condition may be cold and deficient. There will also be more or less oozing from the rash depending on how much dampness has accumulated.

Apart from these general characteristics, each pattern has its own characteristic symptoms.

Phlegm and dampness

- rash often moist and oozing pus
- lots of nasal discharge
- productive cough
- wheezing and rattly chest
- skin has a yellow, sallow hue

Pulse: slippery
Tongue: may be coated or swollen

Heat

- red face
- child is hot to touch or feels hot all the time
- likes to take clothes off, kicks bed clothes off
- restless at night
- thirsty
- good appetite

Pulse: rapid
Tongue: red or pale purple with red dots

Qi and blood deficiency

- rash tends to be less severe and less red
- skin dry and flaky
- child is weak and feeble
- sleep is disturbed, waking many times a night
- limbs like matchsticks
- child has a pale or white face
- often has shadows under the eyes
- appetite is poor
- stools can be loose or normal
- clear white nasal discharge

Pulse: deep, soggy

═══════

In general, the skin may appear to be red and hot due to local stagnation and repeated scratching, although the underlying condition may be cold and deficient. There will also be more or less oozing from the rash depending on how much dampness has accumulated.

═══════

LPF predominates

There are no signs of phlegm, dampness, heat, or deficiency.

- glands in the neck are swollen and often hard
- rash usually very itchy
- skin dry, rash rarely oozes
- child is strong and has good energy
- appetite good, sometimes very good
- limbs are strong and well built
- face is yellow, sometimes with a white forehead
- stools loose or normal, possibly glistening
- green or yellow nasal discharge that is thick and hard to discharge
- eyes are vacant and lack spirit

Pulse: slippery

Accumulation disorder

In addition to there being a lingering pathogenic factor, we often find that a young child will come into the clinic with accumulation disorder. When this occurs you must regulate the digestion before going on to tackle more complex issues, such as the LPF. In theory, accumulation disorder can be the sole cause of the eczema; once it is cleared, so too will the eczema. The reason is found in the consequences of accumulation disorder: phlegm and heat in the body. However, with very few exceptions, there will usually be a LPF underlying the accumulation.

Symptoms associated with accumulation disorder:

- rash is often red and oozing
- child is strong
- red cheeks, green around the mouth
- green nasal discharge
- swollen abdomen
- irregular stools
- foul-smelling stools or stools that smell of apples
- facial color yellow, or if there is a LPF in the Lungs, then yellow with a white forehead

Pulse: slippery, full

Accumulation disorder plus greed

The symptoms are the same as those of accumulation disorder, but the child is also greedy. This makes a difference in clinical practice because one must clear the greed in addition to the accumulation or the problem will return. The greed generally comes from Stomach heat, although it is sometimes part of the essential nature of the child. Stomach heat can be overcome with acupuncture, but essential greed can only be overcome by teaching from the parents.

In addition to the symptoms of accumulation disorder, also look for:

• child often has a large mouth
• entire face may be red
• may sweat on the forehead after meals

TREATMENT

In the case of eczema, it is usually better to treat more than once a week. Quite often there can be relief for a couple of days, after which the child goes back to scratching and misery. If possible, try to treat twice or even three times a week.

Main points

Sp-10 *(xue hai)*
B-40 *(wei zhong)*
LI-11 *(qu chi)*

All of these points benefit the skin and are useful in treating all types of eczema.

It is often beneficial to add Lung points to any prescription to strengthen the Lungs and thereby benefit the skin. Typical points include:

L-5 *(chi ze)*
L-7 *(lie que)*
L-9 *(tai yuan)*

According to pattern

It is important to first clear the predominant pattern—either phlegm and dampness, heat, or deficiency—before proceeding to clear the LPF.

Phlegm and Dampness

S-40 *(feng long)*
CV-12 *(zhong wan)*
Sp-9 *(yin ling quan)*
Sp-6 *(san yin jiao)*

Once the phlegm and dampness have been substantially reduced, then resolve the LPF as described below.

Heat

Liv-2 *(xing jian)*
H-8 *(shao fu)*
LI-4 *(he gu)*

Method: disperse to eliminate the heat

Once the heat symptoms have been reduced, proceed to treat the LPF, as described below.

Qi and Blood Deficiency

First, tonify the child using such points as:

S-36 *(zu san li)*
Sp-6 *(san yin jiao)*
B-20 *(pi shu)*
B-18 *(gan shu)*
B-23 *(shen shu)*
CV-12 *(zhong wan)*

Method: tonify; it is often appropriate to use moxa

Once the child is strong enough, proceed to treat the LPF, as described below.

Accumulation Disorder

Use *si feng* (M-UE-9).

If treating two to three times a week, then add:

CV-12 *(zhong wan)*
S-36 *(zu san li)*
LI-11 *(qu chi)*

Method: use a moving technique at all points

Prognosis: there should be a huge discharge of foul-smelling nappies, and the skin may get a lot worse for a couple of days. The child may shows signs of being angry or distressed.

Accumulation Disorder Plus Greed

Use the same points as for accumulation disorder, plus:

S-44 *(nei ting)*

Treatment principle: clear the accumulated food and the Stomach heat

Prognosis: the results are very similar to the preceding pattern. You must monitor what the child eats and encourage the parents to feed the child less.

Treating underlying LPF

The following points can be used to treat an underlying lingering pathogenic factor:

B-13 *(fei shu)*
B-18 *(gan shu)*

B-20 *(pi shu)*
bai lao (M-HN-30)

According to symptom

It is the symptoms of eczema—the heat and the itching—that cause the child so much distress. In most cases this is what you want to stop, far more that resolving any LPF. Obviously, for a lasting cure you must treat the underlying pathology, but there are points that you can add to help with the immediate problem of the itching and the heat.

Itching

Sp-10 *(xue hai)*
B-40 *(wei zhong)*
LI-11 *(qu chi)*

Calm the Spirit & Regulate the Blood

H-7 *(shen men)*
S-40 *(feng long)*
Sp-6 *(san yin jiao)*

Heat

LI-11 *(qu chi)*
Liv-2 *(xing jian)*

ADVICE

As with many problems, changes in diet and lifestyle are often essential in the treatment of eczema. No matter how inconvenient, parents should be encouraged to make the necessary alterations.

Change the diet

ESSENTIAL

- All phlegm-forming foods, cow's milk, cow's milk products, peanut butter, oranges, and bananas should be cut out of the diet. Even if this has been tried before, make sure that they are cut out over the course of treatment, as the combination of the two are often effective.

LESS ESSENTIAL (BUT STILL IMPORTANT)

- Cut out food colorings and flavorings, or at least keep them to a minimum.
- Sugar should be kept to a minimum.
- The child may have a food allergy. This can be hard to trace, but look out for chocolate, chicken, eggs, and oranges.

Accumulation disorder If the child has accumulation disorder, be sure to provide the necessary advice about diet, regularity of meals, gaps between food, and so forth.

Asthma and eczema Both asthma and eczema have at their base a LPF in the Lung system, which is why they often appear together. In children with both disorders, the Lungs will have been significantly weakened by the LPF. If the child has eczema alone, the Lungs are that much stronger, and this should be regarded as a good thing.

Steroid creams Steroid creams and ointments should be avoided if possible, for there is little doubt that over the long term they aggravate the skin condition. Parents, on the whole, are aware of this. What they may not be so aware of is that steroid creams can push the phlegm deeper into the body: what was previously residing just under the skin migrates to the Lungs, where it can cause asthma.

However, don't be too rigid. There are times when it may actually be the right thing for the child. If there have been countless sleepless nights—the child is exhausted, the mother and father shattered—then some ointment can give the child a good night free of intolerable itching. This can make a big difference to the health of the child.

GUIDELINES FOR PROGNOSIS

It is usually difficult to say, with any degree of reliability, how long eczema will take to cure. This is the hardest thing to explain to a parent, for apart from wanting their child to be free of this misery, the element of doubt is discouraging. Still, it is worth saying that nearly all children receive some benefit from treatment. You should see some improvement after five treatments; however, after the initial improvement, be prepared for a setback, but do keep going.

Usually after ten treatments you will see definite changes for the better, and after twenty, a distinct improvement. Perhaps half of the patients are cured completely in thirty treatments, while others may be greatly improved, showing signs only every now and again, especially when under great stress.

If you do suffer a setback at any stage, carry on. It is only if you see nothing changing after ten to fifteen treatments that you should either question your diagnosis, look at the family dynamics, or try another therapy. That having been said, here are some rough guidelines:

- if the child is weak, then it will take time to build up the qi: fifteen to twenty treatments
- if there is a very strong and deep LPF, then this will take time to clear: thirty-plus treatments
- if there is a strong emotional factor it must be addressed, and you should expect little improvement until this is done
- if the child is reasonably healthy: ten to twenty treatments

A Good Sign

If you are treating a child with a LPF who at first did not have much phlegm, but during the course of treatment starts to develop visible signs of phlegm—such as a cough or runny nose—take this as a good sign. The phlegm that was obstructing the flow of qi and blood is beginning to move and come out.

❖

29 ❖ Failure to Thrive

INTRODUCTION

Failure to thrive is a delightfully loose term, having both the clarity and lack of precision of an earlier period of medicine which one would not expect to find in modern medicine. You can imagine old-fashioned doctors saying, "Well, we all know what is meant by failure to thrive" while modern medicine is hard put to find a precise definition. A commonly used index in modern medicine is weight gain: if a child is seriously under the average weight for its age—say, under the fifth centile—then that would be a strong indication. Yet taken on its own, this is not a reliable indicator, for some children are naturally large, while others are naturally small.

Perhaps the one thing that distinguishes this from other "illnesses" is that no one symptom stands out above all the others. So, for example, the child might have poor appetite, but not so bad that you think it needs treating; or the child may vomit from time to time, but in itself the vomiting is not really a serious problem. It is only when you add up all the little problems that you see something is going seriously wrong.

ETIOLOGY

One of the axioms of traditional Chinese medicine is that the Kidneys control growth, reproduction, and development. Failure to thrive, one of whose symptoms is poor growth and weight gain, is therefore a manifestation of weak Kidney energy. Another axiom is that there are two components to Kidney *jīng* or essence, 'pre-heaven qi' and 'post-heaven qi', which are often loosely translated as inherited energy and acquired energy. Although these translations are not precise, they serve very well in this instance, for they point to the causes of failure to thrive from the perspective of Chinese medicine: weak inherent Kidney energy (i.e., weak constitution) and interference with the acquisition of qi. In our experience, there are two main causes for the latter: either the child is not getting enough qi from its parents, or it may have a lingering pathogenic factor (LPF) which prevents the proper absorption of qi.

To summarize, the three causes of failure to thrive are weak Kidney energy, insufficient qi from parents, and a lingering pathogenic factor (LPF).

SIGNS & SYMPTOMS

In general

The child may present with a number of the following symptoms:

- poor weight gain
- poor appetite
- weak spirit : either a wimp, or always complaining and irritable
- occasional vomiting
- loose stools
- frequent mild infections
- poor sleep, or excessive sleep

According to pattern

Weak Kidney Energy

- eyes may be alert, but there is no energy in them
- small head
- possibly dribbling
- thin bones
- low-set ears
- veins apparent on temple (like varicose veins)
- skin color usually all right

Insufficient Qi from Parents

There are two causes for this. Either the parents themselves are completely exhausted, and you will see:

- really ill parents, just hanging on

or, the parents may be withholding their qi, as described in Chapter 3. In this case you will see:

- parents in radiant health
- child weak and feeble
- child's skin color may be dull

Lingering Pathogenic Factor (LPF)

- child's weight gain was quite satisfactory until it received an immunization or had a bad illness; the child's development then suddenly slowed
- prone to frequent infection
- glands in neck are swollen

TREATMENT

The first stage of treatment is very simple and straightforward. The guiding principle is to tonify the Kidney and Spleen qi (the Spleen because the appetite is usually poor). A typical prescription would be:

S-36 *(zu san li)*
Sp-6 *(san yin jiao)*
CV-12 *(zhong wan)*

Method: tonifying method, with only moxa at CV-12 *(zhong wan)*

In many cases this simple treatment is enough, irrespective of which pattern they have. After only two or three treatments, the appetite improves enormously, and the child will start to grow and put on weight. One child of eighteen months we treated in this manner grew one centimeter each week for three weeks!

Differentiation of patterns is only necessary if nothing much happens after two to three treatments.

According to Pattern

Weak Kidney energy

It is not difficult to choose the points. A typical prescription would be:

B-20 *(pi shu)*
B-23 *(shen shu)*
Sp-6 *(san yin jiao)*

Method: needle all points with the tonifying method, and use moxa on the back points

Treatment is easy; it's the results that are difficult! In perhaps half of the cases the children gradually improve, so that after ten to fifteen treatments they are making significant progress. But in quite a number of other cases, progress is very slow. There just does not seem to be enough energy available, and the child remains small and weedy, in spite of your best attempts. This is particularly likely if the child has a lot of phlegm as well as this very weak Kidney energy.

Insufficient qi from parents

We have met this pattern before. The child is more or less unwanted. Not exactly so, for they do actually want their child, but they also want the child to be good, and they want to save their energy for their careers and their interesting lifestyle.

As we have said before, we do not find it effective to confront parents with our opinion, but we do find it effective to give treatment. By tonifying the child's qi, you give it enough energy to start claiming its rightful energy from its parents. It then has enough energy to make a nuisance of itself, and to avoid being crushed. Usually two to four treatments are enough for this purpose.

However, acupuncture does not always work. Sometimes, after four treatments, you get loud complaints from the parents saying that when they first brought their child it was good tempered, and now it is really annoying, and they find they are having to do drastic things, like lock the child up in its bedroom in order to subdue it. Comments like this from parents always leave us aghast, and we have nothing much more to say. Sometimes we find we can get through to the parents, but often not. Perhaps a way around this is to work together with a family therapist.

Lingering pathogenic factor

What is different here is that the pattern manifests mainly in this condition of "not thriving," rather than just asthma or vomiting. What is happening is that the pathogenic factor sits in the interior, and obstructs the whole production of qi (the *qì jī,* or qi mechanism), rather than producing one rather strong symptom.

The straightforward treatment set forth above is usually enough to start things moving. So, unlike the weak Kidney pattern, you should see something happen after three or four treatments, but you may feel that progress is too slow. In that case it is usually time to change your approach, and adopt a new treatment principle. We suggest the following: treat the major symptoms, and soften hard phlegm.

For example, if the child has a really significant symptom—like a cough which goes on and on—then treat the chronic cough with points such as:

B-13 *(fei shu)*
L-7 *(lie que)*

Likewise, if the child has frequent vomiting attacks of the hot type, then use:

P-6 *(nei guan)*	Stops the vomiting
S-44 *(nei ting)*	Clears the Stomach heat

The other part of the treatment principle—softening the hard phlegm—may be more important. Use such points as:

bai lao (M-HN-30)
B-18 *(gan shu)*
B-20 *(pi shu)*

The effect of this treatment will be much the same as when you treat chronic cough: it may liberate a lot of phlegm, which may then itself need treating.

You may need to continue treating for up to ten treatments if the child has a severe condition, and the LPF has been there for a long time.

Conventional Medical Treatment

The only conventional medical treatment we have heard of is to give injections of human growth hormone. We have no experience with children who have had this treatment, and would be interested to hear from anyone who has. We would be particularly interested to know if this treatment has an effect on tonifying the child's qi.

We do have to admit to a mild prejudice against this treatment, however, for the hormone is extracted from human cadavers, and besides this unsavory thought, there is a real risk of transferring Kreuzfeld-Jakob disease, which rots the brain. Apparently, there is now an alternative medication which is genetically engineered, and so does not have the same risk.

CONCLUSION

Treating failure to thrive is usually very rewarding. Simple treatments often produce startling results, with a child catching up on a year of growth in just a few weeks. At the outset of treatment you can see a weak and feeble child who is often distressed, and at the end you see a radiant, energetic child.

NOTE

- For a case history involving failure to thrive, see Case 17 in Chapter 47.

❖

30 ❖ Learning Difficulties and Mental Retardation

INTRODUCTION

In this chapter we discuss what acupuncture can do to help children who have learning difficulties or are mentally retarded. It is quite common for children to be brought to the clinic with learning difficulties of one sort or another. This may range from the tag 'attention deficit disorder' through 'educationally subnormal' to 'handicapped'— it rather depends on which institution gets hold of the child first. Here we will try to show which sort of learning difficulties can be helped, and which cannot.

In later chapters we will be discussing hyperactivity, and then the special cases of Down's syndrome children (or mongol children, as they used to be called), autism and dyslexia, and cerebral palsy.

Mind

From the Western point of view, learning is a function of the mind, and from the traditional Chinese point of view, of the spirit *(shén)*. Each child's mind is different. Each has certain interests and aptitudes that it is born with, and each child develops at a different rate. Consequently, there are real difficulties in determining whether a child really has a learning difficulty or not, and if so, whether it is pathological.

There is a natural state for each child. Some children have great intelligence and aptitude, while others simply do not. Some bring with them a clear and open character, while others come clouded and disturbed. Some may be highly sensitive, to the point of being oversensitive, while others may be undersensitive, to the point of being slow-witted. These imbalances may be really quite serious, but they may not be pathological, and so may not be amenable to treatment by herbs or acupuncture. Some children are just naturally "intellectually challenged," and medicine is not going to change that.

A full discussion of the mind is beyond the scope of this book. However, it is worth spending a little time looking at the nature of the mind. A good way of analyzing it is in terms of the five phases or elements: each relates to a broad category of functions of the mind, and also to its corresponding organ.

Fire

Fire relates to the Heart, where overall the spirit resides. The function of the mind which particularly relates to fire is consciousness, awareness, and also lateral thinking.

Earth

Earth relates to the Spleen. The function of the mind which particularly relates to earth is gathering, remembering, and handling facts.

Metal

Metal relates to the Lungs. The function of the mind which particularly relates to metal is discrimination, that is, being able to distinguish among different things. It was noted in the *Inner Classic* that metal people make good judges.

Water

Water relates to the Kidneys. The function of the mind which particularly relates to water is mental energy, and the ability to hold ideas without being unduly influenced by others.

Wood

Wood relates to the Liver. The function of the mind which particularly relates to wood is spatial and temporal awareness. Thus, the Liver is characterized as the general in charge of planning.

Spirit *(shén)*

Again, a full discussion of the nature of spirit and its different aspects in Chinese medicine could fill several large tomes, and we do not propose to spend more time on it. Besides, when it comes down to the clinical situation, an understanding of these ideas is not all that important. What *is* important is to understand that thinking, learning, and awareness are all manifestations of spirit, and that the spirit resides in the Heart in normal everyday life. In dreams it leaves the Heart and is free to roam where it will, and in certain illnesses it may be only half-in or half-out of the Heart. Likewise, we will see that phlegm can disturb its function.

Emotions

In Chinese thought and culture, emotions play a different role than they do in the West. In China, emotions can be strong and violent, but after they have come, they go, leaving little trace. Anyone who has seen the sudden and violent outbursts of anger in the Chinese, followed by calm afterwards, will know that their temperament is different. By contrast, we in the West have the ability to hold on to feelings like resentment, guilt, and failure for years and years. This can have a really serious effect on our ability to learn. The influence is not direct, in that emotions are not thought of as residing in the mind; nevertheless, emotions, and subconsciously held thoughts, can have a huge effect on learning ability.

PATTERNS

From the point of view of traditional Chinese medicine there are four main patterns which lead to learning difficulties. It is understood that there can be energetic imbalances which stand in the way of learning and obstruct the mind, and that by righting the imbalance, you open the way for the mind to realize its full potential. There are, of course, many other causes of learning difficulties—insecurity, boredom, fear of teachers, bad teaching at an early age—but these are really non-medical problems, and can only be helped indirectly (if at all) by acupuncture. (If this is an area that interests you, we recommend reading the book *Why Children Fail*.)

The energetic imbalances are:

• Kidney and Spleen deficiency
• qi and blood deficiency
• phlegm-dampness misting the mind
• heat affecting the Heart

Much of the material in this chaper about the first two patterns—Kidney deficiency and qi and blood deficiency—is based on the book *Pediatrics in Traditional Chinese Medicine (Zhong yi er ke xue)* by the Shanghai College of Traditional Chinese Medicine.

ETIOLOGY & PATHOGENESIS

Kidney and Spleen deficiency, qi and blood deficiency

Mental retardation may occur as a result of a genetic defect; because the mother's essence and blood are deficient and weak; or because the womb qi is insufficient. As a result, the Spleen and Kidneys are feeble, and the Heart and spirit are then not properly supported. After birth, the primary cause in China is malnourishment, which leads to deficiency of qi and blood. In the West it is due to a deficient diet, that is, poor quality food, or "junk" food.[1]

Phlegm-dampness

Arises from eating too much cold or damp-producing foods such as ice-cold juice, milk, and cheese; from repeated attacks of external pathogenic factors; or continuous treatment with damp-cold medicines such as antibiotics, or anesthetics given to the mother in childbirth. The phlegm is carried up to the head and brain where it disturbs the pure yang, affecting consciousness. The child's head feels heavy or as though it were wrapped in cotton, and the child has difficulty concentrating.

Heat affecting the Heart

Caused by eating too much hot or "junk" food, or as a result of a febrile disease, or an immunization. Occasionally it is caused by emotional stress in the parents, which is reflected in the child, or by womb toxin. The Heart houses the spirit, and if heat affects the Heart, the spirit and mind become restless. The child thus has difficulty sitting still and concentrating. At about the age of seven a child begins to be able to control itself and behave in a more reasonable manner. When this happens the child may develop Liver qi constraint.

PATTERNS & SYMPTOMS OF DEFICIENCY

Spleen and Kidney deficiency

• head and neck are soft and weak, cannot raise head
• mouth soft and with a tendency to remain open, lips thick
• small-boned
• poor tooth formation: may be late in appearing, crumbly, black
• small, low-set ears
• chews and sucks without strength
• often dribbles saliva
• arms soft and hanging down
• weak and cannot stand
• muscles slack and without strength
• easily tires
• feels light to carry
• not well grounded: easily influenced by the moods of those around, even to the point of being psychic

---

1. In two studies that were published simultaneously in 1993 it was found that school children's performance increased quite considerably by giving them a daily mineral and vitamin pill.

Pulse: deep and with strength (probably from accumulation of dampness)
Finger vein: thin

Treatment principle: tonify the Kidneys and strengthen the Spleen

Sometimes this pattern is accompanied by accumulation of dampness (due to Kidney deficiency) or phlegm (long-term stagnation of dampness). Symptoms then include:

- dribbling at the mouth
- nasal discharge

These symptoms are those of classic Kidney deficiency. They are often seen in clinical practice, and require little explanation, except perhaps the behavior and sensitivity to moods. This sensitivity occurs because the foundation energy (basal qi) is weak. There is no firmness in the foundation, such that even a small outside influence can cause a big disturbance in the child. In other words, there is nothing to stabilize the child.

Another way of looking at this is that the Kidney's function in supporting the Heart is not strong. When the Heart is left unsupported, the spirit is also unsupported, and so becomes unstable.

Qi and blood deficiency

- skin and body are soft and weak
- joints are soft and weak
- cannot sit up straight
- may have history of difficult labor or pregnancy (or in the West, anesthetics given in childbirth)
- spirit dull, stupid or idiotic behavior
- facial color bright white
- cold limbs
- mouth hangs open, tongue hangs out
- poor appetite and digestion
- lips white
- easily bored
- may have dark rings round eyes

Tongue coating: shiny
Pulse: deep, without strength; sometimes full and slippery in the middle positions on both sides
Finger vein: fine

Treatment principle: strengthen the qi and support the blood

TREATMENT

Body acupuncture

GV-14 *(da zhui)*	Strengthens the brain and spinal cord

an mian #2
   (N-HN-22/b)
GV-15 *(ya men)*   ⎫ Strengthens the brain and
GV-13 *(tao dao)*   ⎬ spinal cord
GV-20 *(bai hui)*   ⎭
yin tang (M-HN-30)
P-6 *(nei guan)*   Both points invigorate the circula-
LI-4 *(he gu)*   tion of qi and blood
S-36 *(zu san li)*   Strengthens the Spleen qi and
                         basal qi

Method: tonifying method is used. In any given treatment, some points on the head should be combined with others on the extremities. In addition, points should be added based on the pattern below.

Kidney and Spleen Deficiency

B-23 *(shen shu)*
K-7 *(fu liu)*
Sp-6 *(san yin jiao)*

Result of treatment: there may be quite rapid improvement during the first five to ten treatments, with the child gaining energy and strength. After this, progress is slow, and it is often found that the child slips back if treatment is terminated because it does not have enough energy to cope with daily life.

It is often worth giving weekly treatments for a year, followed by less frequent treatment for another year.

Qi and Blood Deficiency

S-36 *(zu san li)*
Sp-6 *(san yin jiao)*

Result of treatment: there should be a steady improvement, lasting over the course of ten to fifteen treatments—at least in principle. In practice, there are always complicating factors. For example, if the qi is weak then the child may keep getting coughs and colds of one sort or another, which sets the treatment back. Likewise, one often finds that deficient children are just overworked at school, and simply don't have the energy to keep up with what is expected of them. In this case, you may have to continue giving support treatments, say every three to four weeks, for a year or more. At the outset it is hard to predict whether this will happen; it is more likely if the child is unhappy at school or at home.

Other useful points:

B-20 *(pi shu)*
CV-12 *(zhong wan)*

Note

• Some of these children will have signs of heat, possibly from a lingering pathogenic factor. In such cases treatment should alternate between tonifying the Spleen and Kidneys (or qi and blood) and dispersing the heat.

PATTERNS & SYMPTOMS OF EXCESS

Information about the two patterns of excess is drawn from our own clinical experience.

Phlegm-dampness

• speech may be indistinct
• face and lips pale
• watery eyes, dribbling at the mouth, clear nasal discharge
• possibly loose stools, swollen abdomen
• pale or gray face
• rather podgy children, with excess round the tummy, and often with thick legs (from dampness descending and collecting in the muscles)
• heavy-footed
• mind feels "woolly" or "foggy"
• slow reactions
• slow to answer, often answering a different question from the one asked

May also include signs of phlegm, such as:

• breathing through the mouth
• clearing throat from time to time
• nasal discharge
• chronic cough which comes and goes
• often picks nose

Tongue coating: thin and white, or thick and greasy, or more commonly sputum is tenuous and draws out into long threads
Tongue body: pale
Pulse: fine and deep or slippery-soggy

Treatment principle: transform the phlegm and tonify the Spleen

The picture just given is clearly that of a phlegmy child. It must be said that quite often there are only few signs of phlegm, so that if you ask the parents whether there is any catarrh, their answer would be "no." However, you will nearly always find something that leads you to this conclusion, perhaps only the slippery pulse, or the heavy way the child walks, or the stringy nature of the saliva.

Heat affecting the Heart

• difficulty concentrating, short attention span
• difficulty sitting still, restless, fidgety
• possibly irritable
• possibly insomnia with dream-disturbed sleep
• possibly dyslexia
• facial color red, lips red
• plays with something, possibly with fingers

Pulse: a little rapid, usually slippery
Tongue body: red
Tongue coating: possibly thin, yellow
Pulse: rapid, usually slippery

Treatment principle: clear the heat and calm the mind; in older children, also relieve the Liver constraint

TREATMENT

Phlegm-dampness

S-40 *(feng long)*	Transforms the phlegm
Sp-6 *(san yin jiao)*	Tonifies the Spleen and transforms the phlegm
CV-12 *(zhong wan)*	Tonifies the Spleen and transforms the phlegm
S-36 *(zu san li)*	Tonifies the Stomach and Spleen
yin tang (M-HN-30)	Clears the mind

Method: even needle manipulation; moxa, or moxa on garlic, may also be used

Prognosis: progress is usually steady. You may produce quite a strong expulsion of phlegm for a day or two after each of the first few treatments, with symptoms of cough, nasal discharge, and loose stools, but otherwise the child should gradually become more energetic and better able to concentrate. As with the heat pattern, ten to twenty treatments is quite normal.

Advice

As with all phlegm disorders, diet is very important: avoid cow's milk, cow's cheese, peanuts, bananas, oranges. In some children there is a wheat allergy.

Heat affecting the Heart

H-8 *(shao fu)*	Clears heat from the Heart
Liv-2 *(xing jian)*	Clears heat and regulates the Liver qi

GV-20 *(bai hui)*   Clears the mind
yin tang (M-HN-30)   Clears the mind

Method: dispersing method is used, provided it does not scare the child

Other useful points include:

G-34 *(yang ling quan)*
S-44 *(nei ting)*

Prognosis: usually there are no side effects to treatment. The child gradually becomes calmer. After five or six treatments a definite improvement should be noticed, and by ten to fifteen treatments the child should be a lot better. Just occasionally there are some unusual reactions as the heat comes out, maybe as a fever, sometimes as hot, painful diarrhea, sometimes as a rash of red spots on the body or on the head.

Advice

It is essential that the child avoid all sugar and artificial flavorings and colorings during the course of treatment. The child should also be tested for other allergies such as wheat gluten, oranges, eggs, and the like.

Other Prescriptions from the Literature

These are mainly for the deficient patterns.

Ear acupuncture

Points: Heart, Kidney, Spleen, Brainstem, Lower Skin

Method: treat every other day. In general, we do not use much ear acupuncture on children because they wiggle so much and like to pull on their ears. It is suitable for those young children who can cooperate, or older children. The attraction of ear acupuncture is that the needles can be inserted very quickly and left in place for most of the day. This means that patients can be fitted in between other patients, making daily treatments a real possibility.

Point injection therapy

Point: S-36 *(zu san li).* Inject with 0.3 to 0.5ml of 5% Radix Angelicae sinensis *(dang gui)* essence.

Method: treat every other day

Prognosis: ten treatments constitute a course, and many courses may be required

Prescriptions from   FIRST PRESCRIPTION

*Practical Acupuncture
(Shi yong zhen jiu xue)*

ji san xue (M-BW-37) "Three Vertebral Holes"[2]

Method: the six points (bilaterally) are injected with 0.3 to 0.5ml of a 5% ginseng solution. Treat every day. Thirty treatments constitute one course, after which there should be a rest of ten to fifteen days. After the second course, treatment may be given every other day.

SECOND PRESCRIPTION

GV-14 *(da zhui)*
GV-15 *(ya men)*
G-20 *(feng chi)*

Method: these points are injected with a 5% ginseng solution, in the same manner as the prescription above

MIXED PATTERNS

We have presented four patterns above, each of which often appears in the clinic. It is also true that mixed patterns occur, especially heat with phlegm. These two factors are frequently the result of a febrile disease or immunization.

Heat and phlegm

One often finds heat and phlegm together. This is a potentially dangerous combination, and can lead to the 'manic' type of hyperactivity (see Chapter 31). Here, we can point out one key symptom of that disorder: the child does things that it *knows* are wrong. While the brain damaged child may do things that *appear* very wrong, it does so simply because it does not have the ability to distinguish between right and wrong. The manic child, however, does things that it knows are wrong.

*Kidney deficiency
and phlegm*

Kidney deficiency and phlegm are likewise often seen together as a mixed pattern.

TREATMENT

It is usually possible to treat the two factors in the mixed pattern in the same treatment. For example, heat and phlegm can be successfully cleared using a prescription such as:

---

2. These are three points which are needled bilaterally. The first is 1 unit below GV-15 *(ya men)* and 0.5 unit lateral to the spine. The second is 0.5 unit lateral to the spinous process of the second thoracic vertebra, and the third is 0.5 unit lateral to the second lumbar vertebra.

H-8 *(shao hai)*
G-34 *(yang ling quan)*
Liv-2 *(xing jian)*

Likewise, Kidney deficiency and phlegm can be treated by the combination:

B-20 *(pi shu)*
B-23 *(shen shu)*
Sp-6 *(san yin jiao)*

Priorities in Treatment

There are no hard and fast rules about which pattern should be treated first, but from our own experience, we suggest the following:

1. clear heat
2. tonify deficiency
3. clear phlegm

We suggest this order of priority because if heat is present, its effect will become more severe if you strengthen the Kidneys, or resolve phlegm. The child is likely to behave in a much more manic way if you do not clear the heat first.

If both phlegm and Kidney deficiency are present, it is better to treat the deficiency first, because the child needs energy to get rid of the phlegm. If you simply try to reduce the phlegm straightaway, not much will happen.

RELATED DISORDERS

To conclude our discussion of learning difficulties, we will briefly look at brain damage, epilepsy, and boredom.

Brain Damage

If a child suffers from brain damage it will almost certainly have been discovered by conventional medical tests. And from the point of view of conventional medicine, no further explanation is needed to account for the learning difficulties. However, this does *not* mean that there is never any point in treating a child with brain damage. There are two circumstances when it is worthwhile to do so:

• if there is an energetic imbalance
• if the brain damage is recent

Energetic imbalance

Quite often there is an energetic imbalance of the kind described above—heat, phlegm, or Kidney deficiency, or a combination of the three—because the problem that caused the brain damage was a severe illness, such as wind-heat or phlegm-heat leading to febrile convulsions, which has left behind a lingering pathogenic factor (LPF). If you treat the LPF, clear the heat, and strengthen the Kidney energy, it is unlikely that you will cure the brain damage, but it does mean that the part of the brain that *is* functioning will do so much better as a result of your treatment.

Recent brain damage

If the injury to the brain was recent (a month or so) and was not too severe, then treatment by acupuncture can make a big difference in the extent of the recovery. Just as treatment of stroke patients by acupuncture—where the brain is damaged by a cerebrovascular accident—produces astonishing results, with some patients recovering almost completely, so too can brain-damaged children sometimes be helped enormously, provided treatment is given soon enough.

It should be pointed out that frequent treatment should be given, preferably daily for a course of ten treatments, with a five-day break, just as in cases of stroke.

Epilepsy

An epileptic child is very likely to have learning difficulties. These are often aggravated by the anticonvulsive drugs that are frequently prescribed, and which have the effect of dulling the mind.

As we show in Chapter 40, epilepsy can often be treated successfully with acupuncture, although it requires many treatments (fifty to a hundred). The same three syndromes underlying learning difficulties (heat, phlegm, Kidney deficiency) also underlie epilepsy.

Boredom

It seems almost too obvious to mention, but many children are bored most of the time at school. They just don't want to be cooped up in a stuffy classroom or sit at an uncomfortable desk. They find what the teacher has to say quite irrelevant, and sometimes they have an instinctive dislike of their teacher.

This condition is so common that everyone must have suffered from it at one time or another. If it is really serious, and continues for a long time, it can develop into a really serious problem. In the first stage, the problem will be on the mental-psychological level. The child will be slow at learning, bottom of the class, and gradually come to believe it is "no good."

This can lead, in turn, to a physical disease. It commonly takes one of two courses: deficiency or excess. In the deficient type the child shows less and less interest in what is going on around it, and its qi gradually weakens. This can evolve into Spleen qi deficiency, or Lung and Spleen qi deficiency. Alternatively, the child may become more and more rebellious. The feeling of being "no good" or "worthless" is resisted by a strong Kidney yang. The energy must find an outlet, and may at first find expression in disruptive behavior—in class at first, then in destruction and violence outside. Likewise, the pattern may start to produce physical symptoms, especially heat. Sometimes heat and phlegm emerge gradually, and then the stage is set for a really serious problem: for when heat and phlegm are present together, one finds children doing things that they know are wrong. When this is driven by the struggle for a sense of self-worth, the result is disaster.

Obviously, one cannot expect to alter the boredom level that the child experiences in the classroom. However, if there are significant physical imbalances, one can make a big difference. By restoring qi to the deficient child, one may give it enough energy to cope with a boring lesson, and to make its voice heard—that it simply hates school. Similarly with the phlegm and heat types.

When there is no physical imbalance, this itself is a diagnosis. The fact that the qi is flowing well and that there are no significant imbalances points away from a medical solution and toward a solution in the child's life. The two remaining possibilities are that the child really hasn't got much mental ability, or that there are problems at school. These two choices can usually be distinguished fairly easily by looking at the child. If he or she really has low mental ability, there will be a sort of "loopy" look in the eyes: there is something that is not quite all there. As the saying goes, "The spirit appears in the eyes."

On the other hand, if the child has some problem at school, this can be identified by the old adage, "Problem at school, trouble at home; problem at home, trouble at school." So if a child is bored at school, it may behave perfectly well at school, but abominably at home. By the same token, serious upsets at home, such as separation of the parents, is often reflected in bad behavior at school.

CONCLUSION

Difficulty in learning is a complex problem which is a result of the interaction between the spirit and the physical condition. The disorders which are most readily helped by acupuncture are those where there is a significant energetic imbalance that reaches right through and gives rise to significant physical symptoms. By clearing away the imbalance you can clear away the obstacles to learning, and open the way for the child to develop its full potential. Sometimes the result is that the child makes its voice heard for the first time, and may eventually lead to a change of school.

❖

31 ❖ Hyperactivity and Attention Deficit Disorder

INTRODUCTION

Hyperactivity is almost unknown in China, whereas it is now well-recognized in the West as a major problem. The term 'hyperactive' is used to describe a whole spectrum of behavior in children ranging from very energetic to disruptive and rude and to positively violent.

From a Chinese point of view the categories are very clear, and although there may be slight overlaps, the main problem is usually easily identified. This is one of the great strengths of Chinese medicine and is part of the reason that hyperactivity can be treated so well with acupuncture. To be able to identify the cause, and to treat the condition, we can cure the child.

This is in stark contrast to conventional medicine, where the cause is unknown, and there are few tools with which to help these children other than drugs—which do not always work—and possibly some dietary advice.

Having a child who is hyperactive is exhausting for parents. These children can completely disrupt the whole family with their screaming, shouting, throwing tantrums, breaking things, fighting, and so on. Even when they are comparatively "quiet" they don't sit still, are unable to concentrate, and demand constant attention. The problem usually extends to school, and the parents often receive letters telling them of their child's behavior; in extreme cases, the child may be asked to leave.

Two of the most exasperating things for parents are that there seems to be no rhyme or reason for their child being like this, and there is little in the way of reliable treatment. Child psychiatry may help in some cases, but not always, and the drugs prescribed are of limited use. In some cases diet helps, but often these children crave the very thing that makes them worse (sugar, food colorings) and find ways to get hold of the stuff. It is partly because there is so little in the way of help that we see a lot of hyperactive children in the clinic—and also because word soon gets around that acupuncture is very effective in helping these children.

Although it can be very stressful treating such children—they upset other patients, make a lot of noise, kick, scream, bite, wreck the clinic—they are, in some ways, the most rewarding cases to treat. They do not *want* to be like this; they are often desperate to stop their behavior, and are miserable because of it. With your treatment you can actually "bring them back" to their parents and family. They can turn from aggressive, difficult children into happy, lively, and contented kids who are a joy to be with.

From the perspective of traditional Chinese medicine, there are four patterns. The first two are the most commonly seen and are "true" forms of hyperactivity. The third is almost identical to the hyperactive Spleen qi deficiency pattern described in Chapter 3, and is usually seen in older children. The fourth pattern stems from deficiency and is therefore not "true" hyperactivity. The four patterns are:

- heat
- heat plus phlegm (mania)
- weakness in the middle burner
- Kidney deficiency

Heat

These children are hot! They have red faces or lips, get angry, throw tantrums, cannot sit still. They tend to be clingy children. Their sleep is disturbed, as they are restless and tend to wake up early. They are the ones that run about the clinic shouting, screaming, and disturbing all the other practitioners. The cause of the heat is varied. Among the common sources are immunizations, hot-type foods, flavorings, food colorings, or heat transferred from the mother during pregnancy.

Heat and Phlegm

These children are hot too, but they are also full of phlegm and seem to be more aggressive and violent than the pure heat types. Most have red faces (some do not) and have the same irritability, tantrums, and insomnia, but in addition have signs of phlegm and tend to be willfully destructive, and even cruel, to other children. They may also have genital or anal fixations. These children make comments about your privates and try to grab hold of them during treatment. They also delight in destroying your clinic, tearing up clean paper and throwing it all over the floor, pulling the arms and legs off the cuddly toys, and hitting and kicking you during treatment.

Weakness in the Middle Burner

This is a manifestation of hyperactive Spleen qi deficiency. The basis of the pattern is deficiency, even though the child appears to have lots of energy. As with hyperactive Spleen qi derficiency, the parents are often exhausted, while the children are manipulative, and tend to have poor appetites and other signs of Spleen deficiency. However, there are some aspects that are slightly different and put these children into the hyperactive bracket. They tend to be full of "hate." They are the ones that love to play video games with names like "Doom," "Mega-Kill," "Death," and other such jollities. They can be really destructive and nasty, but it is cold and calculating. Unlike the previous two patterns where the child is boiling up with rage, these children are pale or gray in the face, and possibly even cold in energy. But inside there is this terrible hatred. You would expect hatred to be linked with anger, which stagnates the Liver qi and transforms into heat, but this does not seem to happen. (For example, Liv-2 *(xing jian)* does nothing for these children.) Theirs is a cold hatred; one can find oneself quite shocked by them, almost frightened, and they can be very difficult to help.

Kidney Deficiency

This is not a true type of hyperactivity. These children are tall and beautiful, and tend to be frail, and often ill. They have weak Kidney energy, and so become hyperactive when they are tired or excited: the Kidneys cannot hold down the energy, and it rises up to the head. Typically, they do not like to go to bed; even though they are tired they can keep themselves up for ages. They get "hyper" when they are excited—perhaps hysterical—running around, unable to be controlled, although they do not become violent as a rule. By contrast, during the daytime they may be quite weak and floppy.

ETIOLOGY & PATHOGENESIS

Heat

The heat in the body rises up to affect the Heart, which houses the spirit and is easily affected by heat. The spirit becomes disturbed, causing irritability and restlessness. Common causes include:

- food: some foods create heat in the system. Curries, spicy foods, and shellfish are all hot in energy.
- food additives: colorings and flavorings
- womb heat: if the mother has a very hot nature, or if she eats a lot of oranges during pregnancy, heat can transfer across the placenta to the child and it is born hot.
- lingering pathogenic factor (LPF) from an immunization: a lingering pathogenic factor can be hot in nature. Measles and HIB immunizations, in particular, tend to leave heat in the body.
- after a febrile disease: if a hot pathogenic factor is not properly cleared from the body. For example, if antibiotics are used to cool a fever, the heat can remain locked inside the body as a lingering pathogenic factor.
- accumulation disorder: this can be the cause of heat in young children.

Heat and phlegm (mania)

Heat and phlegm rise up and affect the Heart, disturb the spirit, and lead to anger and willful acts of aggression that are characteristic of this type of hyperactivity. The presence of phlegm causes "misting" or clouding of the mind, which can lead children to do things they know to be wrong. Their morals get blotted out. Among the causes of this type of hyperactivity are the following:

- Lingering pathogenic factor (LPF): a lingering pathogenic factor that is hot in nature and causes the formation of a lot of phlegm in the body. Typical examples are LPFs from measles and HIB immunizations.
- Food: a diet that is rich in phlegm-producing foods (dairy products, refined sugar, wheat). In young children the diet can cause accumulation disorder—producing heat and phlegm—and in older children the food itself can be both hot and phlegm producing. It is common for these children to have a gluten allergy; because gluten produces dampness, when they eat wheat a nasty thick goo develops. If taken off wheat, there is often a dramatic improvement.
- Accumulation disorder: diet and regularity of feeding in young children can cause accumulation disorder, which produces heat and phlegm in the body.

Weakness of the middle burner

Hyperactive Spleen qi deficient children must draw their energy from people around them. Usually parents can prevent this by setting up boundaries, thereby forcing the child to get energy for itself—from food. Where there are no such boundaries, the child can help itself to all it wants, commonly from parents, who are nearest at hand. The parents become exhausted and then cannot establish boundaries. This situation seems to promote in the child a sort of greedy, grabbing mentality—selfishness, which then develops into cruelty and hatred. The child becomes demanding out of all proportion (i.e., hyperactive), and furious when it can't get what it wants. This hyperactivity is especially noticeable when the child does not get what it wants *and* the parents withhold their energy.

The pathology of this condition is complex. It seems that the Spleen energy is weak and that the child draws qi from those around it. When qi is withheld for some reason, the child gets angry, probably because it is frightened by the sudden loss of energy. The qi becomes temporarily deficient and the blood does not circulate properly, withholding nourishment from the Heart. The child then gets anxious, restless, fidgety, and cannot sit still. Common causes include:

• Spleen qi deficiency: this can arise from many causes—immunizations, lengthy childbirth, anesthetics in childbirth, and long-term accumulation disorder, to name but a few. It can also stem from drinking too much fruit juice.
• No boundaries: these children seem to be able to manipulate their parents mercilessly. They manage to get their way in most things. In addition, they draw on their parents energy, who in turn become more and more exhausted, and thus less able to stand up to their child.

Kidney deficiency

The *yuán* qi (basal qi) Kidney energy is weak, and rises up to affect the Heart and the mind, resulting in hyperactive behavior. It is more obvious when the child is tired or overstimulated. Causes of Kidney deficiency include:

• constitutional Kidney weakness: the Kidney energy can be weak from birth, usually from weakness in the parents, genetic disorders, or severe illness during pregnancy
• long-term illness: if a child has been ill over the years, the Kidney energy can be weakened
• severe illness: a very severe illness, such as a long febrile disease or meningitis, can deplete the Kidney energy

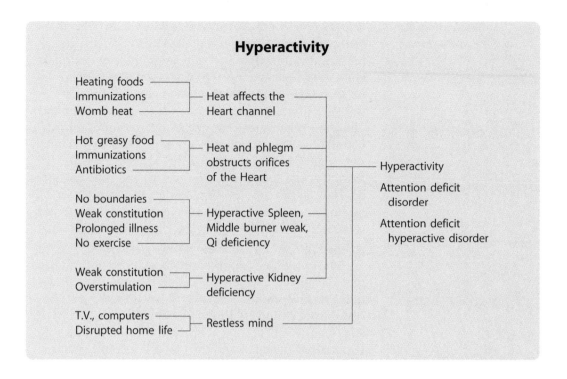

PATTERNS & SYMPTOMS

Heat	In younger children there may be accumulation disorder.

- very active
- restless
- talkative
- may destroy things
- insomnia: wakes up early (5 A.M.) or may be awake for an hour or two in the middle of the night
- red lips
- possibly whole face red

Tongue: red
Pulse: rapid, but hard to take

Heat and phlegm	In younger children there may be accumulation disorder.

- irritability
- restlessness
- shouts
- tantrums
- insomnia: wakes early, restless while sleeping
- violent
- willfully destructive
- may be sexually premature
- possible anal or genital fixation
- cannot concentrate

Tongue: red, possibly yellow coating
Pulse: rapid, slippery, but hard to take

Weakness of middle burner	• gray or pale face
	• dull or resentful eyes
	• lips may be dull
	• appetite poor
	• manipulative
	• sleep is poor, or only needs little sleep
	• often has great thirst and drinks a lot of fruit juice
	• loves to play destructive games: video games, or aggressive games with guns
	• may be cruel to brothers or sisters, and rude to parents

Tongue: pale, possibly with a red tip
Pulse: possibly weak, or wiry

Kidney deficiency	• thin, tall, beautiful
	• pale face
	• frail body
	• often ill
	• eyes are too bright, glittering
	• when overexcited the face may become red
	• hyperactive at the end of the day, when tired
	• hyperactive when overstimulated (e.g., at a party)
	• hyperactive after watching television
	• often terrified of needles

Tongue: may be pale, or red
Pulse: fine, floating

One way to distinguish a child with "false" hyperactivity from one with a "true" type is to feel the back of the child. If it feels weak and is curved, then it is likely that the child is of the Kidney-deficient pattern. If the bone structure is good, and the back straight and strong, then it is more likely to be another type of hyperactivity, if indeed it is pathological at all. The child may just be inquisitive and a bit annoying.

Case History

Master G, age eight, was brought to the clinic because he was behaving badly at school. He had always been demanding, but now was completely out of hand—never sitting still, always wanting attention, and being very difficult if he didn't get it. His mother was very upset. She felt as if she were "losing" her son. They had always been very close, but now he was becoming more and more distant and rude toward her.

Master G fell into the category of weak middle burner—very choosy about food, pale gray face, and manipulative. When it came to treating him he would scream "NO, NO!" at full volume and curl up in a ball on the floor. When I did manage to get a needle in him, he would break out into a big smile! However, the next point was the same—screams and protestations, then a smile when the needle was in. Things were slightly easier if the mother left the room, but still hard.

This ritual was infuriating as it would take a good forty-five minutes to treat him, which is a problem if your clinic is full and you are already running late. One student observing in the clinic was so fed up with him one day that he bribed him: ten pence per point. Master G was not impressed and negotiated twenty pence! After this, provided the rate was agreed beforehand, I was allowed to treat him. After about ten treatments he was noticeably different and we did not even need a bribe. Eventually, we reached the end and he did not have to come anymore. He was always going to be strong-minded, but he was not nearly as rude, and could control his temper much better. His mother was delighted; she felt as if she had "found her son again." I thought Master G himself would be delighted: no more torture! But on the last day he came up to me with a sad look and gave me a very loving hug and a "thank you."

TREATMENT

Treating a child with hyperactivity is no easy task. They can start off by wrecking the clinic, disturbing other patients and practitioners, and then irritating you. During treatment they hit, kick, scream, and make life difficult, to say the least. However, do persevere: the results can be quite astonishing—perhaps not immediate—but gradually the child will calm down.

Taking the pulse: with some children this can be virtually impossible, but hopefully it will not matter, as you should have a pretty good idea of what is going on by having read through the case history.

Advice about advice: try to be realistic about your advice to parents. A long list of "don'ts" is daunting and often unworkable within the structure of the family. Try to provide alternatives so that parents don't have to think too much themselves—they are often exhausted!

Heat | *Treatment principle:* clear the heat and calm the spirit

Main points:

H-7 *(shen men)*		Calms the spirit
Liv-2 *(xing jian)*		Calms the spirit, clears the heat, subdues the manic behavior
S-44 *(nei ting)*		Clears heat from the Stomach

If the main points don't seem to be working, try substituting H-8 *(shao fu)* in place of H-7 *(shen men)*. This point calms the spirit and clears heat from the Heart. Other points might include:

LI-4 *(he gu)*	Clears heat
Liv-3 *(tai chong)*	Calms the spirit, clears heat, and regulates the circulation of qi

Method: use a strong reducing technique

If there is accumulation disorder, use *si feng* (M-UE-9).

Reaction to Treatment

There are two common reactions during treatment with these children. On the one hand they tend to react strongly: they howl and scream, quite often just for effect. On the other hand they do not feel the needles at all, especially if there is a great deal of heat. (The interior heat disrupts the flow of qi to hands and feet, dulling sensation.) Thus, you can tell the child is improving when the drama of the treatment diminishes; and improvement in the condition brings increased response—and screams—to the needles.

In all children with this type of hyperactivity, they can go wild after treatment, as some heat is released. Do warn the parents of this. If you tell them, they can prepare themselves, and they will have faith that you actually know what you are doing!

Prognosis

Generally, ten to fifteen treatments are needed, depending on the severity and the amount of heat. If less severe, perhaps things will improve sooner. There should be gradual improvement in all cases.

Advice

As a matter of course, the child should be taken off all food colorings, additives, dairy products, oranges, orange juice, and sugar. There should be no colored soda pop or junk food. Regular meals, with a well-cooked and a well-balanced diet, are essential. The child should be encouraged to exercise, watch less television, and play fewer video games and the like. If the child has accumulation disorder, advise appropriately.

Phlegm and heat (mania)

Treatment principle: clear heat, resolve phlegm, and calm the spirit

Points:

H-7 *(shen men)*	Calms the spirit
H-8 *(shao fu)*	Calms the spirit and clears heat from the heart
Liv-2 *(xing jian)*	Clears heat, calms the spirit, and subdues the manic behaviour
S-40 *(feng long)*	Transforms the phlegm
G-34 *(yang ling quan)*	Transforms the phlegm
P-5 *(jian shi)*	Calms the spirit and clears the phlegm surrounding the Heart

Method: use a strong reducing technique

Reaction to Treatment

There will, over the course of treatment, be a discharge of phlegm—usually through the bowels and the nose, but it may be vomited. The stools may be loose for one to two months depending on the amount of phlegm present. This is a surprisingly long time, but it seems to be alright. A productive cough may also develop. As with the previous pattern, following treatment, the child may get very angry as heat is released. The reaction during treatment is likewise similar to that in the previous pattern.

Prognosis

Ten to thirty treatments may be required, depending on the severity of the condition. Once all the phlegm and heat has been cleared you may well find an underlying Spleen dysfunction which may need treatment.

Advice

Similar to the previous pattern, and no peanuts or peanut butter.

Weakness in middle burner

Treatment principle: strengthen the middle burner, tonify the Spleen. Encourage the parents to establish boundaries.

Points:

Sp-6 *(san yin jiao)*	Tonifies the Spleen
S-36 *(zu san li)*	Tonifies the Stomach and Spleen
Liv-3 *(tai chong)*	Calms the spirit and regulates the circulation of qi
H-7 *(shen men)*	Calms the spirit
CV-12 *(zhong wan)*	Use moxa

Reaction to Treatment

These children will often scream blue murder! They will cry crocodile tears and make such a noise that even your colleagues will look at you with a "What were you doing to that poor child?" expression. It is somewhat infuriating as you know that it doesn't hurt that much: the child is just being difficult and manipulating its parents! It can reach such a pitch that the parents will begin to doubt you, and may give in and stop bringing the child.

One way around this is to *get the parents to leave the room,* if the child is old enough. In this way the child cannot play up to them so much, and cannot draw so much qi from them. When we have done this, far from being a trauma, the child often becomes very calm.

Prognosis

Quite variable. Possibly ten treatments, and up to thirty. A lot depends on the home situation.

Advice

The main advice is to the parents: they must set boundaries. This is often very difficult because the first few weeks can be hell for the family as the child gets very upset at being told what to do and having all his free energy withheld. Keep off fruit juice and limit consumption of liquids. Also important for these children is to stop them from watching television and playing video games. And—as with the other patterns—diet, exercise, and a regular lifestyle are important.

Kidney deficiency

Treatment principle: tonify the Kidney energy, calm the spirit

These children are usually genuinely afraid of needles, so don't use them. Using needles is actually counterproductive as their fear weakens the Kidney energy further. Herbal medicine is often useful, although they may find it too disgusting to take.

Points:

B-23 *(shen shu)*
K-1 *(yong quan)*
L-8 *(qu quan)*
Sp-6 *(san yin jiao)*

Method: use moxa at all points. You may also advise that they drink teas like limeflower or passiflora.

Reaction to Treatment

If you just use moxa the child should be happy, but if you try to use needles the child may really freak out. You can tell the difference between these children and those with the previous pattern by looking at their eyes and feeling the lower back. If the eyes are bright and glittery and the back is weak, then they fall into this category. If the eyes are intense and the back is reasonably strong, then it is likely they are of the hyperactive weak middle burner type. It is not always easy to tell though.

Prognosis

It takes time for these children to recover. Depending on the severity of the Kidney weakness, you may need to treat for many months.

Advice

The child must be encouraged to rest, early nights, no television or any form of stimulation for a couple of hours before bedtime. They must also avoid sugar, and should take gentle exercise. Suggest something like artistic acting.

NOTES

- Some children are labeled hyperactive and put on drugs when actually they are simply bored with school. Often they are strong, willful, and intelligent children who simply do not want to sit still for long periods, and are easily bored with simple school work. Identifying these children can be hard, but important, especially if they are going to be put on drugs, which simply dampens their enthusiasm for life. Moreover, the drug Ritalin, a derivative of speed which is commonly prescribed for hyperactivity in children, is very damaging to the Spleen. Long-term use inevitably leads to Spleen qi or yang deficiency.

- For an additional case history involving hyperactivity, see Case 22 in Chapter 47.

❖

32 ❖ Down's Syndrome

INTRODUCTION

In this chapter we discuss what can be done for children with Down's syndrome. We will see that acupuncture can make a great difference to a child, and can make the difference between having to spend life in an institution, or living a more or less normal life. I have not found anything in the Chinese literature about it, so this lesson is based entirely on our experience with Western children. This is not because Down's children are not born in China, but perhaps because they are just accepted as part of the scene of normal life. Even in England up until the early part of this century it was common to have a "village idiot," who may well have been a Down's child. In those days when we were closer to the soil, and there was less emphasis on mental agility, there was a place for such people in society—as children and as adults. Now, because of the quick reactions needed even to stay alive in a busy city, there is no place for them. However, as we have said, with acupuncture, a Down's child may be able to function much more effectively in the modern world.

What is Down's syndrome?

Formerly known as "mongolism," there are abnormalities in the chromosomes. These children characteristically have rounded skulls, a flattened face with obliquely set eyes. They have a fresh complexion, and short hands with rather stubby fingers. Often the tongue is fissured, or else sticks out all the time. Often the mouth hangs open, frequently dribbling. The children are nearly always slow and backward. Although they can learn skills, if painstakingly taught, they have difficulty in solving problems.

Causes of Down's Syndrome

In Western medicine Down's syndrome is attributed to a defective gene. This gene is considered responsible for the many symptoms which were first described by Dr. Down of Richmond, England, in the eighteenth century.

In traditional Chinese medicine there is the same idea of something inherited and immutable, but it is put rather differently—insufficiency of essence *(jīng)*. The prenatal energy supplied by the parents is insufficient. Essence is stored in the Kidneys, and also activates the Kidneys, so in traditional Chinese medicine deficiency of essence manifests in the characteristic way of Kidney deficiency: unusual bone development, poor mental ability, poor brain development, imbalance in water metabolism. Having said that, Down's children are really in a special category all their own. There are many signs of Kidney weakness, as we will see, and yet physically they are very strong.

Physical causes

The physical cause of Down's syndrome is weakness of essence supplied by the parents. In the past this was usually because of conception late in the parent's life, when the essence was declining; often, this conception followed earlier, healthy children. In conventional medical books, it is said that Down's syndrome babies are much more commonly born to mothers over thirty-five years of age, with the percentage rising with age.

This pattern seems to be changing. My own observation, and that of practitioners in both conventional and complementary fields, is that Down's syndrome is now more common for mothers in their late twenties. Listed below are some possible reasons for this.

Overwork and exhaustion

One need only walk down the street of any major city in the United Kingdom to see that the majority of men and women of childbearing age are absolutely exhausted. The drive toward greater productivity, and the overstimulation from common entertainments, leads to a depleted state, especially depletion of Kidney energy. So too does reckless indulgence in sex.

Poor food

An indication of the decline of essence available for reproduction is to be found in sperm counts. It has been reported that sperm counts in Europe are now less than half what they were twenty years ago, and that there is a steady decline. It is estimated that if this trend continues, then in twenty years time most men in Europe will be infertile. Both food and pollution of the environment have been blamed for this in conventional medical circles. Food has been considered the cause because nonorganic food is deficient in trace elements needed to maintain health. Although there is a mountain of over-produced food in Europe, most of it is of such poor quality that it has given rise to malnutrition.

Wheat is grown on bare soil only by means of chemical fertilizers. The strains of wheat themselves are selected for productivity, and are poor foods which are difficult to digest. The milk is squeezed from cows by means of hormones, which deplete the cow's energy so that its life is three years instead of twenty.

Thus, one can see that all the foods are drawn from exhausted soil and exhausted animals. From the point of view of Chinese medicine, it is not surprising that milk and meat which comes from exhausted animals leads to a state of deficiency.

Pollution

The effects of pollution are now thought to be much more widespread than originally believed, especially on the reproductive system. It has been shown that pollution as diverse as car fumes and shampoos, growth hormones in meat and pesticides, all contain chemicals that mimic estrogens or progesterones. These chemicals are not easily metabolized in the body, and sit on sites receptive to estrogens and progesterones. Consequently, the whole reproductive system in both men and women is put significantly out of balance.

Contraceptives

For more than thirty years hormonal contraception has been used. When they were developed, no one thought of any long-term problems. But it is now clear that they alter the balance of hormones for many years after their use has been stopped. This is bound to have some effect on the unborn baby.

Causes at the Level of the Spirit

In the traditional description of conception in Chinese medicine it is said that the parents provide prenatal qi from their essence. But it is also said that the spirit comes from the child. Working with children, one is struck again and again with the accuracy of this description. Children look like and behave like their parents—they get their bodies and manners from them—yet each child is an individual. Their genes are inherited, but what they make of their genes, which ones they select, which they switch on or switch off, is up to the individual. Each child has a spirit which is unique. The external manifestation, the thought and behavior, is strongly influenced by the parents, but the core of the spirit is unique. There is something in each child's make-up which comes from nowhere but that individual.

Moreover, it is equally clear that some children bring certain imbalances and illnesses with them. Often mothers ask why their children have certain illnesses, and usually one can find a reason—either in such things as infections or diet, or in some problem of the parents or of the pregnancy. But sometimes there appears to be no obvious reason. A child is just born a certain way. There seems to be no obvious reason why a child has a particular problem, or a particular nature, beyond that it was born that way. This was the pattern that the child brought with it into this world.

This is very much the case with Down's syndrome, for although there is a clear reason (in deficiency of essence) why they should manifest their symptoms, there is no external reason why they should manifest in this particular way, with a mixture of physical sturdiness and Kidney weakness. If it were simply due to Kidney weakness, one would expect a much more sickly child.[1]

It has certainly been observed that there is a disturbance of the spirit in Down's children: they all have great difficulty in solving problems. They appear to have no difficulty in memorizing actions and activities, but the part of their mind concerned with finding new ways and solutions to problems tends to be underdeveloped. To compensate for this, their intuitive faculties are much more highly developed, and they respond strongly to the feelings of those around them. Another universal feature of Down's children is their level of happiness. In contrast to many other types of unbalanced children or brain damaged children, joy and spontaneous love bubbles up from within and affects all who come close to them.

PATTERNS & SYMPTOMS

There are two major constitutional patterns:

• phlegm-dampness
• full heat

You will have no difficulty distinguishing these patterns.

---

1. In fact, these children with straightforward Kidney essence deficiency are now so common in the West that they have been grouped together as 'Noonan's Syndrome'.

The "normal" pattern, that is, the one which they normally show when they come to see you, is the phlegm-dampness pattern. During the course of treatment, this cold, wet, deficient pattern evolves into the full heat pattern.

Phlegm-dampness

- pale face
- puffy face
- nasal discharge pale and watery
- watery eyes
- dribbling from the mouth
- slow, large movements
- rather docile
- prone to frequent infections

Pulse: deep and weak, or slippery and full, or soggy
Tongue: pale, often with white coating

Full heat

- red face
- nasal discharge is yellow, thick
- red tongue
- restless, inquisitive, active
- demanding, insistent, dominating

Pulse: rapid, full, often slippery
Tongue: red

TREATMENT

Everyday Illnesses

Down's syndrome children are prone to all the diseases that other children get: coughs, colds, fevers, indigestion, heat problems, cold problems, wind problems, dampness problems. There is nothing special to be said about treatment of these normal childhood illnesses. The principles and practice of treatment are the same as for any other child. For example, a Down's child was brought recently suffering from repeated chest infections, which developed into pneumonia. The treatment principle was to strengthen the Lungs and protective qi, and to clear the lingering pathogenic factor. Simple points were used, such as L-5 *(chi ze)*, L-9 *(tai yuan)*, and S-40 *(feng long)* in early sessions, followed by B-13 *(fei shu)* later on.

Constitutional Treatment

The constitutional imbalance is deficiency of essence, and it might be thought that nothing can be done after birth. This is not the case. There is one school of thought in traditional Chinese medicine which holds that the child is dependent on the mother for the first three years of life, and continues to receive essence during this time. This certainly seems to be the case and explains, for example, why some women feel "brain dead" and others totally exhausted for two to three years after the birth of a child.

Phlegm-dampness

Simple treatments can be given to tonify the Kidneys, with tonifying method and moxa, or simply moxa alone (usually a moxa stick).

Points:

B-23 *(shen shu)*
K-3 *(tai xi)*
CV-4 *(guan yuan)*

Also select one point from the following list. These points are used to bring the essence to the head and help develop the brain.

GV-16 *(feng fu)*
GV-15 *(ya men)*
B-10 *(tian zhu)*

Treatment is given once (or possibly twice) a week.[2]

Full heat

This pattern usually evolves from the phlegm-dampness pattern. The treatment principle is to clear the heat affecting the Heart.

Points:

Liv-2 *(xing jian)*
H-8 *(shao fu)*
G-20 *(feng chi)*

Method: use even method at all points; quite strong reducing technique can be used.

If the tongue sticks out a lot, add GV-23 *(lian quan),* and change H-8 *(shao fu)* to H-5 *(tong li)*. During the intermediate stage, when there is still some Kidney deficiency but the heat is beginning to emerge, you may also use B-23 *(shen men)* with a tonifying method.

Results of Treatment

If treatment can be given during the first three years, the results of treating in this manner must be seen to be believed. The moon face disappears, the structure of the face changes, with the cheek bones becoming less promi-

2. Of course, the practitioner does not give the child essence, but the treatment opens the way for the mother's essence to flow.

nent, the eyebrows less slanted, the eyes less slit-shaped; thus, the child looks less "mongoloid." Also, the child becomes more alert and quicker at learning. Some of the children that we have treated even develop the ability to solve problems, an ability that these children are not supposed to have. In fact, some children change so much as a result of treatment that it takes an experienced eye to detect any signs which would label them as Down's children.

Case History

This story illustrates what can be done, even without therapy. There is a family in Spain, friends of a Spanish patient of mine (JPS), who had a Down's syndrome baby about forty years ago. They were at first very distressed, because they came from fairly wealthy middle class, and did not like the idea of an "idiot" being born into the family. However, they soon got used to the child being different, and were captivated by his happiness and laughter.

No therapy was available at that time, but they took very great care of him, and did their best to stimulate his mind and body. They were insistent that he go to normal schools, and do everything else that the other children in the town did, as far as possible. This meant that they had to spend a lot of time and influence on the authorities, persuading them and bullying them into accepting their child into a normal school, even though he looked very peculiar. (Since no therapy was then available, he had all the physical marks of a Down's child.) It also meant that they had to spend a lot of time with their child, helping him to learn various tasks, and spending much more time teaching him than one would expect.

Their work paid off, and now, at the age of forty, he is living a happy life. He is married, has a job, and lives in his own house. He is very happy in his job, which (like so many jobs now) is repetitive and mechanical, for he finds problem-solving a bit difficult. This is not to say he cannot solve problems, nor that he cannot face challenges. Last year he gave a talk to 150 normal delegates at an international conference on Down's syndrome about the problems he experienced from having a "mongoloid" face, which puts so many people off.

By contrast, his younger brother (not a Down's child) is very unhappy. Partly as a result of feeling neglected in childhood, partly from a naturally lazy temperament, but mostly from having a quick mind and having to do repetitive work!

What Happens in Practice

All the Down's children brought to us have come with the first pattern—accumulation of phlegm-dampness. This has its roots in Kidney deficiency. After about twenty to thirty treatments, most of the Kidney deficiency has been overcome, and most of the dampness cleared. It is at this stage that one sees the emergence of the full heat pattern. Already the children are very much improved; in fact, by this stage they are so transformed that to look at them, a casual observer may not notice that the child is abnormal. Often the children can go to normal schools and do not require special attention.

This reversal, from cold deficiency to full heat, is surprising. It is certainly worth continuing treatment, for at this stage one often meets a great obstinacy, restlessness, and inquisitiveness that is difficult to live with. Put in common language, these children are "stroppy" most of the time.

What Age to Treat?

The best age to start treating is early in life, preferably during the first three years. One cannot predict with certainty, but it appears that if treatment can be started at this age, the outward signs of Down's syndrome can be almost completely removed, and the child has the best opportunity to develop its full potential.

However, it is certainly worth starting treatment at a later age—at any age, in fact—but the later the treatment begins, the less effect it will have on bone and brain development. So if treatment is given after the age of fourteen, it is unlikely to affect the facial appearance very much, but it can have a very significant effect in clearing dampness and phlegm, and in strengthening resistance to disease.

Other Treatments

We have focused here on acupuncture treatment, but it must be mentioned that practitioners in other fields (e.g., cranial osteopathy, herbal medicine—both Western and Chinese—and homeopathy) also report the huge changes that can come about as a result of their treatment if started before the age of three.

ADVICE TO PARENTS

Diet

Parents should be advised to keep phlegm-producing foods out of the diet as much as possible. During the early stage (cold from deficiency), warming foods and meat are appropriate. In the later stage, when cold and deficiency have given way to heat and excess, the emphasis in the diet should be changed away from meat (which should not be given more than once a week) toward a vegetarian diet.

Activity

The conventional advice is to give Down's children a lot of stimulation and activity, in order to stimulate their brain activity. This is good advice for the cold deficiency stage, but when the child is in the full heat stage, then much less stimulation should be given. At this stage the child is providing itself with all the stimulation it needs, and it should be allowed more time to reflect.

Social Factors

Down's children are very special. They are different from the majority of other children who are born with severe disorders, for they have an openness and a spontaneous happiness which is quite infectious. It is normally quite a shock for the parents, especially the mothers, when a Down's baby is born, but the majority soon bond to the new baby and are able to love it. When this happens, the effect on the family is quite amazing. It seems that the children are great teachers, for they gradually bring about changes in the parents which make them more loving, and value the important things of life, rather than accept the values of society. Mothers no longer see the need to be career orientated at the expense of their families, and fathers no longer feel the need to climb to the top of the career ladder. Both parents start to value the forces of love and harmony more highly than before.

Eugenics

In recent years medical tests have been developed based on amniocentesis which enable one to tell if the unborn child has the defective "deficient" chromosome which gives rise to Down's syndrome. On the basis of this test, many abortions are performed to prevent the birth of a "defective" baby. This test is yet one more of the orthodox tests which brings with it both good and bad, and which brings up yet another moral dilemma. For those who believe in improving the quality of the race, there is no dilemma, and for those who believe that they have a right to give birth to a healthy child and do not want to waste their energy on an unhealthy or deformed child, there is no dilemma. But for most mothers and fathers, the issue is not so simple. They may think with their mind that they would like a perfect baby, and at first be repelled by the thought of anything odd. Yet in their hearts they know that there is new life. They know instinctively that life occurs very early in pregnancy and do not like the thought of killing the unborn child.

There are no easy answers to such a quandary, and certainly orthodox medicine creates the dilemma, but does not solve it. Indeed, there is no answer which is correct for every situation. Each mother must decide for herself what is the best course to take. If she feels she would hate the child and herself for giving birth to a "mongol," then maybe it is kinder to stop the life before it has really begun in earnest.

From the medical point of view, having an abortion may be similar to removing an appendix, but emotionally and spiritually it is quite different. Having an abortion is by no means an easy option, for it can leave scars for a lifetime if nothing is done to help the mother grieve and overcome her ambivalent feelings.

To conclude this survey of the social difficulties generated by the test, we would like to repeat what joy Down's children bring with them. When the family is strong enough to withstand the strains that naturally arise from having a child that needs special attention, then the love and happiness which they bring affects the whole family, and brings love and acceptance where before there was hardness and superficiality. Having a Down's baby is a blessing in disguise. At first it is hard to see anything but the disguise, as it takes time for the blessings to appear.

OTHER POINTS OF VIEW

Chinese Perspective

As mentioned in the introduction, there has not been a Dr. Down in China, so all Down's children come under the category of the "five slows" or mental retardation, discussed in Chapter 30. Some Chinese consider the root cause to be in-breeding, and one of my patients who went to a Chinese herbalist to get herbs to assist my treatment was insulted by the suggestion that her child was the result of incest with her father!

Anthroposophical Perspective

The anthroposophical movement is the work of the great visionary Dr. Rudolf Steiner. He had a wonderful view of how the world should develop, based on love and respect for humanity, and what he called "spiritual science," which is a combination of scientific thought in a spiritual framework. The extraordinary depth and breadth of this vision has led to pioneering work in such diverse fields as farming, education, medicine, banking, art, and architecture, to name a few. In each of these fields he outlined principles and practices which were, and still are, a huge advance over the practice of the time. Although one can find fault with the way some of the "Steiner" institutes are run, the basic truth of his techniques are obvious in the institutions based on his work. Biodynamic farms just feel good to be in, and the cows on the farms are the epitome of "contented cows." Likewise, the banks based on his principles are much more friendly, and see their aims as assisting the community.

Steiner has made a contribution toward the teaching of Down's children. At the time he lived these people were judged to be "village idiots." With his clear insight and compassion, he went to the heart of their problem. He saw them as contented people, basically happy with their lot, who did not, however, have the higher mental faculties that are common to most humans. They can learn, but they have very poor ability in solving problems, and very poor conceptual thought. To compensate for this, they are highly intuitive, and very loving. As such, he considered that these people were in a state of development at the lower end of the human scale, and had, as it were, just made that huge evolutionary step from the top of the animal kingdom to the bottom of the human kingdom.

Whether you agree with this analysis or not, there can be no disagreeing with the homes that have been established for Down's children on the basis of his ideas. The people there are obviously happy. They are given as much autonomy as is possible. In the United States, for example, there are farms which are run almost exclusively by Down's people, with only one or two non-Down's people among forty to fifty Down's, just to do the mental work like accounting. All the important decisions are made by the Down's people themselves.

Buddhist Perspective

There are similarities between the Steiner perspective and that of the Buddhists, although there are differences as well. In the Steiner perspective, souls gradually make their way upward, through the animal kingdom, through the human realm, to eventual union with God. In the Buddhist perspective, successive lives are more like a snakes and ladders game—it is possible to go down a snake to a lower realm, as well as up a ladder to a higher one. Otherwise, there are many similarities. It could be said from the Buddhist perspective that a Down's person must be one who is emerging from a long period in an animal realm. It is a slightly less judgmental attitude, for although it acknowledges the closeness of Down's people to the animal realm, it recognizes that their essential nature is the same as other humans. The person has just had a slightly less favorable rebirth.

SUMMARY

The effect of acupuncture in treating Down's syndrome children must be seen to be believed. Treatment is most effective before the age of three years, when the transformation can be so marked that few of the signs and symptoms normally associated with Down's syndrome remain. Even after three years, however, treatment is still worth giving, and can help the person develop to the stage where they can look after themselves in adult life.

❖

33 ❖ Autism

INTRODUCTION

Autism is a very loose term for a wide variety of problems, and is used as a "diagnosis" for behavioral disorders where a child is rather withdrawn, or fails to interact with other children or adults. It is about as precise a diagnosis as calling someone a metal-type child. The diagnosis includes children who are:

- withdrawn because of shock or terror
- withdrawn because of abandonment
- withdrawn because of brain damage
- withdrawn as a result of serious illness

COMMON SYMPTOMS

Although there is a huge range of conditions included under this heading, they do tend to have some symptoms in common:

- lack of eye contact
- withdrawn behavior
- in extreme cases sits alone, staring into space
- rocking movements

We are asked, from time to time, whether acupuncture can be of help. The answer is emphatically yes. All the children brought to us with "autism" have been helped enormously. This is not to say that they can all be cured, nor that acupuncture should be the only therapy. There are many other therapies which can be of help. For example, if a child has missed out on stages of development, it may need to establish new reflex actions, which can be done with specialized therapy. Likewise, another child may need to learn to speak. However, with Chinese medicine, one can get a picture of how much of the problem is due to physical causes, and how much is due to "psychological" causes, or spirit *(shén)* disturbance, and one can get a clearer idea of the way forward.

We in no way claim to be expert in this field, so the comments set out below are merely a tentative beginning. We would both welcome any contributions and comments from readers who have experience in this area. Indeed, we hope that in time, someone will develop a special interest in this field and provide a much fuller account than ours.

COMMON PATTERNS

There are some common patterns which normally manifest on the physical level, but in some children have an extreme and drastic effect on the spirit. Often, by treating the physical pattern, this enables the spirit to return to a more or less normal state. Certainly it makes it easier if other therapies are being used. The following may be contributory causes to patterns of withdrawn behavior:

• extreme qi deficiency
• lingering pathogenic factor (LPF)
• brain damage
• Kidney weakness
• spirit disturbances

Extreme qi deficiency

This pattern is seen after a febrile disease. During the fever the child will be restless and agitated, and even delirious or convulsive, but when the fever comes down the pendulum swings the other way, and the child may become completely inert. This is quite a common occurrence and normally rights itself; but sometimes the pattern persists and the child is never right again. Instead, it will live in a twilight world, only half there. The spirit somehow never finds its way back to the Heart.

Treatment

S-36 *(zu san li)*	Tonifies the qi
Sp-6 *(san yin jiao)*	Tonifies the qi
GV-26 *(ren zhong)*	Restores the spirit and returns to consciousness
H-7 *(shen men)*	Nourishes the Heart

Effect of Treatment

The qi gradually improves, although it may take some time. It does not guarantee a cure, but it makes it much easier for the child to interact with its surroundings.

Lingering pathogenic factor

This pattern, too, can be caused by a high fever, or alternatively a bad reaction to an immunization. However, the behavior of the child is rather different:

• restless, irritable, cannot settle
• some red on the face, either red lips or cheeks
• may talk to themselves
• unable to concentrate

The pattern here is like hyperactivity, only the effect on the spirit is much more extreme. The heat in the Heart has an extreme effect, and the spirit is just not quiet enough to stay still even for a moment, so the child cannot relate in a normal way.

Treatment

H-8 *(shao fu)*	Clears heat from the Heart
Liv-2 *(xing jian)* or	Clears heat from the body
S-44 *(nei ting)*	Clears heat from the body

Brain damage

Once again, this pattern can follow a high fever where the child convulses for a long time, or it may follow meningitis or an immunization. It can also occur from lack of oxygen to the brain (e.g., during birth or a difficult surgical operation) or from injury to the head. Conventionally speaking, the reason for the autism is that there are parts of the brain which relate to social behavior. In some brain injuries the restraining factor in social interaction is absent, and a child will treat all people as long lost friends, jumping into their laps and giving them slobbery kisses, irrespective of whether they are close family or complete strangers. In autism this trend is reversed, treating close family and complete strangers with equal indifference.

Treatment

Often with brain damage there is underlying Kidney deficiency which must be treated first. When the Kidney energy is stronger, it may be helpful to use scalp acupuncture. Our experience with this pattern is limited. The autistic children that we have seen with brain damage have not been purely brain damaged. There were other things going on—qi deficiency, or a lingering pathogenic factor.

However, even when these disorders had been more or less cured, the child's behavior was very withdrawn, and lacked normal eye contact. The treatment that we gave was B-23 *(shen shu)* because they were Kidney deficient, and GV-16 *(feng fu)*. (It is possible that scalp acupuncture would also be effective.) What happened was that with acupuncture, and the special attention that the child received, it did gradually develop social interaction over the years.

Kidney weakness

This may be attributed to many causes, among them deficiency of Kidney essence from birth, or Kidney qi deficiency due to long illness or overwork. One sees the following symptoms:

- pale face, maybe gray
- weak lumbar back
- feels frail, as though a wind would blow them away
- often sees "ghosts" and talks and interacts with an imaginary world*

Treatment

B-23 *(shen shu)*	Needle plus moxa
CV-4 *(guan yuan)*	Moxa
S-36 *(zu san li)*	

A diet containing red meat may be helpful.

Spirit disturbances

The spirit *(shén)* is so complicated, and there are so many factors which can disturb it, that any description is bound to be a simplification. Moreover, the majority of spirit disturbances are better dealt with by hourly and daily care and love than by weekly acupuncture. There are, however, two patterns we have seen that are appropriately treated with acupuncture. The main characteristic of these patterns is that there are no special physical signs or symptoms.

Shock or Fright

The child has been exposed to a terrifying situation. This disturbs the spirit such that the child does not interact

---

*It is normal for children under seven years to see "ghosts" or "imaginary" beings, that is, beings that those over seven years cannot see. It is especially common for them to be aware of a sort of "guardian angel." My own (JPS) daughter was accompanied by a helpful being at the age of five, and for a few months even insisted that we lay a place at the table for her great friend. In the context of autism, the condition becomes pathological when either the "imaginary" world becomes more important than the "real" one, or when the child cannot make a distinction.

normally with the world around. Sometimes this pattern is accompanied by the tell-tale sign of blue between the eyes.

Treatment

Acupuncture can be effective in bringing back the spirit, with points such as:

GV-26 *(ren zhong)*
H-7 *(shen men)*
S-36 *(zu san li)*

Anger

Anger normally has an upward and outward energy, but if a child is physically abused and neglected, it may find that it suffers yet more abuse or neglect if this anger is allowed to manifest. The anger is then contained, and can react back along the Ke cycle to the metal element (in the controlling cycle of the five phases), causing complete withdrawal.

Treatment

Obviously, the source of the anger has to be removed; if the child is still being abused or neglected, there is little one can do. These children are often removed to homes to get away from the abuse, but neglect may still be there. Acupuncture can be of help, with points such as:

Liv-3 *(tai chong)*	Draws energy away from wood
L-5 *(chi ze)*	Draws energy away from metal, into water
B-18 *(gan shu)*	

=======

At first there may be no reaction at all to treatment, but then one day there may be a sudden and violent outburst, as years of extreme pent-up anger comes flooding out.

=======

NOTE

• For a case history involving autism, see Case 9 in Chapter 47.

❖

34 ❖ Dyslexia

INTRODUCTION

"My child is dyslexic, can you help?" is the cry so often heard. And equally often a sort of blank feeling arises in the practitioner: "Well . . . er . . . I don't know . . . maybe!" And that really is the sum total of it. Maybe you can help with acupuncture, maybe not. In the next few pages we try to show the factors involved, and what to look out for. We will see that the normal patterns which are related to learning difficulties are likely to be present here, but that there are also some special features.

What is It?

Dyslexia is the condition where a child's ability to spell is far behind its other abilities. It can manifest in different ways: just plain bad spelling, or inability to see whether a word is spelled wrongly. A common pattern is to interchange or omit letters in a word, so that "the" may be spelled "hte," or "read" is spelled "wread."

It is only relatively recently that dyslexia has been given a name and an "official" diagnosis. In the past most dyslexic children were classified as either lazy or stupid. Now a child with this diagnosis may be allowed to take special oral exams, rather than written ones, so that he or she may even take a university degree without putting pen to paper!

Why does it happen?

Dyslexia is a peculiarly Western problem, and does not occur in China. It has something to do with our script.

This difference between the two ways of writing is so great that one project in Canada to cure dyslexia involved teaching simple Chinese characters, and giving them Western sounds. At the end of a short course, the pupils could read and write English sentences using Chinese characters. This had such a strengthening effect on their minds that they began to be able to read and write using English letters. My own (JPS) experience is that the mild dyslexia that I have improved significantly when I learned Chinese.

So what is different between the languages? A very big difference has been noted by workers who observe brain waves. It has been found that to write a word in a Roman script, information must go back and forth between the left and right sides of the brain many times. So, for example, suppose you wish to write the word "spoon." First you have to generate the idea of a spoon. This may happen in the left side of the brain. You then need to find the exact sound—"spoon"—which you will find on the other side. You must then look up the spelling, which is stored in the left side. Then you need to look in the right side for the shape of the letters; then back to the left side to output the information into the right hand. (For left-handed people there may be yet another stage, as the information which was intended for the right hand is sent to the left!) In Chinese there is less transfer of information from one side of the brain to the other because there is no spelling, and a word is identified by a *shape* rather than a *sound.*

I may have some of the details wrong in this description, but you get the idea. In order to write, information must be shuttled back and forth between the two halves of the brain. Anything which interferes with this passage of information can cause dyslexia.

Physical Causes

The imbalances that we have clearly described above can interfere with the passage of information, giving rise to the four imbalances, each of which can be a factor in dyslexia:

- heat
- phlegm
- qi deficiency
- Kidney weakness

Heat

With heat, all the information is pushed through too rapidly. All the words come pouring out much too quickly, and in the torrent, some letters get muddled up and come out too soon.

Phlegm	With phlegm, the barrier is the confusing sensation you get when you have a cold. There is a sort of foggy blanket between the parts of the mind, such that letters inserted in one order come out the other side in a different order.
Weakness	With qi deficiency or Kidney weakness, there is not the energy to get things exactly right. The mind lacks precision simply because there is not enough mental energy to keep the mind tidy.

Other Factors

Shock from being dropped

What distinguishes dyslexia from other types of learning difficulty is the pattern of transferred information from one side of the brain to the other. This is very often associated with a left-right imbalance. It may take several forms, such as the qi on one side being much stronger than the other; or lack of real awareness of which side is left and which is right; or of being "wrong-handed": using the left hand when truly right-handed, or using the right hand when truly left-handed.[1]

This can occur in a child who is dropped, especially if dropped onto its bottom, so that the coccyx is injured. The jarring effect can go right up the spine, and cause a serious left-right imbalance. If there is already some physical imbalance of the kind mentioned above, it is very likely that the shock will stay in the system for many, many years. (Those of you with some knowledge of homeopathy will be interested to note that among the indications of the remedy Hypericum are injury to the coccyx and also dyslexia.)

Emotional dropping

Sometimes the pattern can be caused by being emotionally dropped, rather than physically dropped. This lack of sound emotional support may be due to abandonment by one or both parents, or it may be an emotional pattern that is built into family life as a result of abandonment experienced by one of the parents themselves that has not been fully overcome.

Educational Factors

Early learning to read

It used to be the tradition (and still is in some European countries) to send children to school at the age of seven.

---

1. P.F.M. Nogier discusses how to determine intrinsic handedness in *Treatise of Auriculotherapy* (Paris: Maisonneuve, 1972).

Traditionally, they were not expected to begin reading before that age. Now reading lessons may begin at age five or even earlier, in the rush to turn children into little adults as soon as possible. For some children this may result in dyslexia, for it seems that to learn to spell well, a child must develop a clear sense of left and right. For some people this never comes, throughout life, while for others a sense of left and right may come very early indeed. But for the majority of children a clear idea of left and right comes between the ages of about four and six. Below this age you may, for example, see them holding knife and fork in the wrong hand.

Reading and writing are very closely associated with awareness of left and right. For example, words are conventionally written from left to right, and d's and b's are only distinguished by whether the circle is to the left or right of the vertical straight line. (A beautiful example of how difficult children find it to distinguish between d's and b's was provided by a child who spelled the word "blood" as "dlub".)

Insecurity

All sorts of school problems can contribute to dyslexia. On their own they are unlikely to cause it, but together with other factors they can turn a mild problem into a serious one. Among the most prominent are bullying, and being told that one is stupid.

Crawling

Some children have no inclination to crawl, while others are actively encouraged to walk early and curtail the crawling stage. This is a pity, for crawling is one of the best ways of strengthening the connections between the two halves of the brain, so much so that "cross-crawling" is now a major part of dyslexia therapy.

TREATMENT

Body acupuncture

Step One: Treat any Illness

The first step is to treat any imbalance that you see in the child. This is likely to be one of the four patterns discussed above: heat, phlegm, qi deficiency, or Kidney weakness. If you can improve the child's health, then its mind will also improve. Likewise, if there is a serious imbalance, there is little point in treating more subtle imbalances such as left-right energy imbalance.

Step Two: Balance Left and Right

Once you have a reasonably healthy child in front of you, you can investigate left-right imbalance. One way is to feel the overall energy on the two sides, and compare them. A more sophisticated way is to use the Akebani test, where sensitivity to heat (in the form of an incense stick) of the *jīng* (well) point is compared on the two sides. An even more sophisticated test is to compare the electrical resistance or potentials of the *jīng* points.

If there is a significant left-right imbalance, then you can treat this, for example, with points on the Gallbladder and Triple Burner channels, or possibly using the yin and yang heel vessels.

Ear acupuncture

There is an interesting treatment described by Nogier, the founding father of ear acupuncture. He discovered that he could both generate and cure dyslexia by ear acupuncture. He noticed that the polarity of the lobes of the ears was different in dyslexic patients. By altering the polarity (using direct current) in a normal subject he could generate dyslexia, and by restoring polarity, he could cure it.

Other Therapies

There are many other therapies which are used to help dyslexics, a full discussion of which is outside the scope of this book. However, one which has to be mentioned because it is so simple and brings such quick results is "cross-crawling."

Cross-crawling

Cross-crawling is a term which has been coined to describe any activity (including crawling) in which the right arm is moved at the same time as the left leg, and vice versa. A very simple example of this is plain walking, while swinging the arms—marching, in fact. Here the right arm and left leg go forward simultaneously.[2]

A more sophisticated version of this is to lift up the left knee and touch it with the right hand, then lift up the right knee and touch it with the left hand. After about five minutes of this, a child will notice a significant improvement in its dyslexia.

2. You will notice that dyslexic children find it difficult even to walk in a steady manner. They may run and then stop, when taken on a walk, or they may like to carry something so that they do not have to swing their arms.

CONCLUSION

To conclude this chapter, we return to the opening question: can you help dyslexia? As you can see now, the answer is "maybe." The more physical signs there are, the more impact you can make with acupuncture. It is certainly true that acupuncture can be of great help, for the key to curing dyslexia is establishing new pathways between the left and right sides of the brain. Acupuncture can restore the body to health and redress any left-right imbalance, thus opening the way for the pathways to be corrected. This may be enough, or it may be the preliminary that enables other therapies to be effective.

❖

35 ❖ Cerebral Palsy and Infantile Paralysis

INTRODUCTION

Cerebral palsy and infantile paralysis patients can make up quite a large portion of a pediatric acupuncture practice. This may not be because there are all that many patients with these problems, but for two other reasons. First, conventional treatment is quite variable, and is mainly behavioral. The main therapy available—that of repetitive stimulation—is outside the National Health Service (in the United Kingdom anyway). This means that people seek complementary medicines to help their children. The second reason is that once a child has started with acupuncture treatment, it is often worthwhile to continue for a long time.

In this chapter we discuss cerebral palsy and infantile paralysis, and try to give some idea of the effectiveness of acupuncture, what to look out for, when to treat, and so forth. We have included palsy in the same lesson as paralysis, even though their origins are different. From the point of view of conventional medicine, palsy is a problem associated with brain damage, while paralysis is associated with peripheral nerve damage. There is a similar distinction in traditional Chinese medicine: palsy arises from a general condition, usually Kidney weakness, while paralysis is often just a channel problem.

CEREBRAL PALSY: ETIOLOGY

Conventional medicine

Cerebral palsy, as one would expect from the name, is associated with brain injury. In many cases there appears to be a clear reason for brain damage, such as:

- difficult delivery
- forceps delivery, which squashes the brain
- oxygen deprivation due to not breathing at birth, or similar cause
- injury or trauma in pregnancy
- oxygen deprivation due to another cause after birth such as febrile convulsion, asthma attack, heart failure
- meningitis

However, there are times when there does not appear to be any cause. Rather than admit defeat, the virus goddess is invoked, and the mother is assured that either she or her child must at some time have been touched by a mystery virus.

Chinese medicine

The theories and observations of conventional medicine are helpful, but they are clearly not the whole story. They are helpful because the great majority of palsy sufferers do have a history of some external event which would likely damage the brain. Yet this is not the whole story, because there are very many children who do *not* have cerebral palsy, but whose histories are so horrendous that one would feel certain that brain damage must have occurred. We have had more than one child who should, by rights, never have survived. One we treated recently was left for dead, blue and not breathing at all, for fifteen minutes after being born. This happened because the mother was hemorrhaging profusely and needed emergency treatment. During these crucial minutes, all attention was on saving the mother, while the child was neglected. Astonishingly, as soon as the child was resuscitated, it started to live normally. When brought for treatment, the only signs were of cold and qi deficiency (hardly surprising), but with no signs of brain damage.

Case History

Master W was brought to me (JPS) for treatment of paralysis of the right arm. He was an attractive boy of nine months, a bit pale, but with very bright eyes and a strong personality. His ears were unusually large, and well made. The mother was a nurse, and told me the story of the birth. She had wanted to have her baby naturally, without anesthetics, but being a nurse, was quite happy to go into hospital. It is just as well, for first of all she found that the pain was much worse than she had expected, and so she needed anesthetics. But the real trouble started when the boy's head was out. Instead of being able to relax at this time, she suddenly clammed up. Her womb tightened, so that the baby could not move at all. It appears that the doctors and midwives who were attending her (all of whom knew her personally) panicked also, thus compounding her own sense of panic. In the end, they had four strong men assisting in the birth—two to restrain her, and two to pull on the baby's head. Not surprisingly, his head was horribly distorted and dreadfully bruised. However, the only problem from which he suffered (apart from some qi weakness) was paralysis of the right arm due to nerve damage at the shoulder, owing to the pressure and dislocation of the shoulder when he was being pulled out.

Kidney deficiency

So what is the factor that causes some children to be injured by the trauma, while others are unaffected? In our opinion the factor is Kidney deficiency. If a child has strong Kidney energy, accompanied by a strong will to live, then it is much less likely to suffer injury at birth. A weak child is simply more fragile. Likewise, a weak child will be much more susceptible to an infection like meningitis in the first place, and then more likely to suffer brain injury as a result, than a child with strong Kidney energy.

===

The root cause of cerebral palsy is Kidney deficiency. In this context, the child may be strong (spastic) or weak (flaccid).

===

PATTERNS & SYMPTOMS

The root cause of cerebral palsy is Kidney deficiency, usually due to prenatal deficiency of essence (*jīng*). However, cerebral palsy can manifest either as deficiency or excess. The deficient type is flaccid, while the excessive type is spastic.

Flaccid type

• thin body
• pale
• dribbling from the mouth
• completely floppy
• dull eyes
• poor appetite

Spastic type

• face may be pale, but sometimes has good color, and sometimes is bright white
• body may or may not be thin
• limbs are in spasm
• appetite reasonable, although may get fierce abdominal pain
• eyes have some spirit

These symptoms upon which we may differentiate the flaccid and spastic types of cerebral palsy are presented as a guide. There is often a lot of overlap. The key questions to ask are the following:

• are the limbs in spasm, or are they floppy and flaccid?
• is the child deficient in energy, over all, or is there evidence of a strong cold interior condition?

This distinction is really worth making, for, as we will see later, it influences treatment. If there are strong signs of cold, then moxa should be used. It may also be used in the flaccid type, but is not as necessary. Similarly, in the spastic type, quite strong reducing technique can be used, while a much gentler treatment is indicated for the flaccid type.

Similarity to Stroke

Strokes are very common at the end of life, while at the beginning, cerebral palsy, which has very similar symptoms, is common. There are more similarities in that the root cause of both is Kidney deficiency. Also, they both present as a strong type and a weak type—spastic and flaccid. One would like to push the analogy further, but in our experience that is as far as one can go. There is a common Kidney deficiency pattern, but instead of a Liver yang rising pattern (with accompanying heat), one sees a full cold pattern in cerebral palsy. Likewise, it is rare to see phlegm as a real contributing factor in cerebral palsy: it is usually the factor which causes cerebral palsy to manifest as epilepsy.

TREATMENT

Body acupuncture

There are two aspects to treatment with ordinary (body) acupuncture:

• treatment of underlying qi condition
• symptomatic treatment of channels (nerves)

The description of what follows is rather "bitty": there are a lot of little bits to be learned, and to a certain extent it is very symptomatic. This may offend some of the purists among our readers, but we do think it is the right approach. The reason is that when brain damage has occurred, it is very hard to repair. It requires a lot of treatment to get the brain and the damaged nerves working again. So, for example, if the arm is paralyzed due to brain injury, one may have to treat the arm many times, occassionaly upwards of a hundred treatments! There is no way we know of where just a few needles and a few treatments will transform the energy so that the body heals itself. In this respect, it is quite different from (say) insomnia, where carefully thought out treatments can produce wonderful results in a short space of time.

Number of Treatments

As we indicated above, it is worth giving lots and lots of treatments. There are, in fact, two ways of approaching treatment, the first being to bring qi to the affected part. This can be done easily, treating once a week. During the first few weeks, very good results are seen. The arm or leg may become warm when before it was cold; it may become pink when before it was white. But after four or five treatments, improvement often stops. This is because if one is working just at the level of qi, one has done all one can. What is needed at this stage is lots and lots of treatment; in conventional terms, it is nerve stimulation treatment.

The treatment schedule described in Chinese texts is every day for ten days, followed by five days rest. This constitutes one course. To produce good results, one would expect to give five to fifteen courses, which is to say, fifty to a hundred-and-fifty treatments altogether.

Treatment Regimen

The pattern of treatment described—ten days on followed by five days rest—is the same regimen prescribed for stroke patients. It is tempting in the West to replace this regimen with one more suited to Western working patterns, that is, five days treatment followed by two days rest, thereby making up a work week followed by thankful oblivion at the weekend. While this substitute regimen is certainly better than giving only a few treatments, there seems to be some evidence that the ten-day on, five-day rest is really best. The evidence comes from studies on nerve development and learning patterns. It seems that when the nerves are developing—for example, in learning a new skill, as in rehabilitation programs—it is worth repeating the same action or treatment every day for ten days, in order to keep reinforcing the message. Then a five day rest period is needed to consolidate the changes.

However, if you can't face treating your children on Saturdays and Sundays as well as the rest of the week, don't get discouraged. It is certainly worth treating on a five-day on, two-day off schedule. What you should avoid is bargaining with the patient over the number of treatments. All too often a patient will say, "Oh, I can't manage five treatments a week, but I can manage four." Then, when it comes to it, they miss one treatment a week on average, due to "unavoidable circumstances"—public holidays, birthdays, anniversaries, funerals—which all seem to crop up with amazing regularity.

If you find yourself in this position, it may well be kinder to say that you will treat once a week to benefit the overall qi, but if they can't come five days then just stick to one day a week. Don't go for half measures, which leaves everyone dissatisfied.

TREATMENT OF UNDERLYING CONDITION

Flaccid pattern

Treatment is aimed at tonifying the Spleen and Kidneys with such points as:

S-36 *(zu san li)*
Sp-6 *(san yin jiao)*
LI-4 *(he gu)*
B-23 *(shen shu)*
B-20 *(pi shu)*
GV-16 *(feng fu)*

Method: tonifying method is used. Select about three points from the list. Moxa may be used with effect on such points as B-23 *(shen shu),* but is not necessary.

Spastic pattern

Treatment is aimed at stopping the spasms. A good prescription for this are the following points:

LI-4 *(he gu)*
Liv-3 *(tai chong)*

Method: quite strong reducing technique can be used at these points. The stronger the treatment, the more effective the results, so don't be afraid of causing some pain!

In addition to stopping the spasms you may wish to warm up the cold, especially if there is abdominal pain. A good point for this is CV-12 *(zhong wan),* which can be warmed with moxa, or needled followed by moxa.

You may also feel that you want to tonify the qi—but don't do this automatically, without thinking!—in which case the governing *(shū)* points on the back combine well.

Summary

The treatments recommended so far are all "energetic" treatments. They are given as a guide, and are suitable in many cases. Obviously, if you find something different happening with your patient—such as lots of phlegm— then you should treat accordingly. The main thing to understand is that energetic treatment is different from channel treatment. Energetic treatment is effective if given only once a week. Channel treatment is not. Energetic treatment is usually given at the beginning of each session, followed, in the same session, by channel treatment.

CHANNEL TREATMENT

The treatment regimens recommended here are representative treatments. They should, of course, be adjusted to fit the individual patient. These regimens are given in addition to treating the underlying condition.

Number of Points

In contrast to the treatment based on underlying condition, you can use lots of points. Typically, ten to fourteen points are used. If a hemiplegic, then perhaps seven needles on the arm and seven on the leg. If a quadriplegic, then perhaps three on each arm and four on each leg. Generally speaking, try to use the same points for each treatment during a course. That is to say, use the same prescription for all ten treatments in a row. This may go against the grain for some readers. Certainly, when we were taught acupuncture, we were told never to do the same treatment twice. The reasoning was that if the treatment was a success, then the condition would have changed, so the original prescription would no longer be appropriate. Conversely, if the treatment had not been a success, then of course it made sense to alter the prescription.

While there is some validity to this point of view, we feel that one should not stick to any rule rigidly. There are conditions (and times) when one treatment may make an impact, and as such be counted a success. However, the overall balance may be much the same as before. It just needs lots and lots of treatment, all more or less the same.

Points

The points are very similar to those used for stroke patients. Here are some representative selections:

ARM	LEG
L-15 *(jian yu)*	S-31 *(bi guan)*
TB-14 *(jian liao)*	S-34 *(liang qiu)*
L-14 *(bi nao)*	S-36 *(zu san li)*
LI-11 *(qu chi)*	S-39 *(xia ju xu)*
LI-4 *(he gu)*	S-41 *(jie xi)*
TB-5 *(wai guan)*	Sp-10 *(xue hai)*
SI-3 *(hou xi)*	Sp-6 *(yin ling quan)*
	Sp-4 *(gong sun)*
	Liv-8 *(qu quan)*
	Liv-5 *(li gou)*
	Liv-4 *(zhong feng)*
	Liv-3 *(tai chong)*
	K-7 *(fu liu)*
	K-3 *(tai xi)*
	B-54 *(wei zhong)*
	B-57 *(cheng shan)*
	B-60 *(kun lun)*

- Generally, to begin with, select an even distribution of points over the leg, with slightly more nearer the trunk. As treatment progresses, it is common to find that sensation and use return to the upper part of the arm or leg first, then the lower part. As the upper part improves, concentrate on the lower part.
- Select some points on yang channels and some points on yin channels. Never use just yin points or just yang points.

Scalp acupuncture

A paper published in 1993 in the *Shanghai Journal of Acupuncture* reported the use of scalp acupuncture in children with cerebral palsy. The basis of treatment was absolutely straightforward: use the arm area if the arm is paralyzed, and the leg area if the leg is paralyzed. Treatment was given in the same amount as one would use for stroke patients—daily treatment for ten days, with five days rest. Typically, ten to fifteen of such courses would be given, making a total of a hundred to a hundred-and-fifty treatments.

As is so often the case with Chinese research, it is difficult to be quite sure what they actually did, and what the results actually were, but they did show some pretty impressive results: more than eighty percent of children were much better. We don't think one could reproduce these figures exactly, but the results are so impressive that there must be something behind them. In any event, it does seem that using scalp acupuncture is a viable alternative, and may well produce results if you get stuck with body acupuncture.

NEED FOR CENTERS

What is quite clear about the treatment of both paralysis and cerebral palsy is that lots of input is needed. This daily treatment is expensive and time consuming if carried out in a normal acupuncture practice. However, its costs and management would be greatly facilitated if a center were established for the treatment of these problems alone. Treatment would be given by specially trained nurses, who would not need to have taken a full course in acupuncture, as the treatment is relatively straightforward; they could be supervised by a more fully trained practitioner. It would give us both very great satisfaction to see such a center established.

INFANTILE PARALYSIS

Etiology

So far in our discussion we have considered only cerebral palsy. It is now time to turn to the sequelae of infantile paralysis (polio myelitis). The causes of infantile paralysis are two-fold: external and internal. The external factor, the polio epidemic, is the sole factor acknowledged by conventional medicine. It is also recognized in Chinese medicine, as an external pathogenic factor of the wind type. It may present at first as wind-cold, wind-heat, or even wind-dampness. In the early stages there is nothing to distinguish it from any other influenza epidemic. In fact, from the point of view of traditional Chinese medicine, there really is nothing at all to distinguish it from any other infection. To illustrate this, many of my (JPS) generation were not immunized, and yet relatively few got what could be diagnosed as polio. However, by now, most of us have acquired immunity. This means that some time during the past fifty years, many of my contemporaries and I were attacked by the polio virus, but only experienced it as a cold or influenza. Although we were attacked, we repelled the attack before it went deep.

What then is the crucial factor which prevents or permits a pathogenic factor to go deeper? In our opinion there are two factors: weakness of protective qi and weakness of Kidney qi. The protective qi factor is obvious. If it is weak, then it is much easier for a pathogenic factor to invade. This sort of imbalance may occur at any time, and it is more or less impossible to prevent a child's protective qi from becoming weak at one time or another.

Fortunately, it requires more than just weakness of protective qi; it also requires weak Kidney qi. Here we are talking about something slightly different from the insufficiency of Kidney essence which is associated with cerebral palsy. Kidney essence deficiency leads to an overall weakness, a feebleness. Essence deficiency gives rise to poor bone formation, and weak constitution. However, the Kidney qi deficiency which we are talking about for polio is more of an imbalance. The overall constitution may be quite strong, but there may be an imbalance between above and below. Characteristically, one will feel weakness in the lower part of the body and lower back. Likewise, the pulse in the third position may be weak, but not the pulse in other positions.

The overall consequence of this is that the energy is unstable because the Kidneys do not 'grasp' or hold the energy down. It is easy for energy to rush upward. This may be seen in certain characteristics of the child:

• easily excitable
• oversensitive
• exam nerves (or holiday nerves)

It is interesting that this pattern is easily generated at a children's party; it is also typical of children who have eaten too much sugar. There seems to be some evidence that the incidence of polio is much greater if children are exposed to a lot of refined sugar.

Symptoms

Paralysis is sudden, within a day, and accompanies a high fever. The paralyzed limb feels dead and inert.

Treatment

Treatment is very simple: follow the channel treatment set forth above. Like the treatment for cerebral palsy, it is best to treat every day. However, not being quite so deficient, good results may be obtained with only three treatments a week.

When to Treat

The sooner treatment can be given after the attack, the better. Just as in treating stroke, if treatment can be started within three months of the attack, then good results are obtained. If treatment cannot be given within two years of the attack, there is unlikely to be much effect, although it's always worth a try.

Other Treatments

Physical condition

It goes without saying that you should pay attention to the overall physical condition of your patient. In particular, look for:

- Kidney qi deficiency that is still there
- overall qi deficiency
- phlegm, just as you would look for any lingering pathogenic factor

Hua tuo jia ji (M-BW-35) points

In addition to the channel points, some Chinese textbooks advise treating the *hua tuo jia ji* (M-BW-35) points near the site of the spinal lesion. This sounds like a good idea, but we have no experience to report.

❖

36 ❖ Myopia

INTRODUCTION

Many children who are now wearing glasses can be cured of their myopia (shortsightedness). Research conducted at the Guang An Men Hospital in Beijing has recently led to the development of methods which are seventy percent effective in curing myopia, provided that treatment is started before the age of fourteen, and that good reading and writing habits are adopted.

The most common cause of myopia is that the lens which focuses the light on the retina is too strong. In normal eyes the strength of the lens is adjusted by the muscles surrounding the eye, and during the early years of life (up to about five years) the child learns how to focus automatically. Recent research has shown that this really is a learned response, and that a large number of children who have difficulty focusing at the age of three have resolved the problem by the age of five. This means that if a child has mild shortsightedness at the age of three, the best treatment is eye exercises of one sort or another.

Eye exercises are useful in correcting mild shortsightedness. If there is a hereditary component of more than two or three dioptres,* there is little chance that exercises will help.

---

*A dioptre is a unit used in optics to measure the strength of a lens. In ophthalmology it has a slightly different meaning: it measures the amount of the imperfection of the lens of the eye. For example, +1 dioptre would be slightly shortsighted, +2 a bit more shortsighted. To correct short sight of +2 dioptres, a concave lens would be prescribed of -2 dioptres. The mathematical definition of a dioptre is 1 dioptre = $1/$focal length, where the focal length is measured in metres. To give you a practical idea of how strong these lenses are, a magnifying glass of 1 dioptre will focus at 1 metre (about a yard), while a lens of 4 dioptres will focus at 25cms (about 10 inches).

Later onset

The treatments set forth below are effective for later onset of shortsightedness. They are particularly helpful in children whose eyesight was good, but has become poor. This can happen at any time between the ages of about three and fourteen. There are a number of reasons for this, which can be conveniently divided between the physical and the emotional.

Physical reasons for myopia

From the perspective of traditional Chinese medicine, the basic reason for onset of myopia is that something occurs which reduces the normal flow of qi to the eyes. This can be:

• any illness that weakens the qi
• lingering pathogenic factor (from illness or immunization)
• exhaustion from overwork
• exhaustion from rapid growth

Emotional reasons for myopia

• changing schools
• unsuitable school
• bullying
• dislike of teacher
• victimization

Any of these factors can cause the child to withdraw into itself. Shortsightedness is a convenient way to do this. If you cannot see what is going on, then you are to a certain measure protected from emotional hurt.

====

The onset of shortsightedness is a symptom that should be taken seriously. It is always a sign that something is upsetting the child quite badly.

====

TREATMENT

Before starting treatment, the child should be examined by an optometrist or ophthalmologist to confirm that nothing is seriously wrong, such as glaucoma. Also, treatment must be started before the age of fourteen. After this age it is less successful.

Treat the Body

The first thing is to treat the overall body qi. If there is general qi deficiency, then the child simply does not have the energy to do the necessary exercises well. Likewise, if there is great heat, the child will be much too restless to do the exercises.

Treat the Symptom

The principle of treatment is to bring qi to the eyes to help them function better. Once the child can see well, it starts to use its eyes more, and this in itself stimulates the flow of energy to the eyes.

There are four basic treatment methods: massage, improvement of posture, eye exercises, and electric plum blossom needle therapy.

Traditional Chinese massage

A simple eye massage routine is used throughout China for the relief of myopia in school children, and has the effect of directing qi to the eyes. Although the massage is gentle, it is often sufficient to resolve the problem by itself, without any other therapy. In severe cases, however, massage should be supplemented with plum blossom needling (see below). The following techniques should be performed by the child three times a day (Fig. 36.1).

1. Make a fist above the eyes, with the thumb bent at its middle joint. Use this joint to massage around the top of the orbit (just below the eyebrows) thirty to fifty times.
2. Pinch, press, and vibrate B-1 *(jing ming)* with the index finger and thumb about two-hundred times.
3. Massage *tai yang* (M-HN-9). The index fingers should be pressed firmly into these points, and rotated gently about fifty times.
4. Massage G-20 *(feng chi)*. The thumbs should be pressed in firmly on both sides, and rotated about fifty times. This point is often sore, but should be massaged until the soreness goes away.
5. Massage LI-4 *(he gu)*. The thumb of the opposite hand is pressed in and vibrated or rotated about fifty times. Repeat on the other hand.

The exercises should be performed three times a day, and each session should last between five to ten minutes. They should be done by the children, with the parents giving encouragement, although in younger children the massage may be performed by the parents. There is usually no problem in doing the exercises for the first week, but after that the children often complain and resist doing the exercises. At this stage, parents must be encouraged to persist in finding ways of persuading their children to continue. It may help the child if the parents do the exercises along with the child. All this can sometimes seem like too much work to overpressed parents, but if it saves the child from needing glasses, it is certainly worth it.

Immediately before starting the exercises, test the child's eyes, and then test them again immediately after-

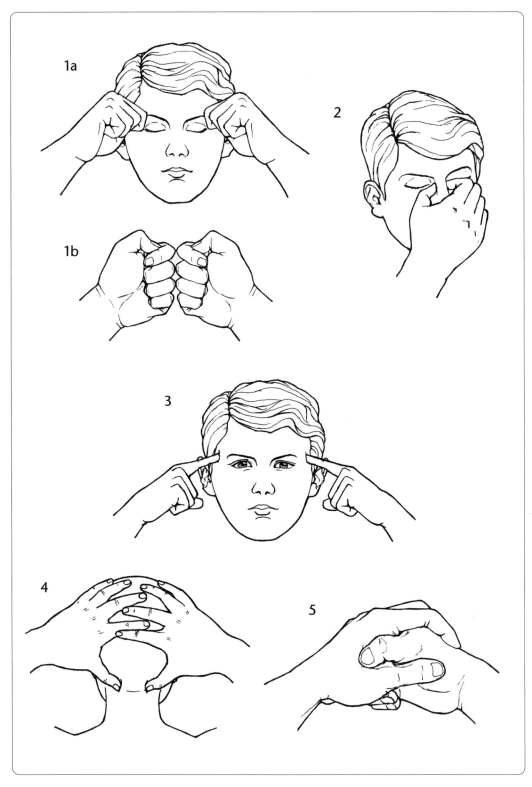

Fig. 36.1   *Eye massage routine*

wards. There should be some significant improvement right away. This is likely to fade over the next few hours, but if the exercises are done three times a day, there should be some lasting improvement after two weeks. It is usually necessary to continue the exercises for six to eight weeks. This may seem like a long time, but it is a worthwhile investment in the future. It may be helpful to play music during the exercises.

Improvement of posture

Poor eyesight may be caused by unnecessary tension and sitting badly when reading and writing. Make sure that:

• the child sits up straight when reading and writing
• books are held at the correct distance.
• the child is not strained when reading and writing

If the child has acquired bad habits in reading and writing, these can often be helped by the Alexander technique.

Eye exercises

Eye exercises are used to encourage the restoration of normal function to the eyes. The exercises used in China are very similar to those devised by W. H. Bates, which are described in his book *Better Eyesight without Glasses.*

Electric plum blossom needle therapy

This treatment was developed at the Guang An Men Hospital in Beijing. In the treatment of myopia, the plum blossom needle is energized by a small electric current, instead of by manual tapping. This makes the stimulation more controllable, and reduces the pain. Basically, the stimulator is set up in a manner similar to that for point detection, with the child holding the ground lead in his or her hand. For plum blossom needles with bone or plastic handles, a wire is wound around the needles and then connected to the stimulator. If the handle is made of metal, the handle itself can be connected to the stimulator, with the part held by the practitioner insulated. (For obvious reasons, it is important that the practitioner not touch any part of the device that is electrically active.)

The needle is rested on the point and the electrical intensity gradually turned up from zero until the child feels the characteristic *deqi* sensation (soreness, numbness, distension). It is then held for approximately twenty seconds. The intensity is turned down all the way between points. This is especially important when a point near the eye is stimulated subsequent to a point on the limbs, as the periorbital points are much more sensitive. The amount of stimulation required to obtain qi on the limbs will cause pain if used around the eye.

Points

B-2 *(zan zhu)*
yu yao (M-HN-6)
TB-23 *(si zhu kong)*
G-20 *(feng chi)*
LI-4 *(he gu)*

In China, treatment is generally given in courses. Each course consists of treatment once daily for ten days, with a rest of five days before beginning the next course. One to three courses are usually sufficient in mild cases. As with the massage exercises, doing a simple eye test before and after treatment will be a source of encouragement to the child and his parents.

When to Use Plum Blossom

Some children take very well to doing the eye exercises. Even quite young children take pride in doing them, and will not let anything get in the way. Others are monstrously lazy, and need cajoling and persuading to do anything that will help their eyesight. For these children, regular treatment, and the status gained by regular visits to a practitioner, can be helpful in giving them the impetus to do at least *some* exercises.

ADVICE

- Always have good light when reading or doing close work. Using the eyes a lot in poor light causes eye strain.

- Don't watch television or do computer games. Both are disastrous for weak eyes, not only due to the flickering, blurred images, but also to the level of tension that results.

- Sit in a good position when doing close work. Reading or writing in a cramped position inhibits the flow of qi to the eyes, and is likely to lead to eyestrain.

- If the child is wearing glasses all the time, spend some time each day without them. Also, gradually *reduce* the strength of the lenses, rather than increasing it.

❖

37 ❖ **Strabismus** (Crossed Eyes)

INTRODUCTION

We continue our discussion of eye problems from the previous chapter. Just as few people realize that anything can
be done for shortsightedness, so also, few people realize
that anything can be done for strabismus. It is often
thought that surgery is the only option; but much more
often, treatment by complementary medicine—and in
particular acupuncture—can cure this disorder. Moreover,
the effect of acupuncture is to strengthen the eyes and so
produce a long-lasting cure. By contrast, surgery weakens
the eyes to a certain extent. Worse still, it is sometimes
found that if an internal strabismus is corrected surgically
in childhood, by adulthood the body changes and an external strabismus may develop! This sort of effect never
happens if complementary medicines are used.

In this chapter we will set forth the causes and treatment of strabismus, and explain when treatment is likely
to be effective, and when to advise surgery.

Need for treatment

Strabismus is so disfiguring that it seems hardly necessary
to provide a reason for treating it. Likewise, binocular
vision is better than monocular, and helps to give a sense
of depth and distance. There is another reason for giving
treatment, especially before the age of eight, and that is
that an eye which is not used at all between the ages of six
and eight becomes blind. When a child is born, its eyes do
not function properly. It cannot focus the eyes, and they
are not coordinated. As the years pass the child gradually
learns how to use its eyes, so that by the age of five its eyesight should be perfect. During these crucial years it seems
that important connections are made in the brain; thus, if

the child only registers what it sees through one eye, and ignores what it sees through the lazy eye, then after the age of eight the lazy eye is ignored completely, and there is little chance of bringing back vision at a later date.

This time factor is important to bear in mind when treating. The clock is ticking, and if you want to save the lazy eye you must get some results in a reasonable time. If you find you are not getting reasonable results, then surgery may well be indicated. We will return to this subject later.

Causes of strabismus

Western anatomy is helpful in understanding strabismus, as it provides an insight into the mechanics of vision. We can then look to see how the functioning of the mechanical system of the eye is affected by the condition of the body.

Mechanics

The eye is moved by three pairs of muscles (Fig. 37.1). The two which concern us are the horizontal ones. They can only contract. To move the eye left or right, only one of these muscles is needed. When the eye is at rest, all the muscles are relaxed, and the eye points forward. After moving the eye in a particular direction by contracting the muscle, relaxing the muscle allows the eye to spring back to central position.

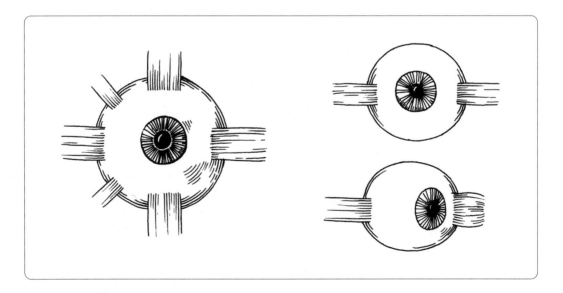

Fig. 37.1

Mechanical Defects

1. Shortened muscle

In Western medicine a strabismus is regarded as just a mechanical defect: one of the muscles (usually the inward-pulling muscle) is too short. Surgical correction is seen as the only solution. The muscle which is too short is cut in a zig-zag fashion to make it slightly longer.

2. Paralyzed muscle

Another defect is paralysis of one of the eye muscles. It happens from time to time that just one of the eye muscles becomes paralyzed. When this occurs, the eye does not have a normal strabismus, for the movement is good in all directions except in the one relating to the paralyzed muscle. We will return to this later.

ETIOLOGY & PATHOGENESIS

There are four main patterns for strabismus:

• congenital
• hot lingering pathogenic factor
• overstimulation and overexcitement
• paralyzed muscle

Congenital strabismus

Congenital simply means that the child is born with a strabismus. Here we really mean quite a bad strabismus. It is rather common for children under the age of three to show some degree of strabismus, for it takes time for them to learn to use their eyes. Just as the focus goes in and out, so binocular vision goes in and out in a young baby. Using one eye is difficult enough; using two, impossible! However, when a baby is relaxed, the eyes should be pointing in more or less the same direction. Sometimes babies are born with eyes pointing severely inward. This would correspond to being born with a significantly shorter muscle. It may simply be a birth defect, but in many cases it is due to womb heat or womb toxin, that is, heat or toxin passed to the child from the mother.

Lingering pathogenic factor

A disturbance in the normal functioning of the eye muscles can occur as a result of a lingering pathogenic factor (LPF). For example, if a child catches a febrile disease and is more or less cured, some effect from the disease may remain behind, in this case a reduction in energy to one or more of the eye muscles. In traditional Chinese medicine this is attributed to the lingering pathogenic factor in the channels, which is blocking the normal flow of qi. This can occur after any high fever, or it may occur after an immunization, such as those for polio or pertussis. It may be helpful to think of this in terms of the fever leaving behind a mild inflammation in the nervous system. For some reason which is not clear to us, a hot LPF can affect just one of the muscles, nearly always the one drawing the eye inward, shortening it.

Overexcitement

On an energetic level, overexcitement corresponds to fire flaring up. It has very similar effects to a hot LPF, the difference being that it is not real fire, but false fire. When a child comes with this condition, it looks to you exactly like the two previously described disorders. Like the LPF pattern, the child would have been born with normally working eyes, and acquired the strabismus later on. The difference here is that there is no history of immunization or fever. Moreover, the child will appear overexcited (maybe shy at first, but soon rowdy), and the parents may notice that the strabismus varies a little according to how tired the child is.

Paralysis of eye muscles

It is surprising that just a single muscle becomes paralyzed. The way this happens is the same way that a single muscle becomes shortened. The etiology is the same, but the effect is more severe: fire blazing upward affects one or more of the channels surrounding the eyes. In mild cases, when the fire subsides, a LPF remains in the channels causing shortening of the muscle. In extreme cases, the fire consumes the yin, and leaves the muscle paralyzed. It is then a localized form of *wéi* (paralysis) syndrome. It is commonly seen after a high fever (as in the Lung heat pattern of *wéi* syndrome[1]) or after an immunization, especially the polio immunization, because polio itself causes paralysis.

Thus, the history of a child with paralysis of an eye muscle will be the same as one with a LPF—the problem occurs soon after a high fever or an immunization.

PATTERNS & SYMPTOMS

Congenital

This is determined by the history: the child is born with a severe strabismus or 'cast' in one eye, and the movement of this eye is severely restricted.

---

1. For discussion of *wéi* syndrome, see *Essentials of Acupuncture* (Beijing: Foreign Language Press, 1980).

Lingering pathogenic factor	The child is born with eyes which are coordinated, but after an illness or immunization (often between the ages of one and three) the strabismus is noticed. In some cases the child alternately uses one eye and then the other, while in other cases the child uses just one eye for seeing, and does not look with the other at all. The eyes are coordinated and move together, but are angled in relation to each other, rather than being parallel. In these cases the angle between the eyes remains constant when the eyes move. Other signs of a lingering pathogenic factor include:

- insomnia
- poor appetite
- swollen glands
- signs of red on the face, such as red cheeks or lips
- possibly red tongue or red tip to the tongue
- irritable, restless

Overexcitement	The pattern of eye movement is similar to that associated with a lingering pathogenic factor in that the eyes move together, but the child only sees through one eye at a time. Moreover, in this type there is usually no clear onset. The strabismus may become worse at times of stress and excitement, such as when the child is overly tired, or has gone to a party, or consumed a lot of sweets. The parents report that the child is easily overexcited. These children may be restless, but they are not irritable so much as irritating to you as the practitioner. This is because they like to get high on excitement, and once they have gotten to know you, they try to provoke you too into being overexcited.

Other signs and symptoms:

- child is born with good eyes, and then develops a strabismus
- often red cheeks
- lower back is often weak
- child is shy at first, then playful and overexcited
- tongue may be red, or may be pale
- pulse rate varies with excitement
- these children are often attractive or beautiful, the 'water-not-controlling-fire' children

Paralysis of eye muscles	When one or more of the eye muscles is paralyzed, the movement of those muscles is restricted. In such cases it will be found that in certain directions the two eyes move together, but in other directions one eye will move, while the other doesn't follow. Another common pattern is that the eyes will move together when looking to one side, but

when looking in the opposite direction the eyes cannot move past the midpoint (Figs. 37.3~37.5).

If this paralysis occurs in children (particularly those over eight years) who have already learned to use their eyes together, they may suffer from dizziness and nausea. This is because the two eyes give different information about the state of the horizon, and so they suffer from a sort of 'sea sickness'.

There are many similarities between this pattern and the LPF, for the simple reason that they both result from fever. In this pattern the fever has gone deeper and caused the paralysis. So one often sees exactly the same symptoms, the only difference being in the movement of the eyes.

However, one does sometimes see an alternative pattern—qi deficiency—with the following signs and symptoms:

• pale face
• tired, floppy
• poor appetite
• sleeps a lot
• dull spirit in the eyes

Other aspects of diagnosis

In the majority of cases the overall flow of qi in the body is good, but is restricted in the region of the eyes. An attempt should be made to assess the local level of qi. Look for:

• quality of energy emanating from the eye (its brilliance)
• color of skin around the eye
• texture and tone of skin around the eye

Misleading signs

Orientals have a fold of skin over the eye which can give the appearance of strabismus, when in fact there is none.

Here is a drawing of an Oriental child. She would be (rightly) most insulted if you suggested that she had strabismus. And yet if she were Caucasian, that look would mean cross-eyed. What is going on?

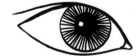 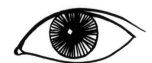

Fig. 37.2

What is misleading is that some Orientals have a fold of skin on the eyelid which makes it look as if they have strabismus. When you are in doubt, the way to be sure is to shine a small flashlight into the eyes, and see where the reflection falls. If the eyes are straight, the spot of light (which is the reflection of your light) should fall at exactly the same place on the iris. If the eyes are crossed, the spot will fall at a different place. I have tried to illustrate this in Fig. 37.3.

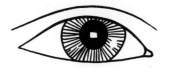 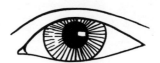

Fig. 37.3

The child below really does have strabismus (Fig. 37.4). Her problem is due to a lingering pathogenic factor. Were the photo in color, you could see the LPF in the excessive redness of the lips, and the rather healthy coloring of the face. (Ignore the water below her left eye. This is merely the after effect of an acupuncture treatment!)

Fig. 37.4

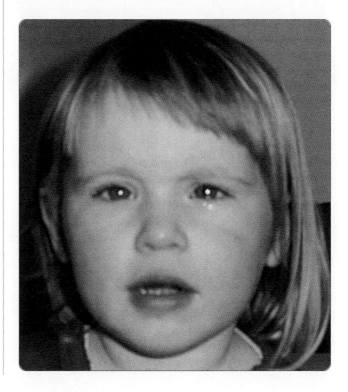

When you look at the enlarged picture of her eyes (Fig. 37.5), you can see that the reflection of the flash comes in a different place on the two eyes. In the left one (her right eye), the white circle is almost central to the pupil. In the right one (her left eye), you can see a crescent of black to the left of the white circle.

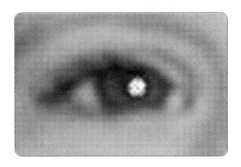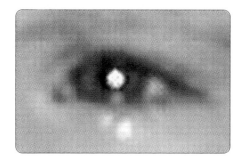

Fig. 37.5

How to Tell if a Child has Strabismus

In Fig. 37.6 you are looking at the left eye. The reflection of the flashlight comes (in this case) at the top of the pupil.

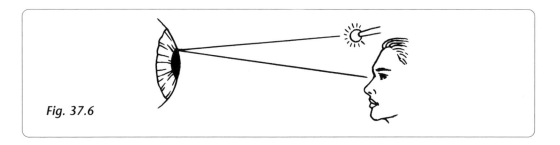

Fig. 37.6

In Fig 37.7 you are looking at the right eye, which we have drawn very deviated. The reflection of the flashlight is well outside the pupil.

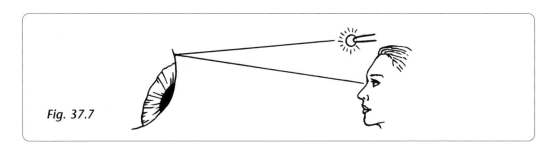

Fig. 37.7

Figs. 37.8 and 37.9 are meant to illustrate what the eyes would look like. Fig. 37.8 corresponds to the eye in Fig. 37.6. The black dot is the reflection of the flashlight. Fig. 37.9 corresponds to the eye in Fig. 37.7. The reflection of the flashlight comes in a different place on the eye.

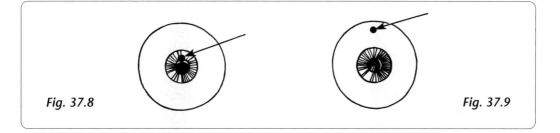

Fig. 37.8   *Fig. 37.9*

Differentiating Between Strabismus and Paralyzed Muscle

In the accompanying figures we illustrate the difference in eye movements between a child who has a genuine strabismus (due to "shortened muscle") and a child who has paralysis of an eye muscle. You can see that the child who has a strabismus can move both eyes together, but they never point in the same direction. It is similar to a motor car where the two front wheels have been set wrong. Both the wheels change direction when the steering wheel is turned, but they are always at the same angle to each other, and never parallel.

If a child has a paralyzed muscle, the movement is quite different. Looking one way, the eyes move perfectly together. Attempting to look the other way, one eye moves, but one eye gets stuck just past the mid-point.

SHORTENED MUSCLE (Figs. 37.10~37.12)

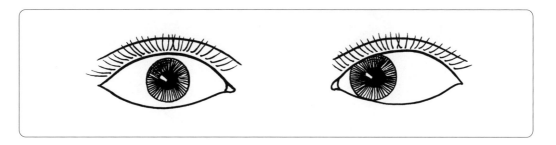

Fig. 37.10   Look right

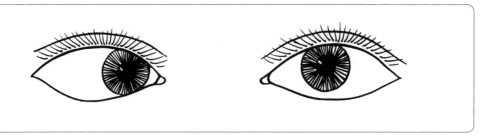

Fig. 37.11 Look straight ahead

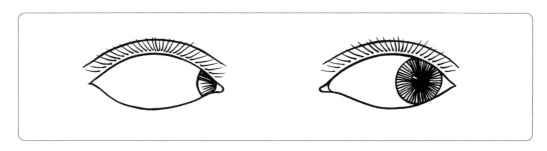

Fig. 37.12 Look left: there is no vision in R eye, so it almost disappears

PARALYSIS (Figs. 37.13~37.16)

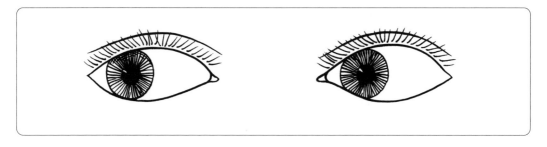

Fig. 37.13 Look right: eyes okay

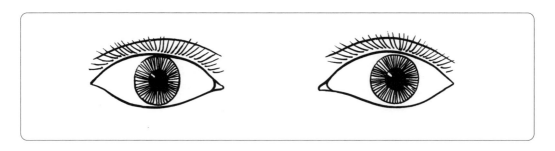

Fig. 37.14 Look straight ahead: eyes okay

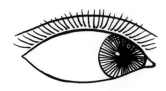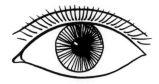

Fig. 37.15   Look left: left eye is stuck at mid-point

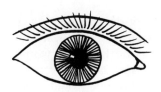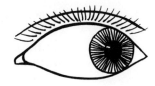

Fig. 37.16   Look left: right eye is stuck at mid-point

TREATMENT

For all types of strabismus

MAIN POINTS

G-20 *(feng chi)* If possible, the needle sensation should travel through to the eye
LI-4 *(he gu)*

For medial strabismus, add:
qiu hou (M-HN-8)[2]
G-1 *(tong zi liao)*
wai ming (N-HN-6)[3]

For lateral strabismus, add:
B-1 *(jing ming)*

Note: the depth of needle insertion at eye points in children should be only 0.2 to 0.3 unit. This is much shallower than in adults because it is simply not possible to needle these points deeply in a child.

Congenital

Generally speaking, there is not much that acupuncture can do for this type of strabismus. The child is born with a

---

2. Located at the inferior border of the orbit, about one-fourth the distance from the outer to the medial side of the orbit.

3. Located about 0.3 unit above the outer canthus.

muscle that is too short. There are, however, two ways that conventional medicine can help:

1. surgery, as described above
2. strongly magnifying glasses. This seems like a strange thing to do, but it does appear to be effective. The reasoning behind it is that when you try to focus the eyes on something close, they naturally tend to converge and cause a slight strabismus. Putting strong glasses on the child will tend to make it longsighted, and so the reflex action will work in the opposite direction and cause divergence, thus helping to correct the strabismus.

Is acupuncture ever appropriate for treating congenital strabismus? Yes, when there is a significant heat imbalance in the baby at the time of birth, that is, womb heat. The treatment would be the same as that given for a hot lingering pathogenic factor, but one would expect the results to be slower.

Prognosis: variable, depending on the severity of the case. Acupuncture can be helpful in regulating the qi, but it takes months or years for the shortened muscle to grow to the right length, and the situation must therefore be continuously evaluated.

Lingering pathogenic factor

Treatment principle: clear the pathogenic factor and brighten the eyes

MAIN POINTS

A prescription that we have found useful many times:

P-7 *(da ling)*	Both points clear the heat and
Liv-2 *(xing jian)*	brighten the eyes

Other useful points include GV-14 *(da zhui)*, LI-11 *(qu chi)*, and LI-4 *(he gu)*, as well as the general points which directly affect the eyes, listed above.

Method: even technique, treating once or twice a week

Prognosis: if the diagnosis is clear, these points alone are sufficient and the condition should be cured within ten to fifteen treatments. In some cases, however, after the pathogenic factor has been cleared, it may be necessary to bring the qi to the eyes by needling such points as G-20 *(feng chi)*.

For medial strabismus, add:
qiu hou (M-HN-8)
G-1 *(tong zi liao)*
wai ming (N-HN-6)

For lateral strabismus, add:
B-1 *(jing ming)*

Overexcitement

Straightforward treatment of the strabismus may or may not be effective. The few children who have been brought to us with this pattern have all been of the panicky type. One glimpse at the needle and they burst into panic-stricken weeping, and then rush out of the room! The only treatment we have managed to give has been to gently moxa B-23 *(shen shu)* and K-1 *(yong quan)* with the aim of strengthening the water. However, one of my colleagues reported treating a child in China who had developed a very severe squint after watching too much television over Chinese New Year. Treatment was given every day.

The most important part of treatment is the advice that is given to the parents. It is absolutely essential that the child's level of stimulation be reduced. This may mean drastic measures such as no television, avoiding playing with friends who get them overexcited, and staying in and pursuing quiet activities such as drawing, rather than going out for activities. Some children have to avoid playing with certain other children who "wind them up"! In addition, the child must be kept away from stimulating foods, especially sugar. These measures often sound repressive when first suggested, but when they are tried, parents are so encouraged by their beneficial effects and the general increase in happiness all round that they find it relatively easy to continue.

Number of treatments: it is always worthwhile giving some tonic treatments to strengthen the water and calm down overexcitement. It is also worthwhile arranging several appointments (say, five) so that you can monitor progress and support parents in their attempts to reduce the stimulation of their child. It is all very well giving good advice at the first appointment, but without several follow-up visits, the advice is unlikely to be acted upon.

Prognosis: a marked improvement is usually seen after changing the child's level of stimulation. Further improvement can be obtained by bringing qi to the eyes. The self-massage routines described in the previous chapter (myopia) are usually preferable to acupuncture, as these children often resist acupuncture, and quite a long course of treatment is required. The exercises often must be performed for two to three months on a regular basis, and for another year on an intermittent basis.

Paralysis of eye muscles

Treatment principle: clear the channels and brighten the eyes

MAIN POINT

G-20 *(feng chi)*

For medial strabismus, add:
M-HN-8 *(qiu hou)*
G-1 *(tong zi liao)*
wai ming (N-HN-6)

For lateral strabismus, add:
B-1 *(jing ming)*

Method: even method, treating daily or every other day

Prognosis: if you remember that this is a form of *wei* syndrome, you will realize that you must give lots of treatments, and as soon as possible after the onset of paralysis. Just as in treating paralysis after a stroke, treatment is very effective if started within three months. If two years have elapsed since the onset, you may then be lucky and get miraculous results (they do happen), but more likely very little at all will change as a result of treatment.

Number of treatments: treatment ideally should be given every day for ten days, followed by a five-day rest before resuming treatment. Each course of ten treatments counts as one unit of treatment, and you may need five to ten units—a lot of treatment, and an amount that few parents are prepared to undertake, even if you decide out of good will to charge only a nominal fee. However, to my knowledge, acupuncture is one of the very few modalities that has a chance of curing paralysis in an eye muscle.

If you can't get the patient to come every day for ten days, or every weekday (five out of seven), it is still worth treating if they only come three times a week. If they can only manage to come once or twice a week, it is generally not worth planning a long course of treatment. It may still be worth giving a few treatments, however, as this will bring qi to the eyes, and may produce a miracle; but as far as the standard treatment to bring back the use of a paralyzed muscle is concerned, three treatments a week is the minimum.

Summary

Strabismus is the result of contracture in one of the eye muscles. As such, it can very often be treated effectively with acupuncture, thus avoiding the need for surgery. To maintain vision in both eyes it is important that they both be used during the crucial years of six to eight. If an eye is not used during this time, the sight in that eye may be lost forever. This sometimes means that surgery is the preferred option, in order to get quick results.

NOTES

• For all types of strabismus, the massage exercises described in the previous chapter (myopia) are also beneficial.

• It can be helpful to put a patch over the good eye to encourage the use of the lazy eye. However, it is quite difficult to get children to do this for any length of time. Strangely, it is sometimes just as effective putting the patch over the lazy eye, which seems to encourage the flow of qi to both the eyes. It also accords with the old acupuncture principle of treating the good side to benefit the bad.

• In severe cases of congenital strabismus, surgery may be beneficial. Strabismus which occurs later in life should not be treated in this way, as a significant proportion of patients who have undergone surgery to shorten a muscle find that the muscle shortens further at some later date. Thus, what may have started as medial strabismus and was corrected by surgery becomes lateral strabismus some years later.

• Some cases of apparent strabismus are in reality cases of farsightedness (hyperopia). These children need to work very hard to focus and accommodate; this leads to one or both eyes turning in. The eyes turn in more erratically than those discussed above. Fig. 37.17 on the following page identifies useful points for treating this disorder.

❖

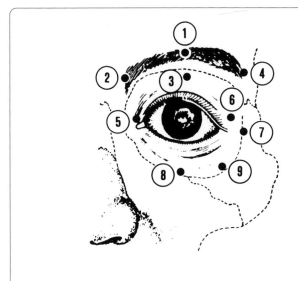

1. *yu yao* (M-HN-6)
2. B-2 *(zan zhu)*
3. *shang ming* (N-HN-4)
4. TB-23 *(si zhu kong)*
5. B-1 *(jing ming)*
6. *wai ming* (N-HN-6)
7. G-1 *(tong zi liao)*
8. S-1 *(cheng qi)*
9. *qiu hou* (M-HN-8)

Fig. 37.17   *Points in vicinity of eye*

38 ❖ Strong Convulsions and Fits (including Meningitis)

INTRODUCTION

Traditional Chinese medicine regards convulsions as one of four major disorders affecting children, along with measles, childhood nutritional impairment, and smallpox. In recent times, as a result of improved living conditions, the other three have declined in importance, but convulsions remain a serious problem. Even today in Britain, five percent of all children suffer convulsions. Brain damage and epilepsy can result from a severe attack, and convulsions can even be life-threatening. That is why Western medicine justifies its rather brutal treatment of administering large doses of such drugs as corticosteroids or barbiturates. Acupuncture, by contrast, is a very gentle form of treatment, and is usually very effective in treating convulsions. In China today, acupuncture is regarded as the treatment of choice, above all other therapies, because of its speed of action.

Convulsions are traditionally divided into acute and chronic patterns (literally 'fast' and 'slow'), but this translation is misleading, for the distinction in Chinese medicine has little to do with the duration of the disease. The 'acute' pattern is a violent one, with rapid jerking movements of great strength. The child is often red-faced, cries out with a loud voice, and thrashes around. The 'chronic' pattern is a weak one in which the child does not have the strength to thrash around violently, and is often pale-faced, with a rather feeble cry. The convulsions themselves are more in the nature of twitching and gentle writhing.

Both patterns start and stop suddenly, and either may be of brief or long duration depending on the condition of the child. The difference between the two patterns is thus

445

one of intensity, and they could more accurately be named 'strong' and 'weak'. A prolonged attack of the 'strong' type may gradually transform into the 'weak' type.

There is a saying in Chinese medicine, "Phlegm and heat [together cause] convulsive wind." This sums up the pathology of febrile or 'acute' convulsions. In most children there is already some phlegm (because of children's weak digestion) and some heat (because children are naturally hot, and their yin is often insufficient). It therefore only takes a relatively small additional factor to cause convulsions. The differentiation of patterns discussed below describes those factors that can readily generate the extra phlegm or heat.

In the first three patterns, heat is caused by external pathogenic factors: external wind (usually wind-heat), summerheat, and epidemic convulsions, which refers to encephalitis and epidemic meningitis.

Phlegm is produced in the two phlegm-heat patterns either from excessive food injuring the Spleen (or in Western children, disturbance of the Spleen during teething), or from an attack of dysentery.

In the fright pattern, convulsions are due to a disturbance of the spirit. The fright may be produced by a shock, or, in those patients who have another illness such as abdominal pain, the fright may be a reaction to the sudden incidence of violent pain. If the fright remains in the child for a long time without being treated, there is often accumulation of heat as well. This is because the circulation of qi is affected.

ETIOLOGY & PATHOGENESIS

External Pathogenic Factors

Wind

This pattern is often seen in summer from attack of wind-heat, and also in winter when wind-cold transforms into heat. Children's skin is soft and weak and therefore vulnerable to external pathogenic wind, which can penetrate to the interior, cause obstruction, and thus transform into heat. Severe heat may in turn transform into fire, which produces phlegm by congealing the body fluids. The extreme heat and phlegm create wind, which rises up rebelliously, manifesting as fever, headache, opisthotonos, and twitching. In severe cases the Pericardium is affected, giving rise to delirium or even coma.

Surnmerheat

The summer and autumn are very hot in China, a time when 'summerheat blazes upward.' The basal *(yuán)* or source qi in children is weak and soft and their yin is in-sufficient, so they are easily affected. Summerheat is a yang pathogenic factor which may transform into fire, disturb-ing the pure yang and giving rise to high fever, vomiting, wheezing and gurgling, delirium, loss of consciousness, and convulsions.

Epidemic type

There is also an epidemic type of convulsions, which pro-ceeds so fast that it is known as 'galloping convulsions'. Heat and fire develop very quickly with symptoms char-acteristic of heat from excess obstructed in the interior, Liver wind, and of a pathogenic factor lodged in the Peri-cardium. This pattern encompasses such biomedically-defined illnesses as viral encephalitis, meningitis, and measles encephalitis.

Phlegm-Heat

The Livers of children often have surplus and their Spleens are often insufficient, so heat and phlegm readily accumu-late. Alternatively, irregular feeding or the ingestion of indigestible or contaminated foods (often together with teething in Western children) can give rise to dampness and heat, which collect in and block the Intestines and Stomach and obscure the yang. The regulation of the qi mechanism is disrupted, and the Liver is affected. Accord-ing to a Chinese adage, "Qi in excess readily transforms into fire." Thus, phlegm-fire and turbid dampness rise up and attack the Pericardium, and Liver wind rises up strongly.

Fright and Shock

The qi of a child's spirit is timid and weak, its basal or source qi is without a strong foundation, and phlegm often interferes with the internal pathways. When a child sees something frightening, hears a loud noise, or is sud-denly startled, fright attacks the spirit and fear attacks the mind, disturbing their peace. Should turbid phlegm there-upon rise up, it clouds the sensory orifices and induces Liver wind and convulsions.

PATTERNS & SYMPTOMS

General

Although acute convulsions usually attack suddenly, there are often prodromal symptoms which give warning, such as the following:

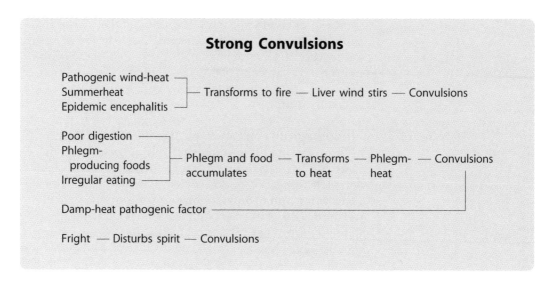

- fever
- vomiting
- restlessness and irritability
- shakes head and plays with tongue
- frightened and cries out
- may fall into extremely deep sleep

At the time of the attack, symptoms may include:

- body very hot, with typical heat signs
- profuse phlegm
- limbs twitching
- convulsive spasms
- opisthotonos (arched back)
- eyes turned up showing only whites
- clenched teeth
- mouth and lips burning and dry
- convulsions and loss of consciousness

These symptoms are characteristic of phlegm-heat causing convulsions.

During the acute stage the focus of treatment is to stop the convulsions, and at other times to treat the underlying pattern. In severe cases a combination of Western and traditional Chinese medicine is indicated.

Convulsions Due to External Pathogenic Factors

Wind

- fever with much sweating
- throat red
- headache

- restlessness and irritability
- loss of consciousness
- convulsions

Tongue coating: thick, yellow
Pulse: floating, rapid

Treatment principle: scatter the wind and clear the heat, clear the sensory orifices and calm the convulsions

Summerheat

- fever
- vomiting
- neck is tense and rigid
- convulsions

Tongue coating: thick and greasy, possibly yellow
Pulse: slippery, rapid

Treatment principle: expel the summerheat and clear the heat, open the sensory orifices and stop the convulsions

Epidemic type

QI AND NUTRITIVE LEVELS AFFECTED

- disease occurs suddenly
- high fever
- restlessness
- thirst
- delirium
- high-pitched shrieks like a bird
- loss of consciousness
- convulsions

Note: this pattern corresponds to meningitis

Tongue coating: thin, yellow
Tongue body: red or purple
Pulse: overflowing

Treatment principle: clear the heat and resolve the toxicity, cool the blood and subdue the wind

HEAT INVADES THE NUTRITIVE LEVEL OF THE HEART

- coma, unconsciousness
- limbs twitching
- body hot, limbs cold, but palms of hands and soles of feet hot
- possibly spots and rashes on the body

Tongue body: red, crimson
Pulse: wiry, fine, rapid

Treatment principle: clear the Heart and open the sensory orifices, cool the nutritive and blood levels, and subdue the wind

Phlegm-Heat Convulsions

Obstruction from retention of food (accumulation disorder)

- feeling of fullness
- vomiting
- abdominal distention
- abdominal pain
- constipation
- fever
- gurgling noise in throat
- spirit dull
- bluish facial color
- convulsions

In Western children this disorder can be brought on by teething, in which case there will be such characteristic symptoms as:

- one cheek red
- putting fingers in the mouth
- irritability and restlessness
- possibly yellow nasal discharge

Tongue coating: dirty, greasy, and yellow
Pulse: rapid

Treatment principle: reduce the food stagnation and resolve the blockage, clear out the filth and open the sensory orifices

Damp-Heat Stagnation and Knotted Convulsions

- high fever
- delirium
- vomiting
- abdominal pain
- stools stinking like rotten fish; may contain pus and blood
- spirit confused
- intermittent convulsions

Tongue coating: yellow, greasy
Tongue body: red
Pulse: slippery, rapid

Treatment principle: clear the heat and transform the dampness, resolve the toxicity and calm the convulsions

Fright and Shock Convulsions

- body rather weak
- no fever, or only slight fever

- movements are restless (fidgety, hyperactive)
- possibly a coma
- generally on waking seems stuporous and twitches
- facial color green or red
- stools green

Tongue coating: thin
Pulse: deep
Finger vein: blue-purple

Treatment principle: reduce the fear and calm the spirit

TREATMENT

Emergency Treatment for Strong Convulsions

When you see convulsions for the first time, you want to do something quickly. There are some simple treatments which can be applied without a second thought.

Emergency treatment #1

LI-4 *(he gu)*
Liv-3 *(tai chong)*

Emergency treatment #2

GV-14 *(da zhui)*
LI-11 *(qu chi)*
LI-4 *(he gu)*

Emergency treatment #3

For those awkward times when you don't have needles: pinch hard on the heels, inside the Achilles tendon, that is, at K-3 *(tai xi)* and B-60 *(kun lun)*

Emergency treatment #4

If the child is unconscious:
GV-26 *(ren zhong)*
P-6 *(nei guan)*

Non-Emergency Treatment

Main points

GV-14 *(da zhui)*
LI-11 *(qu chi)*
L1-4 *(he gu)*

Together, these points clear heat from the body and subdue internal wind.

Method: dispersing method, with no retention of needles; treatment is given every two hours

According to Symptom

Violent spasms in upper half of body

Needle LI-4 *(he gu)* through to SI-3 *(hou xi)*

Violent spasms in lower half of body

Needle Liv-3 *(tai chong)* through to K-1 *(yong quan)*

Limbs twitching

SI-3 *(hou xi)* and B-62 *(shen mai)*. This symptom is caused by wind entering the governing vessel, on which these are the master and coupled points respectively.

Opisthotonos (arched back)

GV-12 *(shen zhu)* and GV-3 *(yao yang guan)* to clear wind from the governing vessel; K-1 *(yong quan)*, P-8 *(lao gong)*, and GV-26 *(ren zhong)* are a frequently-used combination for restoring consciousness

Clenched teeth

S-6 *(jia che)* [local point]

Excessive sputum

S-40 *(feng long)*, L-7 *(lie que)*, CV-17 *(shan zhong)*

According to Pattern

Convulsions due to external pathogenic factors

WIND

Use the main points listed above ("non-emergency treatment").

Prognosis: one to three treatments to clear the convulsions

SUMMERHEAT

Use the main points plus P-3 *(qu ze)* and B-40 *(wei zhong)*, which are commonly used for summerheat.

Method: use the triangular needle to draw a few drops of blood at these points

Prognosis: one to three treatments to clear the main symptoms

EPIDEMIC TYPE

Use the main points plus *shi xuan* (M-UE-1) and GV-20 *(bai hui)* to clear heat from the head and restore consciousness.

Method: use the triangular needle to draw a few drops of blood at these points

Prognosis: acupuncture can reduce the severity of the attacks and give the patient a greater chance of surviving without brain damage; should be combined with Western medicine

Phlegm-heat convulsions

RETENTION OF FOOD (ACCUMULATION DISORDER)

Use the main points ("non-emergency treatment") during an attack. At other times, select from the following:

si feng (M-UE-9) *Note:* do not use this point during an acute attack, as the resulting discharge of food can make the convulsions even worse.

CV-12 *(zhong wan)*	Benefits the transportive and transformative functions of the Spleen
G-34 *(yang ling quan)*	Strengthens the Gallbladder function of assisting digestion
S-43 *(xian gu)*	Induces the food to descend
S-25 *(tian shu)*	Promotes movement in the Intestines
S-40 *(feng long)*	Promotes movement in the Stomach and transforms phlegm

If the child is teething, add LI-4 *(he gu)*.

Prognosis: one to three treatments are usually sufficient; follow-up treatments may be necessary to ensure that there is no recurrence, especially when the next teeth erupt

DAMP-HEAT

Use the main points during the attack. At other times, select from the following:

S-25 *(tian shu)*	Stops the diarrhea
Sp-9 *(yin ling quan)*	Resolves damp-heat
S-40 *(feng long)*	Transforms phlegm
S-44 *(nei ting)*	Clears heat from the Stomach and Intestines

Prognosis: success depends on the severity of the damp-heat; some cases of dysentery are very hard to cure, but the convulsions should be resolved after a few treatments

Fright and shock convulsions

Use the main points during an attack. At other times select from the following, all of which have the effect of calming the spirit:

H-7 *(shen men)*
P-7 *(da ling)*
P-6 *(nei guan)*
Liv-3 *(tai chong)*

Method: very gentle needle manipulation is used to avoid startling the child

Prognosis: variable; often one to three treatments are sufficient, but if the baby has been badly frightened, five to ten treatments may be required

Prevention

Unless you are working in a hospital you will rarely see acute convulsions, but you are quite likely to see children who have had them, and parents who want you to stop their children from having them again. If you understand the causes of convulsions you will have no trouble. Above all, remember the catch phrase, "Phlegm and heat cause convulsions." In our experience there are two underlying conditions which are often seen. Both are easily treated: heat from a lingering pathogenic factor, and heat and phlegm from accumulation disorder.

Heat from lingering pathogenic factor

For the early stages of this disorder, use such points as:

L-10 *(yu ji)*
S-44 *(nei ting)*

Later on, when most signs of phlegm have disappeared, use such points as:

bai lao (M-HN-30)
L-13 *(fei shu)*
B-18 *(gan shu)*
B-20 *(pi shu)*

Heat and phlegm from accumulation disorder

si feng (M-UE-9)
LI-4 *(he gu)*
S-40 *(feng long)*

NOTES

• Pay attention to the diet. Avoid foods that are warming such as spices, fried foods, and red meats. Avoid phlegm-producing foods such as milk, cheese, and peanuts. Watch out for allergies, and avoid artificial food additives. Avoid rough foods, over-feeding, and irregular feeding, all of which are likely to cause accumulation disorder. In patients who only suffer from occasional attacks of convulsions, these precautions will usually be sufficient to prevent further attacks.

• Living habits: keep the child calm, avoid any stimulation, avoid television, and no computer games or flashing lights.

- First aid: teach the parents elementary first aid on how to treat fevers, either homeopathy, herbs, or tui-na.

- There is often an atmosphere of panic surrounding a child with convulsions. It is very beneficial to the mother and child if you can keep calm yourself.

- Treatment should be given every two hours during acute attacks.

- For those who feel faint-hearted about giving treatment during convulsions, we offer encouragement. Acupuncture is a very safe therapy, and by treating during an attack you may be able to spare the child the complications of brain damage. This means that the child will be able to live an ordinary life, rather than spending it in an institution.

❖

39 ❖ Weak or Chronic Convulsions (Chorea)

INTRODUCTION

Chronic or 'slow' convulsions is a condition of deficiency which occurs because of general weakness in the body, especially the Spleen. The traditional explanation is that when the body becomes very weak and empty, wind begins to stir, just as wind stirs in empty, desolate places. This disorder is generally translated as 'chronic Spleen wind', but might be better described as mild twitching due to weakness of the Spleen. It is easy to distinguish from acute convulsions in that the movements are without great force and are more like the writhing and twitching that are sometimes described as chorea. They may be accompanied by 'absences', that is, momentary losses of consciousness, and thus are sometimes diagnosed as petit mal epilepsy in Western medicine.

Chronic convulsions can be caused by any factor which weakens the child's body. This is especially true of dysentery and longlasting febrile convulsions, but any long-term disease can cause the weakness, as can treatment with too much 'cold' medicine. This includes the cold substances of Chinese herbal medicine as well as antibiotics and the anticonvulsive drugs used in the treatment of epilepsy.

As with all diseases of weakness, herbs are preferred to other methods of treatment because of their nourishing effect, but acupuncture is nonetheless very effective. In the differentiation of patterns, the Spleen yang deficiency type is broadly the same as the waning Spleen and Kidney yang type, the latter being a more severe or advanced stage of the former. The Spleen yang deficiency pattern is the one that is most commonly seen in the West. A third type, Liver and Kidney yin deficiency, is a hot pattern. Due to the widespread use of antibiotics, febrile diseases are not allowed to persist for long, and this pattern is thus rarely seen in the West.

The most important distinction here is between hot and cold patterns.

ETIOLOGY & PATHOGENESIS

Spleen yang deficiency

Arises from a bad attack of vomiting and/or diarrhea,* or from acute convulsions that continue without being resolved, with the result that the Spleen yang is injured. May also result from constitutional weakness of the Spleen and Stomach, with frequent attacks of indigestion. The support and nutrient systems become unbalanced, and the Spleen and Stomach become weak and soft. The deficiency of earth (Spleen and Stomach) is unable to check wood (Liver), which flares up as Liver wind, manifested in such symptoms as yellow face, weak spirit, and intermittent twitching.

Waning Spleen and Kidney yang

Caused by prolonged vomiting or diarrhea, or from a lengthy recuperation after an illness. As a result of this constant siege against the Spleen and Stomach, the Kidney yang is injured. With the Kidney yang weakened and waning, yin cold prevails in the interior and is unable to support the Spleen, causing further injury to the Spleen yang. This manifests in symptoms which are characteristic of chronic Spleen wind, including a translucent quality in the face, cold limbs, and twitching without any force.

Exhausted Liver and Kidney yin

Follows acute convulsions, or a damp-heat disease without proper recuperation. The lingering heat attacks the yin and body fluids; the Kidney yin is injured and exhausted and cannot support Liver wood. The Liver blood in turn is insufficient, depriving the muscles and tendons of moisture. Wind from yin deficiency thereupon arises, manifested in such symptoms as red cheeks and muscle spasms, among other symptoms.

PATTERNS & SYMPTOMS

Chronic convulsions are a form of cold from deficiency. Typical symptoms include:

---

*In Western medicine it is understood that there are some types of bacterial dysentery which lead to the production of toxins which can affect the nervous system.

Weak or Chronic Convulsions

Vomiting and diarrhea — Spleen deficiency ⎤

Long-term diarrhea ⎤
Any protracted disease ⎦ — Spleen and Kidney deficiency ——— Wind from
deficiency stirs

Prolonged acute convulsions ⎤
Damp-heat disease — Body exhausted ⎦ — Liver and Kidney
yin exhausted

Spleen yang deficiency

- spirit weak and tired
- much sleeping, or even coma
- yellow facial color
- cold limbs, possibly hot palms and soles
- weak breathing
- fontanel sunken
- shaking head and rolling eyes
- 'absences' (momentary losses of consciousness, 'spells')
- mild twitching and jerking of arms and legs

Treatment principle: the general treatment principle for chronic convulsions is to strengthen the body

- spirit weak and feeble
- likes sleeping and may have periods of 'absence'
- whites of eyes appear during sleep
- yellow facial color
- stools watery and thin
- limbs cold
- twitches from time to time

Tongue coating: white
Tongue body: pale
Pulse: deep, soft

Treatment principle: warm the middle and disperse the wind, support and restore the Spleen yang

Waning Spleen and Kidney yang

- spirit weak and soft
- white facial color
- spontaneous sweating
- limbs damp and cold
- deep sleep to the point of coma
- limbs wriggling (a relatively gentle and continuous motion)
- stools like water

Tongue coating: thin, white

Tongue body: pale
Pulse: deep, fine

Treatment principle: warm and tonify the Spleen and Kidneys, restore the yang, and expel the cold

Exhausted Liver and Kidney yin

- weak
- irritable
- tired and feeble
- cheeks red
- body hot, thin, and emaciated
- palms and soles hot
- limbs and body inflexible and in spasm, either strongly contracted or merely twitching
- stools dry, or constipation

Tongue: shiny without coating
Tongue body: red and dry
Pulse: deep, fine, rapid

Treatment principle: restore the yin and calm the yang, benefit the Liver and extinguish the wind

TREATMENT

Spleen yang deficiency

CV-12 *(zhong wan)*	Tonifies the Spleen yang
CV-6 *(qi hai)*	Tonifies the Spleen yang
S-25 *(tian shu)*	Regulates the Spleen
S-36 *(zu san li)*	Tonifies the Spleen yang
Sp-6 *(san yin jiao)*	Tonifies the Spleen
B-20 *(pi shu)*	Tonifies the Spleen yang
GV-14 *(da zhui)*	Stops convulsions

Method: the abdominal and back points should be tonified. The points may be treated with moxa alone, or moxa on ginger; or, if you are sure of your technique, then they may be needled. Needling these points should be avoided by the inexperienced practitioner because of the risk of unintentional dispersing effect.

Prognosis: five to ten treatments should resolve most of the symptoms, provided the child is not too weakened. Further treatments are advised to restore the child to health. If the child is taking medication, many more treatments will be needed to wean the child from the medication.

Waning Spleen and Kidney yang

B-20 *(pi shu)*	Tonifies the Spleen yang
B-23 *(shen shu)*	Tonifies the Kidney yang
K-3 *(tai xi)*	Tonifies the Kidney yang (often used for convulsions)

CV-12 (zhong wan)	Tonifies the Spleen yang
CV-6 (qi hai)	Tonifies the Spleen and Kidney yang
S-25 (tian shu)	Tonifies the Spleen yang
GV-4 (ming men)	Tonifies the Kidney yang

Method: either moxa alone, or moxa on ginger, should be used at the abdominal points

Prognosis: ten to twenty treatments may resolve this disorder; however, if the child is really depleted, acupuncture alone may not be sufficient

Exhausted Liver and Kidney yin

The following points together regulate the Liver, Gallbladder, Spleen, and Stomach, and support the Kidney yin:

B-19 (dan shu)
B-20 (pi shu)
B-22 (san jiao shu)
B-23 (shen shu)

Method: treat every six hours during acute attack. For needling, use the tonifying method, taking great care not to overstimulate. Despite the fact that this is a yin deficiency pattern, if the legs and feet are cold, the points on the limbs may be treated with moxa, which will have the effect of drawing the heat downward.

Additional points for all types of chronic convulsions

P-6 (nei guan)
LI-11 (qu chi)
LI-4 (he gu)
B-57 (cheng shan)
Liv-3 (tai chong)

Prognosis

Because of the wide range of severity, it is difficult to make general statements about the number of treatments that will be needed. A typical course might run as follows: for the first ten treatments, very little change may be noticed in the symptoms, but slight changes should be seen in the energy of the child. There will also be slight changes in minor symptoms such as the amount of sleep, and the looseness of stools.

Over the next ten to fifteen sessions, some significant changes in the frequency and duration of the fits will be noticed. It is also common for a very thick nasal discharge to appear during this time. This is a good sign, for it shows that the child is getting strong enough to start expelling the phlegm that was there all along.

Over the next twenty-five or so treatments it is possible to reduce the drugs the child is taking, so that at the end of fifty to seventy treatments, the child is more or less well. Treatment should continue every two to three weeks for another six months to consolidate the result.

This may sound like a lot of treatments—indeed it is. But the results are wonderful. You are, in effect, bringing a child back to life. The life it had before, and to which it was destined, was merely a "twilight life," only half-conscious, and heavily sedated.

Other Results of Treatment

It does happen from time to time that the child's health traces back through the original disease. That is to say, weak convulsions are replaced by strong convulsions. This in itself is not a bad thing, provided you recognize what is happening: tonifying a deficient disorder transforms it into one of excess. The new condition is easily treated—some prescriptions were provided in the previous chapter—but DO TAKE CARE. Always remember to ask the parents how the child has been, even if you are in a hurry!

Coming Off Medication

As you get improvement in the frequency of the fits, the parents will start to ask when they can take their child off medication. Of course, this should be done in cooperation with the practitioner who prescribed them, if at all possible. But basically, you are in charge. The time to start this is when you have made significant improvement—in the frequency of fits, and in the child's general health. Since you are reducing the drugs, it is to be expected that there might be a slight increase in the number of fits, but there is actually another phenomenon to beware of: it can happen that *any* change in the dosage provokes a fit. In other words, a reduction in the dose of drugs may produce fits, but so can an *increase* in dosage. This can produce alarming effects if the dosage is frequently changed. Put another way, it is important to be steady in reducing medication. Reduce by only a small amount at a time, and when you do reduce, give extra treatments—up to three treatments per week—to help the child through to the next level of medication.

NOTES

• If the child has suffered from a long bout of diarrhea, treatment can be reinforced by replenishing the body's electrolytes with fluids that are available over-the-counter at any pharmacy.

• Some epileptic children with this type of traditional Chinese diagnosis are on a very high dosage of anticonvulsive drugs. This occurs because the physician has an incomplete understanding of these drugs. They are usually cold in nature, which aggravates the disorder. This results in an increase in the twitching, which in turn leads to an increase in the dosage, and so on, in a vicious circle. When this happens it may take up to two years of acupuncture treatment to restore these children to health.

❖

Case History

A-MD-M was one of those patients that you grow fond of. You try to keep them slightly at arm's length, but if you go on seeing them for a long time, inevitably you become part of their life, and they of yours.

When she first came to the clinic, she was really in a bad way. She had had some very bad fits when she first started teething. Each time a tooth came through she would have really violent fits, becoming unconscious for a good five minutes at a time. Consequently, she had been put on anticonvulsive drugs.

A-MD-M was quite a sensitive girl, so when she first started taking the drugs she immediately had a fit (due to the sudden change in drug level). A week later, when she was taken back to the pediatrician, the fits that she had when she first started taking the drugs were regarded as a sign that she was not yet "stabilized," and so the dose was increased. Result: more fits. Result of that: more medication. And so the cycle went on for a month or more, until she was taking large doses of anti-convulsants.

The consequence of all these drugs was that, from being a robust, red-faced girl, she was now pale-faced and dull-witted, with frequent absences.

When she was a one-year-old, A-MD-M was brought for acupuncture treatment, which consisted of tonifying the Spleen. The points S-36 *(zu san li)*, Sp-6 *(san yin jiao)*, and CV-12 *(zhong wan)* [with moxa] were used again and again. After about fifteen treatments, she started to show a bit more life, and also got a continuous sticky nasal discharge.

And so the treatment continued, until by the end of a year she was really quite healthy. But still she kept on getting fits, although they had changed in quality. Before, they were trembling movements during the day, all day. Now they were violent, and came shortly after going to sleep. It seemed to the parents that when she fell asleep she met something frightening, and started wrestling with it. The struggle would end in her having quite a big fit in her sleep. Sometimes she would wake up, sometimes not.

I (JPS) was confused by this, for by now she was really quite healthy, and did not have enough wrong with her to cause fits. After trying all the obvious points, I decided that there must be a spiritual component to the problem. Perhaps it was some strange spirit that she was wrestling with . . . so I decided to do the outer Liver *shū* point, B-47 *(hun men)*.

Result: miracle. Sleep perfect for six days, but then back again. So it *was* a spirit then! London, as you may know, is full of all sorts of spiritual garbage accumulated since the Romans first settled.

The way that the problem was finally solved was for the parents to pray over the child as she went to sleep. Neither of them was particularly religious, although both were vaguely conscious of something "out there." It was difficult for them to pray at first, for they had not prayed since Sunday school (which they both loathed). But after a few days they got into it, and the child stopped her fits.

40 ❖ Epilepsy

INTRODUCTION

Epilepsy is the common translation of the two Chinese characters *diān xián*   . The first character is also found in the phrase *diān kuáng*   , which means madness, insanity, or more specifically, the withdrawal-mania disorder. This character thus means both madness and withdrawal, and represents the two apparently contradictory notions of rushing around wildly and standing still. The character consists of two parts. The classifier is *nì*   , which means disease and is supposed to show a sick man lying on a bed. The other part is *diān*   , which is related to the idea of divination and oracles, and it is this which provides the link between the two contradictory meanings, that is, the behavior of a person in a trance of divination.

There is a remarkable parallel between the Chinese and the ancient Greek ideas of epilepsy. The Greeks called it the 'sacred disease' not only because of its similarity to the trance of divine inspiration, but because those who suffer from epilepsy often see visions when undergoing an attack. In traditional Chinese medicine another name for epilepsy is 'goat madness wind' *(yáng diān fēng   )*, 'goat' because of the noise that the patient makes during an attack, and 'wind' because of the sudden, shaking nature of the seizure.

Traditional Chinese medicine, and acupuncture in particular, has long been used for treating epilepsy, both during an acute attack and for the underlying cause. We believe that acupuncture is far more useful, particularly in children, than is Western medicine, which at best merely controls the symptoms at the cost of taking drugs for many years or even one's entire life. This is in stark contrast to acupuncture, where a few treatments may be enough to cure a patient if under the age of three.

In principle, there are three distinct categories of epilepsy: the congenital type, the phlegm type, and the blood stasis type. In practice, however, the distinctions among the three types are sometimes difficult to make, and there may be a history which points to more than one cause.

In all types of epilepsy it is important to keep the child calm and to avoid overstimulation. The child should also avoid dairy and other phlegm-producing foods, as well as stimulating foods such as sugar and food additives.

As noted in the previous chapter, some types of epilepsy (Western-defined) would be diagnosed in Chinese medicine as a form of chronic convulsions. Acute convulsions, however, are different from epilepsy in that they involve an immediate precipitant cause, such as an attack of wind, an acute heat process in the body, or (in Western children) intense teething. Epilepsy is attributed to deeper, more ingrained causes and occurs without such a precipitating event. Most children who suffer acute convulsions will eventually get better without treatment; this is not true of epilepsy, which often gets worse.

When is it Epilepsy? When is it a fit?

The symptoms of epilepsy and febrile convulsions are identical, so it is worth pausing for a moment to consider when you would call it 'fits' and when 'epilepsy'. This has great significance, for usually children grow out of fits as they get older and stronger, but most do not grow out of epilepsy. It is thus much more important to treat epilepsy.

The main difference, as we see it, is that febrile convulsions are triggered primarily by a fever, while the key symptom of epilepsy is that the attacks come despite the absence of fever. So fits always have a clearly identifiable trigger, while epilepsy comes somewhat unpredictably.

However, like all distinctions, when you look closely at the boundary you find there is no clear line between fits and epilepsy. A child who has some heat from a lingering pathogenic factor, and who has a fit in hot weather, or when startled, or when exposed to flashing lights, could be classified as either one or the other.

Strong (Excessive) and Weak (Deficient) Epilepsy

The patterns of epilepsy are very similar to those of convulsive fits, and, like fits, there are strong violent attacks, and weak trembling attacks.[1] They are quite different from the nature of fits, and the treatment required is also quite different.

Patterns

In Chinese textbooks the patterns of epilepsy are described as being completely distinct from one another, with no overlap. In clinical practice, however, while you do occasionally see the pure patterns, much more often the child comes with a mixture of all of the patterns. At this stage we will just give a thumbnail sketch of the patterns, so that you can understand the causes of illness.

Pattern	Typical Symptoms
STRONG (EXCESSIVE)	
Fright & yin deficiency	Jumpy, nervous, thin, gray
Phlegm	Snotty, dull, podgy
Blood stasis	Brain injury, no other special signs
WEAK (DEFICIENT)	
Spleen & Kidney yang deficiency	White, staring, vacant, podgy
Liver & Kidney yin deficiency	Thin, staring, red cheeks

ETIOLOGY & PATHOGENESIS

Epilepsy doesn't just come out of the blue. It is a deeply-rooted disease which progresses from an earlier imbalance. Sometimes parents are unaware of the imbalance before epilepsy is diagnosed, but more often than not they are well aware that it has developed from a mild condition to a deeper disorder. For example, they may be aware of frequent infections in their child before epilepsy occurs, or repeated attacks of febrile convulsions prior to the epilepsy.

---

1. We meet another old friend, the problem of translating Chinese. The words *diān xián* are correctly translated as epilepsy. However, they refer to the strong or excessive pattern—like the traditional Western popular perception of an epileptic, throwing themselves down, kicking and foaming at the mouth. However, Western medicine has moved on from there, and epilepsy is now defined in terms of a characteristic dysfunction of the brain. This widens the scope of epilepsy to include the dreamlike state with 'absences,' which in former years would have been labelled "village idiot." In traditional Chinese medicine, this pattern would be classified as weak or deficient convulsions.

In order to understand how epilepsy occurs, we have divided the causes into two categories: internal and external.

Internal Factors

There are three internal factors which can lead to acute epilepsy. They may be present in varying degrees, but only one is necessary:

• weak basal (source) qi
• phlegm obstructs the sensory orifices
• blood stasis/brain injury

Weak basal qi

This is the hereditary factor. In Western parlance we would say that the child had 'weak nerves', or a 'delicate constitution'. Traditional Chinese medicine describes it as a weak *yuán* or foundation for health. The origin of this weakness is weak 'pre-heaven' (prenatal) qi, described further in our discussion of failure to thrive (see Chapter 29). The reason why weak basal qi contributes to epilepsy is that such children are more easily startled, and suffer more lasting injury afterward, than do children with stronger basal qi. Or, in Chinese medical terms, the five spirits *(shén)* are more readily scattered because they are not held firmly in place.

Chinese textbooks say that there are two principal causes of epilepsy that occur before birth: shock in utero and insufficiency of basal yin. Since ancient times both have been thought to cause the same condition. Thus, Chapter 47 of *Basic Questions* observes, "As a result of a big fright to the mother while the baby is in utero, the qi rises up and disturbs the pure yang, giving rise to epilepsy." And in a book by Zhou Zhi-Gan from the early Ming dynasty entitled *Discreet Gift of Alms (Zhen zhai yi shu)* it is noted, "Goat madness wind arises from prenatal basal yin insufficiency; the Liver pathogenically overcomes earth and injures the Heart." This is interpreted to mean that because the Liver and Kidney yin is insufficient, the qi of the Heart and Liver is readily injured; Liver qi thereupon rises up and disturbs the spirit, with such symptoms as twitching, dizziness, and loss of consciousness.

Phlegm obstructs the sensory orifices

There are many reasons for the development of phlegm in the system. But what it contributes to epilepsy is its stickiness. This means that once a child has developed a certain pattern, it gets "stuck" there and cannot find its way back. Phlegm also 'mists the Heart,' which leads to loss of consciousness, one of the characteristics of epilepsy.

Chinese textbooks say that phlegm collects in the region of the diaphragm. After obstructing the great connecting vessel of the Spleen, it rises up and blocks the sensory orifices, cutting off the pathways of the qi mechanism. This can lead to a failure of communication between the yin and yang, which hides and obscures the pure yang.

Blood stasis/brain injury

The brain can be injured as a result of a difficult delivery, resuscitation at birth, or because the child falls forward onto its head. The stasis of blood in the brain obstructs the sensory orifices. This can affect the spirit *(shén)* and mind *(zhì)*, and cause dizziness and loss of consciousness, a condition known as blood stasis epilepsy.

Here, 'blood stasis' refers to a body condition, one where the body has difficulty healing, and in which it is easy for blood to stagnate. This means that if a child suffers injury to the head, it is easy for blood clots to develop and so cause brain damage. This subtle distinction between the clot in the brain and the resulting damage is not especially important for us as acupuncturists; it is more important for herbalists.

Other factors

Chinese textbooks say that phlegm can arise because of deficient Spleen qi, or because an attack of acute or chronic convulsions leads to accumulation of wind-phlegm. In such cases the seizures are often precipitated by an attack of external wind-cold, or the consumption of cold food. Liver and Kidney yin deficiency can also arise as a sequela of another illness which has persisted for a long time without proper treatment.

External Factors

By themselves, the internal factors listed above are not enough to cause epilepsy. Something else is needed, such as:

• repeated attacks of febrile convulsions
• immunizations
• sudden shock
• brain injury
• diarrhea
• inappropriate drug therapy

Repeated attacks of febrile convulsions

This is one of the most common ways for epilepsy to develop. The febrile convulsions may start during a fever, or after an immunization. They then become more and more frequent. In the beginning it requires a high fever for the convulsions to occur, but as the habit develops, a lower and lower fever will suffice, until finally the convulsions happen quite spontaneously, without any apparent precipitating factor. At this stage it is epilepsy.

From the point of view of conventional medicine this pattern is thought to develop because each attack of convulsions causes a little brain damage. After repeated convulsions, the amount of brain damage accumulates until finally epilepsy develops. This is certainly true in some children, especially those who have very bad fits where they are unconscious for minutes at a time. However, there are other children where this pattern develops more as a habit. There may not be significant brain damage, but the child becomes familiar with the fits.

Immunizations

Sometimes epilepsy develops immediately after an immunization. As we have seen, it is relatively common to develop some convulsions; occasionally the pathogenic factor goes deeper and causes epilepsy. From the point of view of conventional medicine, the brain damage is caused by a toxic reaction to the drug. From the point of view of Chinese medicine, it is the external pathogenic factor that causes the wind and heat, because the child is already yin deficient.

Sudden shock

If a child already has the weak nerves that are characteristic of yin deficiency, a sudden shock or frightening event can cause the fright pattern of epilepsy to develop. You will see an example of this in the case histories. Typical situations include being in a car accident, or seeing a sudden death.

Brain injury

An injury to the head can easily cause brain damage, which can lead to the blood stagnation pattern of epilepsy. As far as conventional medicine is concerned, the detection of damage in the brain becomes in itself almost positive proof of epilepsy. Typical causes of brain injury are a blow to the head, injury to the head during childbirth, and oxygen starvation of the brain either by asphyxia or from violent, prolonged febrile convulsions.

However, it is interesting to note that in babies, none of these events will necessarily cause epilepsy. There are tales of new-born babies being left for twenty minutes without breathing, of babies' heads being squashed beyond recognition during birth, of falling out of windows twelve feet high onto their heads—with no illness developing. It would seem almost certain that one of the predisposing conditions is necessary for epilepsy to develop.

Diarrhea

A bad attack of diarrhea, especially one accompanied by great abdominal pain, can develop into the deficient type of epilepsy. Previously, we saw how spleen deficiency can cause wind, and then develop into convulsions. If, in addition, the child is very frightened by, for example, fierce abdominal cramps, then epilepsy can develop.

Inappropriate drug therapy

As previously explained, the illness defined as 'chronic convulsions' in Chinese medicine includes the biomedical disease of epilepsy, and that one of the causes of weak convulsions is described by the proverb "Excessively cold medicine causes Spleen wind." This applies also to epilepsy. Here, cold medicine can mean cold Chinese medicines, or cold Western drugs.

Epilepsy

Shock in utero — Disturbs spirit ⎤

Phlegm accumulates — Rises to block — Spirit cannot ⎥— Epilepsy
                sensory orifices   move freely

Blood stasis ⎦

Aggravating factors:

Spleen deficiency — Creates phlegm
Chronic convulsions — Generates wind
Protracted febrile disease — Liver and Kidney yin deficienccy

---

PATTERNS & SYMPTOMS

Strong (Excessive) Patterns

General symptoms

Before the attack there are usually prodromal symptoms:

- dizziness
- mouth falls open
- stifling sensation in chest
- palpitations
- staring eyes
- numbness and tingling in the limbs

The attack itself may be mild or severe. Symptoms of a mild case include:

- short duration of attack (about thirty seconds)
- twitching is mild and gentle
- eyes may rise upward

- shakes head
- child does not cry out, but may forget what has happened immediately before the attack

In severe cases, the symptoms include:

- convulsions and violent shaking and twitching
- clenches teeth
- attacks last a long time, perhaps tens of minutes
- attacks are rather frequent, perhaps every day or two

Fright type

- may be brought on by a sudden noise, flashing lights, or anything which frightens the child or makes it nervous; the child is oversensitive
- cries out in sleep
- clings to mother and likes to be rocked in her arms
- stools greenish, with hard pieces
- urine scanty, yellow
- facial color may be red, sometimes white; sometimes gray-blue; sometimes there is only just a blue coloring between the eyes
- possibly signs of weak constitution
- generally, it is the *absence* of symptoms which characterizes this pattern

Tongue body: maybe red (but not necessarily)
Tongue coating: white
Pulse: wiry, rapid, or wiry and slippery; varies with level of anxiety

Treatment principle: sedate the Heart and calm the spirit

Phlegm type (symptoms are seen between attacks)

- all the orifices are blocked by phlegm
- gurgling noise of phlegm in the throat
- vomits "water" or dirty fluid from time to time
- yellow facial color

Tongue coating: should be thick (but often is not)
Pulse: should be slippery, rapid (but often is rather weak)

Treatment principle: transform the phlegm and clear the sensory orifices

Blood stasis type

- blue dots on the tongue or skin
- history of trauma and damage to the brain

Note: the blue dots on the tongue are rarely seen, even though brain damage is frequent. If blue dots *are* there, it is a good sign, for it means that the blood stasis is a general body condition. This means that if you can change the overall body condition, there is a good chance of changing the blood stasis (or clot) in the brain.

Pulse: fine, choppy
Finger vein: deep, broad

Treatment principle: move the blood and transform the stasis, regulate the sensory orifices and stop the attacks

General

Chinese textbooks say that if the epilepsy is allowed to continue for a long time, or if the child's body is weak, or if the child suffers from nervous exhaustion, and there are additional symptoms such as poor appetite, weak spirit, dull facial color, back and knees sore and painful, pulse weak and fine, these are signs of injury to the Liver and Kidneys, with qi and blood scattered. The treatment principle in such cases is to reinforce the Liver and Kidney yin.

Epilepsy does not develop in quite the same way in the West. It is true that the Liver and Kidney yin do become depleted by long-term illness, lack of appetite, or consumption of junk food, but it is rare to see back and knees sore and painful. Much more common is a very thin child who is either a bit hyperactive, or else drugged out of his or her mind. It is the thinness which is the key sign, and it is a bad sign. It means that there is very little basal *(yuán)* qi, and so it will be difficult to cure.

TREATMENT OF STRONG (EXCESSIVE) PATTERNS

Treatment principle: restore consciousness

During an Attack

Main points

GV-26 *(ren zhong)*
LI-4 *(he gu)*
P-6 *(nei guan)*
Liv-3 *(tai chong)*

Other useful points include *shi xuan* (M-UE-1) and K-1 *(yong quan)*. These points help bring down heat from the head and clear the sensory orifices.

Method: dispersing method is used; manipulate needles vigorously until the attack ends

Between Attacks

GV-26 *(ren zhong)*   Restores consciousness
H-7 *(shen men)*   Calms the spirit

yao qi (M-BW-29)[2]	Special point used for epilepsy

Of these three points, GV-26 *(ren zhong)* and H-7 *(shen men)* are the most widely used. According to some sources, however, epilepsy cannot be successfully treated without using *yao qi* (M-BW-29), in which the needle sensation must be felt to move up the spinal cord. While this is indeed a very effective point, it is nevertheless possible to treat epilepsy successfully without it.

Fright type

P-6 *(nei guan)*	Calms the spirit
Liv-3 *(tai chong)*	Calms the spirit, stops the spasms, and regulates the Liver

Or, if there are signs of heat, use the following points:

Liv-2 *(xing jian)*	Calms the spirit, clears the heat, and regulates the Liver
B-15 *(xin shu)*	Calms the spirit [moxa]
GV-20 *(bai hui)*	Calms the spirit and clears the sensory orifices
K-1 *(yong quan)*	Calms the spirit and clears the sensory orifices [moxa]
B-18 *(gan shu)*	Regulates the Liver
B-23 *(shen shu)*	Tonifies the Kidney yin

Method: treatment should be given three times a week. We used to think you could successfully treat epilepsy by treating once a week, but now we don't think so. Occasionally you get good results, particularly if there are very clear signs of one or another pattern, but typically not. Take care to avoid overstimulation and causing further shock.

Prognosis: if the epilepsy is purely due to fright, three to ten treatments may suffice for children under three years. The older the child and the longer the disease has lasted, the greater the number of treatments required. What is much more common is that there is something else going on—one of the other patterns as well, or weak basal qi—and it is common to give many more treatments. In fact, you may find that after fifty treatments you are still making slow progress.

Phlegm type

Here the treatment principle is to transform the phlegm, and stop the epilepsy. We have never seen a pure phlegm pattern, and we are not sure it exists! All the cases we have

---

2. There are two methods of locating this point, both on the posterior median line: 2 units superior to the tip of the coccyx; or below the spinous process of the second sacral vertebra. It should be needled to a depth of 2-3 units.

seen have had Kidney deficiency as well. At first sight we were unaware of the Kidney deficiency, but it became apparent when we examined the back, which turned out to be quite concave in the lumbar region

Therefore, the proper principle of treatment is to resolve the phlegm, tonify the Kidneys, and stop the convulsions.

CV-14 *(ju que)*	Tonifies the Spleen and transforms the phlegm
S-40 *(feng long)* G-34 *(yang ling quan)* Sp-6 *(san yin jiao)*	Even method
B-23 *(shen shu)*	Tonifying method: needle plus moxa

Additional points to help the spasms and contractions:

LI-4 *(he gu)*
Liv-3 *(tai chong)*

Method: even method; treat every day or every other day

Prognosis: results are variable. With phlegm, there is usually another pathogenic factor which has penetrated right to the governing channel. What often happens is that the child gets a lot better from the first ten or so treatments—which has the effect of reducing the phlegm—but after that, progress is very slow. It is quite common to require fifty to a hundred treatments.

Sometimes a lingering pathogenic factor suddenly stirs up and the child has a fever (with a rash), but sometimes not, and although the child is much better, it is not always possible to effect a complete cure. It may be that a combination of acupuncture and homeopathy can help here. Homeopathy appears to be good at bringing heat to the surface.

Blood stasis type

Again, we have not seen this pattern by itself. We have seen it with Kidney deficiency, and also with phlegm. So the principle of treatment is much the same as in the other two patterns, with the difference being that treatment should be directed toward clearing the local blood stagnation, with such points as:

GV-14 *(da zhui)* GV-16 *(feng fu)* GV-20 *(bai hui)*	Clears the sensory orifices
ashi points on the head Site of blood clot, if known	
Liv-2 *(xing jian)* Liv-3 *(tai chong)* B-17 *(ge shu)*	Transforms blood stasis

Method: even method is used. Treat every day or every other day. After ten treatments there should be a period of seven to ten days before treatment is resumed.

Prognosis: once again, one occasionally gets miracle results, with the child being cured after about ten treatments, but more often it takes fifty to a hundred sessions. When there is definite brain damage, but without signs of blood stagnation, then you will be lucky if you make any significant progress. What we usually recommend with these patients is that they measure the results not after each single treatment, but after each ten treatments.

Ear Acupuncture

Liver, Spleen, Heart, Sympathetic, Endocrine, Brain

Method: select three points for each treatment. After obtaining a sore or numb sensation, leave the needles in place for two hours. (If intradermal needles are used, the patient may leave the clinic with the needles in place, and remove them two hours later.) Treat one side one day and the opposite side the next. This method has been used with excellent results in China, and is very attractive in terms of saving time for the patient and practitioner. However, it is not suitable for younger children, since it is virtually impossible to leave the needles in place for such a long period of time.

Comment

What we have described so far have been disorders that were relatively strong or excessive in nature, and you would expect from what has been said that epileptics would, in general, be strong children. In fact, this is by no means the case. Often you get a child who fits nicely into one of the patterns, but one look at the child and you know straight away that it is a weak child—thin body, weak bone structure, and so forth. When you see this, you know that you've got difficulties on your hands. When a child is weak or deficient like this, it may just not have the overall strength to throw off such a deeply-rooted disease as epilepsy.

Another situation you may encounter is that the child does not seem to have any of the predisposing factors at all—no special weakness, not much phlegm, no history of brain damage. When this happens, then the chances of a cure are much lower.

NOTES

• Patients suffering from epilepsy should avoid over-stimulation and loud music with a pronounced rhythm. They should especially avoid watching television and other media with flickering lights.

• Phlegm-producing foods, such as milk, cheese, and peanuts, and irritating foods, such as spices and artificial flavorings and colors, should be avoided.

• When treating children under medication, the dosage should not be reduced until significant improvement is seen; and when a reduction is attempted, it should only be in small increments, and not more frequently than once every two weeks. It is often found that a child suffers a mild attack about five to six days after changing the level of medication. This is true whether the change is a reduction or an increase in dosage.

Weak (Deficient) Patterns

General symptoms
• child is dull-witted and stares blankly
• during attacks, may lose consciousness for just a second or two
• in more severe cases, may tremble like a leaf
• in more severe cases still, may fall down

Spleen and Kidney yang deficiency
• white faced
• often much phlegm
• movements often heavy

Liver and Kidney yin deficiency
• much less frequently seen
• child is thin
• red cheeks
• frightened, easily upset
• may have other signs of heat, such as sweating, insomnia

TREATMENT OF WEAK (DEFICIENT) PATTERNS

The treatment regimen for weak (deficient) patterns is quite different from that used in treating strong (excessive) patterns. The guiding principle is to tonify. For the yang-deficient type, tonify the Spleen and Kidney yang.

Spleen and Kidney yang deficiency

Treatment principle: tonify Spleen and Kidney yang

S-36 *(zu san li)*
Sp-6 *(san yin jiao)*

CV-12 *(zhong wan)*
B-20 *(pi shu)*

Method: tonifying method at all points, plus moxa at CV-12 *(zhong wan)* and B-20 *(pi shu)*

Results of Treatment

There are three major unexpected effects of treatment:

- a lot of phlegm starts to appear, after about ten treatments
- the child starts to get strong attacks instead of weak ones
- from being cold and damp, the child begins to exhibit signs of heat

You must alter your treatments accordingly.

Liver and Kidney yin deficiency

Treatment principle: for yin-deficient patterns, the treatment principle is to tonify Liver and Kidney yin

K-3 *(tai xi)*
B-18 *(gan shu)*
B-23 *(shen shu)*

Results of Treatment

We don't know, because we have never seen this type of epilepsy. However, we would expect the treatment to be difficult since Kidney yin-deficient types don't like being needled!

Problems Arising during Treatment

Non-attendance

As we have indicated, it takes a long time and many treatments to cure epilepsy. In our opinion it is worth it, for you have the opportunity of overcoming an illness which would otherwise be there for life; but it does require commitment and dedication on the part of the parents. As we have said, it is best if treatment can be given twice or three times a week. But this is rarely possible. In our experience, the children with epilepsy all seem to live two hours' drive away from the clinic, with parents who either have no money or no time or both! Such families find coming even once every two weeks difficult to cope with. They are often eager to commit themselves at the beginning of the course of treatment, thinking that no sacrifice is too great to cure their child, but quite soon they realize that it is going to take more energy than they have to spare, and start missing appointments. When this happens, it is usually best to stop treatment then and there, and ask them to resume treatment only when they have sorted out their lives. (In actual practice, of course, we find this hard to do, and rarely manage to be so clear-cut.)

Coming off medication

There is a real problem in getting children off medication. It is a fact that each time you *change* the dosage of drugs they are taking, there is likelihood of an attack; it does not matter if you increase or decrease the dosage. Thus, two or three days after the drugs are reduced, the child has an attack. This completely freaks out parents, since it has been some time since their child has had an attack, and they have forgotten how frightening it is to see. Also, all the misery and despair comes welling up again. What happens next is that they increase the dosage to what it was before. This is the worst possible thing they could do, because it is another change, and is very likely to precipitate another attack!

The only way around this problem is to warn the parents beforehand, and to insist that they maintain the changed dosage for at least ten days. Point out to them that a few fits are not a disaster, and at the end of ten days the wave of fits will have subsided. This worthy advice can be supported by the practical measure of giving them more frequent treatments—three, four, or even five times a week for two weeks.

The logical conclusion to this is that the child should only consider reducing drugs at a time when you will be around to give extra treatments. Don't try this just before you go on holiday!

Psychic interference

In a small minority of children there is active psychic interference. Whatever you do, somehow you are unable to cure the child. A typical pattern is given in the case history below. In epilepsy, perhaps more than in any other illness, the psychic factor has to be taken into account. As we mentioned in the introduction, the ancients believed that a sufferer was taken over by the gods during an attack. Modern opinion in psychic circles is rather that it is a very negative psychic force that takes over a child during an attack. My own experience, as exemplified in the case history at the end of this chapter, would confirm this.

Symptoms of psychic disturbance

The key sign that a child is psychically disturbed is the strange look they have in their eyes. There is an odd, sullen look there. It is a crafty, watching look, almost as though another being—other than the child—were looking through their eyes. This look is present in a lot of epilepsy patients at the outset, to a varying degree. But as treatment progresses it should disappear. However, if this odd, sinister look is there strongly, and persists throughout your first ten or so treatments, then it is unlikely you will cure the child.

Common effects

The effects of psychic interference are strange, and they tend to block all progress in treatment. A typical pattern is that you start to get some results, so that after about eight sessions you are sufficiently pleased with the progress that you point this out to the parents. Then, mysteriously, in between this treatment and the next, something happens which screws up all the progress you have made and puts you back to square one. It is usually something seemingly unconnected, such as a car accident, a family crisis, a routine visit to the hospital. At first you think it is just chance, but when it has happened three times, you begin to wonder.

Spiritual Treatment

We live in dark times, spiritually. Large numbers of people have no spiritual beliefs, and are so deeply wedded to the beliefs of materialistic science that they are outraged and frightened at even the mention of the spiritual nature of man and his diseases. Therefore many of your patients will not be receptive to the idea of the necessity to address the psychic and spiritual problem. Of those who do accept the need, the majority have a real problem accepting any form of orthodox religion, and yet have not found a substitute. For the minority who are already practitioners of religion, help is at hand in the form of exorcists or banishers of spirits, and even in simple rites like baptism. For those who cannot accept this sort of help, it is more difficult. Some can accept the idea of praying for their child, while others prefer simply to visualize their child bathed in a purifying light. In this area, some ingenuity is required.

Caution

The psychic forces surrounding an epileptic are sometimes very powerful. Do not attempt to do any spiritual work on your own, without someone who has experience and can guide you if things go wrong.

NOTE

• For two additional case histories involving epilepsy, see Cases 18 and 19 in Chapter 47.

❖

Case History

The first time I came across the psychic forces that are involved in epilepsy was with a boy of about four years of age. I did not know much about epilepsy then, and certainly could not recognize the different patterns. Now, I would classify him as a weak child, with the blood stasis and phlegm patterns. I did not know that at the time! Nevertheless, I charged in and started treating. What I did notice was that he had a weird look in his eyes. I can remember it to this day.

Since the phlegm was obvious, I thought the the best way to approach the problem would be to clear some of the phlegm. I was lucky with treatments, and after five or six (weekly!) treatments had made some progress—the fits were less severe and less frequent. I mentioned this to the parents, who seemed quite pleased.

For some strange reason, the boy did not come the following week or the week after. It turned out that his grandfather had died. He was very attached to his grandfather, and naturally had been upset, and unfortunately this had put him back to square one with his epilepsy attacks. So I started again, and after about five or six treatments had again made some progress, which I mentioned to the parents.

Once again, he did not come the following week. This time it turned out that the family had been riding in the car while the father had a minor traffic accident. Not surprisingly, our boy was upset by this, and all the improvement that I had made in his epilepsy had again been wiped out.

Undeterred, I started once more. And again, I made progress, perhaps a little more slowly than before. However, after about ten treatments his fits had decreased so much that I advised the parents that they could consider reducing his anticonvulsive drugs. By a happy coincidence, he was due to go for his quarterly check-up at the hospital, so I advised them to ask about the possibility of a reduction.

And so, the following week? You've guessed it: the following week a zombie came in, still with the same weird look in his eyes. The consultant had decided not to reduce the amount of drugs he was taking, but to double them! Not surprisingly, during the days after doubling the drugs he had lots and lots of fits. And also not surprisingly, about this time the parents lost heart, and started coming less and less frequently.

41 ❖ Nocturnal Enuresis

INTRODUCTION

Nocturnal enuresis, or bedwetting, is quite common, and there is relatively little in the way of treatment in Western medicine. By contrast, Chinese medicine, and especially acupuncture, is often very successful in treating this problem. With the advent of washing machines and disposable diapers, the problem is not quite such a burden on families as it used to be in the West, and still is in China.

Chinese textbooks are all rather vague about its etiology, for it relates to Kidney weakness, which in Chinese medicine is supposed to arise mainly from overwork or too much sex—problems which should not affect those under seven! Sometimes one can trace a congenital Kidney weakness or hereditary damp-heat disorder, and frequently one can detect a feeling of insecurity in the child. This insecurity may be due to the child's own nature, or it may have its origin in family quarrels or troubles at school. In some cases, however, no clear cause can be found.

The section on patterns below is based on a translation of *Pediatrics in Traditional Chinese Medicine (Zhong yi er ke xue)* and *Clinical Handbook of Pediatrics in Traditional Chinese Medicine (Zhong yi er ke lin chuang shou ce)*, with some additions and adaptations drawn from our experience in the clinic.

There are four main patterns associated with enuresis:

- weakness in the lower gate
- Spleen and Lung qi deficiency
- damp-heat in the Liver channel
- lingering pathogenic factor plus an emotional factor

Although we describe four patterns, it is important to understand that in *all* children with enuresis there will be

481

some measure of weakness in the lower gate *(xià guān)*, that is, weakness of the Kidney qi. If this were not the case, there would be no enuresis. Weakness in the lower gate allows fluids to leak out. The weakness—Lung and Spleen qi deficiency, for example—would manifest in another way, say as asthma. Even when there are signs of heat or damp-heat in the lower burner, one will also find weakness in the lower gate.

Weakness in the lower gate

It is said that this pattern can be distinguished from the others by the large amounts of urine passed during sleep. There tend to be two different types of children who have this pattern. The first is a typical yang-deficient child who is slow, inattentive, floppy, overweight, and cold. The other type of child tends to be thinner and slightly jumpy and nervous, possibly even hyperactive, in the evening or when overstimulated. In both types the lower gate is weak. The timbre of the voice—which is related to the health of the Kidneys—is an important sign in these children. Genuine cases of deficiency are often distinguishable by rather gruff, low-pitched voices, or voices of a cavernous nature. Note that the term 'base' *(yuán)* refers to the constitutional energy of the body, which resides in the lower abdomen. Often these children are constitutionally weak.

Spleen and Lung qi deficiency

This is really two patterns. In the first the child is basically healthy but has some aspects of weakness in the lower gate. When the child catches a cough the fluid metabolism is disrupted, as the function of the Lung and Spleen is impaired by the pathogenic factor, and the child has a temporary bout of enuresis until the illness is gone. Often, the child will then recover by itself.

The second pattern is seen in children where the Lung and Spleen are chronically weak and the lower gate is weak. These children will wet the bed and get repeated infections due to the weak Lung and Spleen energy. In order to cure these children, you must tonify both the Lung and Spleen as well as the lower gate.

Damp-heat in the Liver channel

This pattern is rarely seen by itself. The urinary incontinence occurs because the urine is somewhat stinging and irritates the urinary tract, causing the child to pass water. These children tend to be hot and are often angry, naughty, or disruptive. There may be a greenish color around the mouth. Although such children may show many signs of heat from excess, there is an underlying deficiency of the lower gate which must be tonified, in addition to dispersing the damp-heat. During the course of treatment the child often has yellow-green discharges from the urethra, vagina, or nose, which is characteristic of damp-heat.

Lingering pathogenic factor plus emotional factor

This is a complex pattern. There is a lingering pathogenic factor (LPF) which disturbs the flow of fluids in the body, and is the physical factor underlying the enuresis. Children with this pattern may not urinate at all during the day and then wet the bed at night. They may be strong or weak children—there is no real pattern. On top of this, there is some sort of emotional factor. This is a bit difficult to define; it is usually not as straightforward as in the last pattern, and it is an intrinsic part of a LPF. In Chapter 3 we explained how a LPF has a subtle effect on the child's emotional balance, which makes problems difficult to deal with. The slightest thing can really distress these children and result in tears or tantrums. Very often they find home life difficult to deal with for one reason or another, possibly for good reason. These are the children who may stop wetting the bed when they are away from home.

Sleep

In all of the patterns there may be heavy sleep, which prevents the child from waking up to urinate. If this is the case, it is essential to use points like GV-20 *(bai hui)* to help lighten sleep; otherwise, no matter how strong the signal from the bladder that it is full, they will not wake up to urinate.

Pulse

The pulse in children is usually a reliable indicator of what is happening. For example, if the pulse is strong and slippery then the child is usually full of phlegm and strong; if the pulse is weak then the child is usually weak. In enuresis the pulse should be weak or soft, especially in the third position; in these cases the problem is usually straightforward and can be successfully treated with acupuncture. In about half the cases that come to our clinic, however, the pulse is opposite to the symptoms, that is, the pulse is strong and slippery. In these patients the lymph glands in the groin are usually swollen, indicating a lingering pathogenic factor, combined with a deficient condition. This condition is more very difficult to treat with any success, for besides the straightforward physical problem there is usually a complex emotional tangle. The child may wet its bed to attract attention, and may also be experiencing the insecurity of one of the parents, or expressing a strain in the relationship between the parents. If the enuresis persists past the age of seven it is even more difficult to cure.

ETIOLOGY & PATHOGENESIS

Weakness in the lower gate

The Kidney qi governs the two yin—the anus and the urethra—and has an internal/external relationship with the Bladder. If the Kidney qi is weak then the lower burner will not be strong, and the two yin orifices will be unable to hold the fluids; hence the functions of storage and retention of fluids is impaired. The situation is further aggravated because the Kidney qi is unable to support the Bladder qi, and its function of regulating the water passages fails as well. These two factors cause enuresis.

The underlying causes of this pattern are thus quite straightforward:

• constitutional weakness
• long-term illness
• severe illness

Often, children with this pattern are insecure. This may be due to the child's own nature, or to its surroundings—family squabbles, school, and so forth.

Lung and Spleen qi deficiency

Both of these patterns have a similar pathology. Like all children with enuresis, we begin with some weakness in the lower burner. In addition, the Lungs govern the qi and rule the water passages, sending fluids to the Kidneys and Bladder, while the Spleen controls the transportation and transformation of fluids. If both organs are weak, control over the fluids is lost, and, coupled with the weakness in the lower burner, enuresis results. Quite often the water is not excreted properly during the daytime, and these children may hardly go to the toilet at all. At night, however, when energy returns to the organs, the water starts to drain out. This pattern is caused by any factor that depletes the Lung and Spleen qi such as repeated coughs and colds, immunizations, inappropriate use of medicines, or inappropriate diet. It may also occur after an illness.

Damp-heat in the Liver channel

Dampness and heat collect in the Liver channel and pour down to the Bladder. The dampness and heat irritate the urethra and prevent the Bladder from transforming the fluids efficiently, resulting in enuresis. There is also some measure of weakness in the lower burner, but this may not be a major factor. Common causes of this pattern are constraint of the Liver qi by emotional factors, which generates heat that collects in the channel; poor diet consisting of spicy junk foods; and possibly an external invasion of cold in the Liver channel which transforms into heat.

Lingering pathogenic factor plus emotional factor

This is a combination of things. The presence of a LPF can be attributed to many factors, common ones being repeated infections that have not been properly cleared, use of inappropriate medicines, and immunizations. The LPF disrupts the flow of fluids in the body, which gives rise to a thick phlegm which is characteristic of a LPF, which in turn further hinders the circulation of fluids. Fluid circulation can be so disrupted in some children that they may urinate very little during the day, but wet the bed at night. In addition, as in all cases of enuresis, the lower gate is weak; coupled with the effects of the LPF, enuresis ensues.

In a straightforward case these may be the only factors, but we usually find that this is not so, because of the subtle changes that a LPF makes in a child. When the qi is not flowing properly for any length of time—and sometimes the LPF has been there for nearly all the child's life—then it appears that the emotional balance is disturbed. This results in the child being unable to cope with stressful situations. In all children's lives there are tears and tantrums; this can be a normal and healthy response. However, when the child cries at the slightest thing, or flies into a rage all the time, then this is not normal, and is very often the result of a LPF. Such children just cannot cope. This is very distressing to the parents and the child, and causes great stress in the family—often never discussed. This added stress exacerbates the enuresis.

It may be that the home life is good but the child will still find some reason to get upset or angry. On the other hand, the home life or life at school may be very upsetting; even in a healthy child this may cause problems, but in these children the problem becomes insurmountable and completely disrupts their lives.

There are two other situations that you may see in clinic, and which should be mentioned here:

• habitual enuresis
• urinary tract infection

Habitual enuresis

In some cases the child has no underlying pathology but is simply not trained properly, or not looked after. The child starts to urinate at night and over a long period this becomes a habit. Acupuncture is of no use in such cases.

Urinary tract infection

When a child has a urinary tract infection there is more likelihood of urinating at night. This should be considered if the enuresis is of recent onset, or if the enuresis comes and goes. This falls under the heading of damp-heat and is treated as damp-heat in the Liver channel.

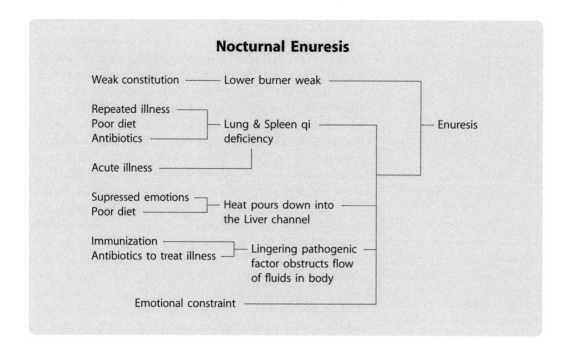

Nocturnal Enuresis

Weak constitution ——— Lower burner weak ————————————┐
                                                      │
Repeated illness ┐   │
Poor diet   ├─ Lung & Spleen qi ——————┐   ├— Enuresis
Antibiotics ─────┘   deficiency   │   │
                                            │   │
Acute illness ──────────────────┘   │   │

Supressed emotions ┐   │
Poor diet ─────────┴─ Heat pours down into ──────┐   │
                      the Liver channel   │   │
                                                  │   │
Immunization ──────────────┐   │   │
Antibiotics to treat illness ┴─ Lingering pathogenic ──┘
                               factor obstructs flow
                               of fluids in body

Emotional constraint ——————————————————————————┘

PATTERNS & SYMPTOMS

Weakness in the lower gate

• urinates a large amount every night during sleep, then wakes up
• facial color bright
• possibly dull-witted, inattentive, a bit incoherent when answering questions
• younger children are floppy
• possibly thin, jumpy, and nervous child
• possibly hyperactive
• back and knees are weak and sore
• daytime urination is clear, copious, and frequent
• in extreme cases the limbs are cold and there is aversion to cold
• tongue is pale
• pulse is deep, slow, and forceless

Lung and Spleen qi deficiency

There are two possibilities here. In the first situation, the child just wets the bed when he or she has an infection. Look for:

• signs of an external pathogenic attack
• may occur after another illness
• urinates while sleeping, but does not pass a large amount
• facial color white
• weak spirit
• limbs are weak

- poor appetite and little thirst
- stools are loose
- tongue is pale
- pulse is slow or deep or fine or floating

The second situation is a chronic condition, where the above symptoms persist:

- history of Lung and Spleen problems
- recurrent illnesses, especially of the Lung

Damp-heat in the Liver channel

This pattern is rarely seen by itself. There is usually some inflammation of the urethra or the vagina. Other symptoms include:

- urinates while sleeping: yellow and foul-smelling, hot, scalding urine
- easily angered and temperamental
- grinds teeth at night
- face and lips are red
- pulse is wiry, slippery

Lingering pathogenic factor

- usually a complex of factors
- history of repeated infections treated with antibiotics or immunizations
- swollen glands in the neck and stomach
- often an emotional factor involved
- may not urinate much in the day at all, but wets the bed at night
- pulse is full and slippery

GENERAL ADVICE

The following advice can be offered to all children who come for treatment of enuresis.

- Children should not be given anything to drink after 4 P.M. If there is a great thirst, this is a sign of internal heat and should be treated with acupuncture. If the usual points do not work, try using CV-23 *(lian quan)*.
- Children with heat signs should be kept off heating foods.
- If the child is deficient, they should be encouraged to rest.
- Some factors in a child's life tend to cause the qi to leave the lower burner and rise up to the head: reading, school work, television, computer games, and the like. Also anything that makes the child want to "escape from the world": an emotional crisis, family disputes, or sexual abuse. The withdrawal of qi from the lower burner can aggravate or cause enuresis.

• Some children often wet the bed when staying away from home. This is sometimes due to the unfamiliar smell of a strange bed. A simple way of overcoming this problem is for the child to take unwashed sheets and pillows to put on the unfamiliar bed. In other words, take a homely smell with them if staying away from home.

TREATMENT

General points

There are three points that can be used in all cases of enuresis. We have found them to be useful regardless of the pattern. However, in order for there to be a lasting cure, additional points must be used to treat the underlying condition.

CV-3 *(zhong ji)*	Tonifies the lower gate
Sp-6 *(san yin jiao)*	Tonifies the three leg yin
Liv-8 *(qu quan)*	Tonifies the three leg yin; benefits the Bladder

These points work in all cases because they strengthen the lower burner and the Bladder. In treating the first pattern, this is sufficient. However, for the other patterns you must treat the additional problems as well. Just strengthening the lower burner will help, but when the child gets tired the bedwetting is likely to start all over again. Or, in the second pattern, if the Lung and Spleen are not treated, then, when the next cough comes along, the child will be weakened and the bedwetting will start again.

In addition, sometimes it must be pointed out to parents that even though the bedwetting has stopped, extra treatments may be needed to consolidate the result or it will return.

Method: CV-3 *(zhong ji)* is treated with needle and moxa. Try and get the sensation to move up the legs from Sp-6 *(san yin jiao)* and Liv-8 *(qu quan)*. Chinese texts say that the treatment is more effective if it goes all the way up to the perineum. In practice, however, it usually goes only about half way up the leg.

According to Pattern

In addition to the general points above, other points should be added according to the particular pattern.

Weakness of the lower gate

Treatment principle: tonify the lower gate, strengthen the Bladder

B-23 *(shen shu)*	⎫ Strengthens the back and tonifies
B-25 *(da chang shu)*	⎬ the lower gate
B-28 *(pang guang shu)*	⎭
K-3 *(tai xi)*	Strengthens the Kidney and Bladder qi
K-1 *(yong quan)*	Strengthens the Kidney and Bladder qi [moxa only]
CV-6 *(qi hai)*	Tonifies the qi of the whole body

Bedwetting (hand point) On the palmar surface of the little finger in the middle of the transverse crease of the distal interphalangeal joint [moxa with 3-7 cones]

Method: moxa may be used at all the points. The governing *(shū)* points on the back should be treated only with moxa until the child is stronger, since, like all Kidney-deficient patients, it will fear the needles, and especially those on the back. Sometimes you will have to start by using only moxa at *all* points until the Kidney qi is stronger. In any event, needles are never used at K-1 *(yong quan)* in children.

Prognosis: the time required to cure these children depends on the extent of the deficiency. In a reasonably strong child, three to four treatments will be sufficient, but in a weaker child, many more.

Lung and Spleen qi deficiency

Treatment principle: strengthen the lower gate, tonify the Lungs and the Spleen

   Use the general points, plus the following:

S-36 *(zu san li)*	Strengthens the Spleen qi and tonifies the basal qi
CV-12 *(zhong wan)*	Strengthens the Spleen qi
L-7 *(lie que)*	Tonifies the Lung qi and regulates the water pathways
Sp-9 *(yin ling quan)*	Tonifies the Spleen qi and resolves dampness
Liv-1 *(da dun)*	Strengthens the retaining function of the Bladder [moxa only]
B-13 *(fei shu)*	Tonifies the Lung qi
B-20 *(pi shu)*	Tonifies the Spleen

Use moxa at CV-3 *(zhong ji)* and CV-12 *(zhong wan)*.

Prognosis: if the child is reasonably strong and just has enuresis with a cough or cold, then one to three treatments may be enough to aid recovery. If the child is weak and feeble, wets the bed all the time, and gets repeated infections, then many more treatments may be necessary—up to thirty for a lasting curing, although you should see a marked improvement in the bedwetting much sooner.

Damp-heat in the Liver channel

Treatment principle: strengthen the lower burner and clear heat from the Liver channel

Use the general points above, plus the following:

Liv-11 *(yin lian)*   Local point
Liv-3 *(tai chong)*   Regulates the Liver channel and calms the spirit
H-7 *(shen men)*   Calms the spirit
Sp-9 *(yin ling quan)*   Clears damp-heat
Liv-8 *(qu quan)*   Clears damp-heat

These additional points are important for treating this type of enuresis, since the damp-heat must be cleared from the Liver channel. Liv-3 *(tai chong)* has the additional advantage of spreading Liver qi and releasing constrained emotions. H-7 *(shen men)* is added if there is a significant emotional factor.

Prognosis: the number of treatments is variable, depending on the cause and the level of emotional disharmony in the child's life. If the cause is diet or an external attack of wind-cold, then, with the necessary changes, a cure can be effected in five treatments. If the cause is more emotional, or a combination of factors, it will take longer.

Lingering pathogenic factor plus emotion

Treatment principle: resolve the lingering pathogenic factor and strengthen the lower burner

The general points above will usually bring some immediate respite. However, nearly always the bedwetting will return when the next emotional crisis arises. Therefore, add the points below, as appropriate.

If the child is weak, use the following points to tonify:

S-36 *(zu san li)*
CV-12 *(zhong wan)*

Method: add moxa

When the qi is strong enough to expel the lingering pathogenic factor, use:

GV-20 *(bai lao)*
B-18 *(gan shu)*
B-20 *(pi shu)*
B-23 *(shen shu)*

Prognosis: the length of time needed to cure this condition is quite variable. In a strong child where the LPF is obvious and of fairly recent origin, only ten to fifteen treatments are needed. If the child is weak and the LPF has been around for a long time, then thirty-plus treatments are needed. However, if you can persuade the parents to continue treatment, you will surely help a lot. If there is a real emotional problem (e.g., family disputes) you may suggest some form of counseling for the whole family. In such cases it is unlikely that acupuncture will succeed by itself.

According to Symptom

Heavy sleep   GV-20 *(bai hui)*
Irritability   H-7 *(shen men)*, Liv-3 *(tai chong)*

NOTE

• For a case history involving noctural enuresis, see Case 20 in Chapter 47.

❖

42 ❖ Urinary Tract Infection

INTRODUCTION

Urinary tract infection includes urethritis, cystitis, and diaper rash. Traditional Chinese medicine divides it into acute and chronic types. Acupuncture is usually very effective in treating acute attacks in children, and is also effective in treating some chronic conditions; however, in chronic cases the prognosis is more variable because the basis is usually a lingering pathogenic factor. In acute attacks there is frequently involvement of a pathogenic factor (associated with a bacterial or viral infection in biomedicine), but the predisposing factors are varied, and thus the patterns and treatment are different. In examining the patient, the abdomen and back should be palpated carefully to determine the site of inflammation.

In the following discussion we will treat acute UTI first, and then chronic.

CHINESE VERSUS WESTERN

Compared to the rather complex Western (biomedical) analysis of urinary tract infection, the traditional Chinese perspective is far simpler and often far more useful, for in most cases acupuncture is extremely effective. In "simple" cases of bacterial infection a cure is virtually guaranteed. Even where there is a renal abnormality or dysfunction for which surgery is suggested, it may well be worth trying acupuncture first, as it can still help.

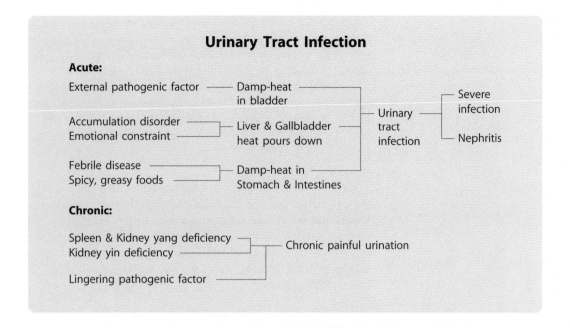

Urinary Tract Infection

Acute:

External pathogenic factor ——— Damp-heat in bladder

Accumulation disorder ——— Liver & Gallbladder
Emotional constraint ——— heat pours down

Febrile disease ——— Damp-heat in
Spicy, greasy foods ——— Stomach & Intestines

— Urinary tract infection — Severe infection / Nephritis

Chronic:

Spleen & Kidney yang deficiency ——— Chronic painful urination
Kidney yin deficiency ———

Lingering pathogenic factor ———

PATTERNS & SYMPTOMS

Acute Attack

Urinary tract infections occur because of pathogenic damp-heat, which collects in the lower burner and obstructs the flow of qi in the Bladder. The damp-heat is associated with three different causes, and depends on predisposing factors in the child. This gives rise to the three patterns:

- damp-heat in the Bladder
- damp-heat in the Liver channel
- damp-heat in the Stomach and Intestines

Damp-heat in the Bladder

This is caused by an invasion of an external pathogenic factor—usually pathogenic damp-cold—which transforms into damp-heat. The common cause is the child getting cold and wet while swimming. You may also see this in an acute flare-up of a chronic infection.

Symptoms

- urinary urgency
- possible increase in frequency of urination
- urine is yellow and painful to pass
- lower abdomen is distended and painful
- young child will cry out, is restless, and clings to mother

Tongue: yellow and greasy, or white and greasy
Pulse: soggy and rapid

Damp-heat in the Liver channel

This is caused by interior heat from excess that has accumulated in the body and then enters the Liver channel and pours down to the Bladder. In contrast to damp-heat in the Bladder, there is no external pathogenic factor present. In conventional biomedicine this may correspond to nonspecific urethritis. It occurs because the urine itself is irritating and scalding.

A common cause of the heat in babies and toddler is accumulation disorder. In older children there is often some emotional constraint that causes heat in the Liver. It is also seen when heat is being expelled from the body in the course of treating another disease with antibiotics or acupuncture. The heat is expelled in the urine and this causes inflammation.

Symptoms

- difficulty and pain in urinating
- urination frequent, and possibly yellow
- fever with aversion to cold
- possible bitter taste in mouth
- feeling of fullness and possible vomiting
- vexation, irritability, and restlessness
- diaper rash

Tongue: yellow coating
Pulse: wiry, rapid
Finger vein: purple

Damp-heat in the Stomach and Intestines

This is the result of damp-heat in the Stomach and Intestines pouring down into the Bladder. The most common cause in children is a consequence of yang-ming fever, for example, influenza where the intense heat in the middle burner passes to the Bladder. Thus, this pattern is really a further development of another disease.

Symptoms

- high fever that is not relieved by sweating
- foul breath
- thirst with desire to drink
- abdominal pain and constipation
- urine scanty and yellow

Tongue: yellow, greasy coating
Pulse: overflowing, rapid

Complications

General complications

With all urinary tract infections, as the damp-heat accumulates, the pathogenic factor and normal qi engage in battle. This gives rise to chills and fever.

Regardless of where the damp-heat originated, it can accumulate in the middle burner and obstruct the Stomach and the Spleen causing vomiting, nausea, diarrhea, and a feeling of fullness.

If the heat rises up to the Heart, the child will become restless and irritable.

Nephritis

The Bladder has an interior-exterior relationship with the Kidneys. If damp-heat accumulates in the Bladder and is not treated, it can easily pass to the Kidneys, resulting in a serious organ disease. The main signs to watch out for include:

- frequent, urgent, and painful urination
- back pain
- child will scream and cling to the parent; there may also be fever and restlessness
- nausea, vomiting, diarrhea
- headache

Nephritis can be treated with acupuncture, but this must be done quickly and often in order to prevent serious complications. It may be preferable to take the child to hospital to be treated.

TREATMENT

Main points

In the treatment of acute urinary tract infection, you can always use any of the following four points:

CV-3 *(zhong ji)*	Alarm *(mù)* point of the Bladder
B-28 *(pang guang shu)*	Back *(shū)* point of the Bladder
Sp-6 *(san yin jiao)*	Benefits the three leg yin channels
Liv-8 *(qu quan)*	Clears damp-heat and benefits the Bladder

Use CV-3 *(zhong ji)* and *ashi* points on the abdomen. Look for *ashi* points along the surface projection of the urinary tract, as far up as the kidneys. These may be spontaneously painful or may require gentle palpation to discover.

Liv-8 *(qu quan)* should be used when there is pain in the Bladder.

If there are chills, and the pain improves with warmth, then you can use moxa. This is in sharp contrast to herbal medicine where the use of warming herbs should be avoided.

According to Symptom

Vomiting	P-6 *(nei guan)*	Stops the vomiting
Diarrhea	Liv-13 *(zhang men)*	Regulates the Spleen
	S-25 *(tian shu)*	Regulates the Spleen
Irritability	H-8 *(shao fu)*	Calms the spirit, clears heat in the Heart and damp-heat

According to Pattern

Damp-heat in the Bladder

Use the main points, plus:

B-58 *(fei yang)*	For Bladder infections
Sp-9 *(yin ling quan)*	Clears damp-heat

Prognosis: one to three treatments if the child is strong. If the child is weak, you may need further treatments to build up the qi.

Damp-heat in Liver channel

For accumulation disorder:

si feng (M-UE-9), and possibly Liv-8 *(qu quan)*

In older children, use the main points, especially Liv-8 *(qu quan),* and choose from the following:

Sp-9 *(yin ling quan)*	Clears damp-heat
Liv-2 *(xing jian)*	Clears heat form the Liver, especially when inflammation affects external genitals
G-25 *(jing men)*	Benefits the Kidneys and Bladder, and regulates the Liver and Gall Bladder

Prognosis: one to three treatments are usually enough in young babies with accumulation disorder. In older children, one to three treatments as well, but if the cause is stress, the condition may recur if the stress is not resolved.

Damp-heat in the Stomach and Intestines

Use the main points, plus the following to reduce the fever:

GV-14 *(da zhui)*
LI-11 *(qu chi)*
LI-4 *(he gu)*

Treat every six hours while the fever is high. Further treatment should then be given to help recovery. Moxibustion should not be used when there is a high fever.

Encourage the child to drink a lot of fluids. If constipated, give a purgative.

Prognosis: the urinary tract infection will clear when the fever has come down. The prognosis will be the same as for influenza.

Chronic Patterns

Chronic urinary tract infections are due to pathogenic damp-heat together with an underlying deficiency. It is often associated with a lingering pathogenic factor. Chronic urinary tract infection in children is not all that different from adult patterns.

There are two subcategories reflecting two different types of child with different underlying pathologies. The first is more a yang-deficient type, and the other more yin-deficient. There are no rigid boundaries here, but this division is generally adequate for the purpose of treatment. The two patterns are:

• Spleen and Kidney yang deficiency
• Kidney yin deficiency

Chronic urinary tract infection is usually seen when the true or upright *(zhèng)* qi has been injured. The damp-heat remains in the body causing the urination to be painful and difficult. In Chinese medicine this is known as painful urinary dysfunction *(lín zhèng)*.

Spleen and Kidney yang deficiency

This is usually a deficient-type child. There are repeated urinary tract infections because the protective and true qi are weak. These infections are often treated inappropriately with antibiotics, or not really treated at all, since they may only be mild. This then gives rise to a damp-heat lingering pathogenic factor that lurks in the lower burner. The chronic damp-heat can also come from food that is not properly digested. In older children, when the Spleen is weak it cannot digest food properly. If the child continues eating too much or inappropriate food—common in the West but not in China—then the food tends to rot in the Stomach, turning to heat. The dampness and heat so formed can pour down to the Bladder.

Although the disease itself is damp and hot in nature, these children are cold and yang-deficient. The reason for this is that the pathogenic damp-heat is localized in the Bladder or lower burner, while the Spleen and the Kidney energies of the child remain cold and weak.

This pattern can show itself in two forms: the "normal" one in which the child is characteristically weak, and the hyperactive one in which the child is deficient yet appears to be hyperactive.

Symptoms

- urination is sometimes painful and possibly difficult, but other times there is no problem
- no energy
- breathless
- little speaking
- slow and dull responses
- watery stools
- weak back

Tongue: pale body and thin, white coating
Pulse: deep and fine, weak

For hyperactive Spleen and Kidney yang deficiency, symptoms are the same, except:

- child appears to have lots of energy
- parents are often exhausted

Kidney yin deficiency

These children are also deficient, but instead of being cold and weak, they are actually yin-deficient. This is not very common, but may occur in older children or in those who have had a very high fever. It is listed here for the sake of completeness; you are unlikely to see it. The nearest pattern that is commonly seen in the West is the hyperactive Kidney deficient types—the jumpy, nervous children.

Symptoms

- urination is sometimes normal, sometimes difficult and painful
- dizziness and tinnitus
- back pain
- low grade fevers
- night sweats
- mouth dry, lips parched
- possibly hyperactive when excited

Tongue: red with little or no coating
Pulse: fine, rapid

TREATMENT

Spleen and Kidney yang deficiency

Treatment principle: strengthen the Spleen and Kidneys and dispel dampness

S-36 *(zu san li)*
Sp-6 *(san yin jiao)*
B-20 *(pi shu)*
CV-4 *(guan yuan)*

B-28 *(pang guang shu)*
Sp-9 *(yin ling quan)*

Moxa may also be used.

If there is rotting food in the Stomach, add Sp-4 *(gong sun)* and CV-12 *(zhong wan)*.

Prognosis: speed of recovery depends on the general health of the child: the weaker the child, the more the treatments. Requires between five and twenty treatments.

Kidney yin deficiency

Treatment principle: tonify the yin and clear the damp-heat

Liv-8 *(qu quan)*
Sp-6 *(san yin jiao)*
CV-3 *(zhong ji)*
B-28 *(pang guang shu)*
H-8 *(shao fu)*
K-3 *(tai xi)*
B-23 *(shen shu)*

Prognosis: once again, the time required to cure will depend on the overall health of the child:

• if the child is recovering from a fever that has been cured, one to three treatments
• if the child is exhausted, twenty or more treatments will be needed. In this case you may be unable to use needles, as the child will be frightened of them. Use moxa instead
• if the child is of the hyperactive type, advice should be given and you may have to play at various games to get the child to accept treatment

NOTES

• Use points along the Liver channel when the external genitals are affected.

• In cases where there is heat from excess, try to encourage the child to drink a lot of water. Contrary to much advice, this is not true in all cases of urinary tract infection. If the basis is yang deficiency, more water will make matters worse as it further weakens the Spleen.

• If the child has a lingering pathogenic factor and is obviously deficient in energy, but the pulse is wiry or full and slippery, this is not a good sign. These children are often unhappy and frequently difficult to treat.

- Urinary tract infection can be a sign that the child is being sexually abused. When this is the case it is always well disguised; possibly the only inkling you will get is that your treatment is not working. (Of course, your treatment may not work for a multitude of other reasons as well!)

- Diaper rash is not given extensive treatment here, as it usually responds to attention to hygiene (i.e., keeping the lower regions scrupulously clean). If it does not respond to this, the reason is either that the excreted urine is somewhat corrosive, or that the stools are corrosive, in which case one should look to the accumulation disorder.

❖

43 ❖ Stages of Growth and Problems at Puberty

INTRODUCTION

In this chapter we discuss the causes of some common ill-nesses that face children after about the age of four. The period up to four years has been dealt with in Chapter 1, which covers such problems as weaning, learning to walk, teething, and so forth. After about the age of four, things settle down gradually, leading up to the seven-year transi-tion. This is quite a big change, when it is more common to grow out of an illness than to develop one; thus, the years between about eight and twelve are usually the healthiest of life. The childhood problems are behind, and the adult problems have not yet started.

The next transition, at fourteen years, is momentous. It is the beginning of the turbulent years of puberty, when the sexual energy bursts forth. The changes that take place at this time are so great that this transition is considered to be a major 'gate of life' for both men and women.

The following topics will be discussed in this chapter:

- two important transitions: seven and fourteen years
- illnesses and beneficial changes associated with each transition
- expulsion of lingering pathogenic factors
- growth spurts
- rashes at puberty
- knee problems
- BCG immunizations (immunization against tuberculosis)
- TB miasm
- special problems facing girls at puberty
- supporting treatments

501

TWO IMPORTANT TRANSITIONS

In the *Inner Classic* it is noted that boys have an eight-year cycle and girls a seven-year cycle. In our experience this is not quite right. It is true that girls develop intellectually and emotionally more quickly than boys, but it appears in clinical practice that the ages of seven and fourteen years are important transitions for boys and girls alike. These transitions have clinical significance because old diseases can be cleared out and new diseases can appear.

The Seven-Year Transition

The big change that takes place at around seven years is an awareness of emotions as being something distinct and separate. For the first time the child begins to realize that she is not identical with her emotions. So, for example, a four-year-old child could say that *it* is happy, *it* is the same as happiness; in other words, the happiness and the child are one, indistinguishable, inseparable. Likewise with anger. An angry child is the very embodiment of anger. There is no restraint, no observation, no awareness of the anger, because the anger is so all-consuming. At seven years of age this changes. For the first time a child may notice that anger is something different from itself. This is the beginning of a separation between the mind and the emotions.

With this separation comes an awareness of something else, which remains constant throughout the storm of anger. This was expressed by my (JPS) daughter as, "Mummy, I am not the same as my anger, am I?" This has great significance for the cause of disease. Not at first, but after a few years, for with an awareness of emotions as something separate comes an ability to control them. In particular, there comes a desire to control the feelings of anger, and to override the feeling of exhaustion. (What is said about anger applies equally to all other emotions.)

A four-year-old who is exhausted will simply stop and collapse. If she becomes tired while crossing a road, she just sits down then and there—never mind that there are huge vehicles bearing down on mother and child! At seven years this changes. The child recognizes that she is exhausted and finds that it is possible to override her feelings.

Thus, for the first time, one commonly sees the occurrence of two major patterns:

• stagnation of Liver qi
• exhaustion from overwork, leading to Kidney deficiency

The first pattern, stagnation of Liver qi, comes about from suppressing restlessness and anger, while the second pattern, exhaustion from overwork, occurs from ignoring the feelings of tiredness. An example of a child overriding her feelings of tiredness is a case from our practice, a ten-year-old child who wished to be a champion swimmer. Every night after school she swam at least half a mile. Her body must have been crying out from exhaustion—judging from her pulse, her continuous sore throat, and the weakness of her back. But in spite of this, her determination to be tops kept her ploughing up and down the pool, night after night.

What other effects does this important transition have? One which has a bearing on treatment is that if there is a physical imbalance before the transition, then after the transition it becomes a physical and emotional imbalance. Thus, the whole vibration of the child in its imbalanced state becomes set or solidified in its emotional make-up as well as its physical one. An illness which persists through the seven-year transition becomes not just one illness, but two—a physical *and* an emotional imbalance.

So, for example, a child that has a hot imbalance (e.g., due to a lingering pathogenic factor) will be restless, irritable, or fidgety before the transition, but generally will not be expected or even able to control this behavior. In extreme cases such a child might be labelled 'hyperactive'. After the seven-year transition the imbalance is still there, so the child receives the same impulses from the body—the same desire to fidget, the same irritability—but instead of venting these feelings, the child will suppress them, and try to sit still. This may give rise to constraint of Liver qi, which may persist throughout the child's life.

An illness which persists through the seven-year transition becomes not just one illness, but two— a physical imbalance and an emotional imbalance.

Illnesses that Appear at this Time

There are three common illness that will now appear: headaches, asthma, and hay fever.

Headaches

You will notice that there is no chapter devoted to headaches in this book. This is because children under the age of seven should not have headaches. Headaches arise for a variety of causes. The main one is thinking too much. But the underlying condition may be one of deficiency (often Spleen and Stomach), or a lingering pathogenic factor, or blocked sinuses; or it may be a condition of excess from stagnation of Liver qi, or even Liver yang rising. So the condition of headache should be treated according to the presentation. But the reason for the headaches appearing at this age is that the child can now override its feelings of mental weariness, and continue doing what it is expected to do, long after it should have stopped.

Asthma

When asthma appears at this age it usually comes to children who previously suffered from chronic cough or asthma, but have grown out of it. When they reach this age, the combined effects of weak Lungs and Liver qi stagnation can develop into asthma

Hay fever

Hay fever and asthma are very closely related, with hay fever residing more in the channels, and asthma in the organ. The special thing about hay fever is that it has to do with one of the sensory organs, and as such, the troubles only occur when the child has to control its reaction to the messages it receives from the sensory organ. For the first time in its life, irritation at the emotional level may find expression in nose irritation.

The Fourteen-Year Transition

The transition that occurs around fourteen years is, if anything, more important than the seven-year transition, with effects that can last a lifetime. In traditional Chinese medicine this transition is one of the 'gates of life',* a time when health can take a big turn for the better or for the worse.

In the next few pages we will describe the other changes that may take place at this transition—for better or for worse.

What happens

On the developmental level, the child's individuality starts to come through. This is not the first time that individuality makes its appearance—each child shows its own characteristics from the moment of birth—but between the ages of fourteen and twenty-one the child begins to distance itself from its parents; in modern jargon, it "becomes its own person." It starts to develop its

---

*This is the only gate for men. It is said that women have three others: marriage (which traditionally coincided with their first sexual experience and moving away from home), childbirth, and menopause.

own ideas. There is the beginning of an awareness that it wants to do something different in life, often something very different from what the parents do. If all goes well, the parents will recognize this and gradually give the child more freedom so that the separation process can take place.

On the physical level there is another huge driving force, which is what can make the teenage years so turbulent: sexual energy is awakened for the first time. In terms of traditional Chinese medicine this energy originates in the Kidney yang, and finds its expression through the Liver. In a vigorous child this uprising force is immensely strong, so that if there is the least obstruction to the free flow of qi, it can severely tax the free-flowing function of the Liver, with corresponding outbursts of anger.

Effect of lingering pathogenic factor

We have seen that an illness that persists through the seven-year transition imbeds itself, and becomes a deeper disease. It becomes both a physical and emotional imbalance. If the lingering pathogenic factor continues to persist through the fourteen-year transition, it moves deeper still. Not only does it leave a physical and emotional imbalance, it affects the way in which the individual relates to others. The whole personality is affected.

An illness which persists through the seven- and fourteen-year transitions becomes not just one illness, but three: a physical imbalance, an emotional imbalance, and a personality imbalance.

To help understand this, it may be helpful to consider the case of a hot lingering pathogenic factor that a child acquires when very young. Before seven years this will give rise to symptoms of heat such as thirst, insomnia, and a red face. If it persists through the seven-year transition, the child will make a great effort to control the restlessness and irritability, and this effort will cause stagnation of Liver qi. If it continues to persist through the fourteen-year transition, it is likely to color the child's relations with everyone around. Stagnation of Liver qi means that the teenager will be much more moody, is likely to have difficult relationships, tackle problems in an aggressive manner, and get into difficult situations. An illness which persists through the seven- and fourteen-year transitions becomes not just one illness, but three: a physical imbalance, an emotional imbalance, and a personality imbalance.

Beneficial Changes that May Occur

If properly directed, the enormous outpouring of yang energy from the Kidneys can have very beneficial effects. On the physical level there are two common effects: expulsion of a lingering pathogenic factor, and expulsion of heat poison.

Expulsion of a lingering pathogenic factor

Puberty is a wonderful opportunity for expelling a pathogenic factor, which may have been there for most of the child's life. The energy which surges up at this time flows through the channels, pushing out any obstruction. Before then there is often just not enough energy to throw out the thick phlegm which flows in the channels (manifesting as swollen glands), but this tidal wave of energy can be strong enough to expel the last traces. As far as the child's nature is concerned, one may find that a child that was prone to sniffles and colds, and who was rather depressed before puberty, now becomes more vigorous, outgoing, and positive. Likewise a child who was restless and fidgety due to a hot lingering pathogenic factor becomes more confident and calm.

How do these changes occur?

These changes may occur gradually over a period of one or two years, or they may occur quite suddenly and manifest as disease. For example, a hot lingering pathogenic factor might clear out quite suddenly in the form of a fever: the child will have a temperature for a week or so, be utterly exhausted by it, but feel much better afterwards. Likewise with a cold lingering pathogenic factor: the child might have a huge outpouring of phlegm, with loose stools and a bad cough, which continues for several weeks. Often the illness will seem like a rerun of the original pathogenic factor that invaded many years ago. For example, a child with a lingering pathogenic factor from whooping cough may get a very harsh cough, possibly with vomiting, as the pathogenic factor is finally expelled.

Expulsion of heat poison

When we discussed the problems that could arise from pregnancy, we saw that there was something that all children bring into the world with them: heat poison. We saw how this was linked to a fierce sense of individuality and self-importance, which is in fact necessary for the survival of the infant. We also saw how the physical manifestation of this is a red purulent rash, which is a characteristic of measles. In Chapter 20 we saw the changes in a child's temperament that occur with measles, and how a rather selfish and self-centered child can become more open-hearted and outgoing after an attack of measles. We saw, in fact, how there are many beneficial effects of measles, provided the attack is well-managed and nursed, and that the child is not actually injured by the attack.

In the past it was common for every child to get measles. Now, with mass immunization, many children do not get measles, at least not before puberty. This means that they approach puberty with the heat poison (and its corresponding self-centeredness) still in the system. As just noted, the transition that occurs at puberty is closely connected with the development of the self, and thus with the heat poison. This means that puberty is an excellent opportunity to expel the poison that in another age would have been expressed as an attack of measles. It often happens that a healthy child will develop a measles-like rash, not as extensive in area or as pronounced as genuine measles, but continuing for many months, and even a year or two. If you see this in clinical practice, its significance should be explained to the mother.

Treatment of measles-like rash in puberty

The principle of treatment is to support the Kidney yang where necessary with points like B-23 *(shen shu),* and to assist in the transformation of the heat poison with points such as GV-10 *(ling tai),* B-18 *(gan shu),* and Liv-3 *(tai chong).*

A rash in puberty may be the sign of a healthy body expelling heat poison.

Looking After the Child

The fourteen-year transition is difficult. For one thing, the child needs Kidney yang energy to expel any lingering pathogenic factors, and it may simply not have enough energy to do this. Also, if the lingering pathogenic factor is expelled in an illness such as a cough or fever, there is a possibility that the child's protective qi will not be strong enough to overcome the pathogenic factor and expel it completely. Equally possible in our society is for the child to be treated with suppressive remedies such as antibiotics.

From such things as these we can see the kind of support that we as acupuncturists can provide children to help them through puberty. In the year or two before onset, the Kidney yang energy may need to be supported, especially in children whose Kidney energy is constitutionally weak, and those who still have quite a strong lingering pathogenic factor. Similar support may be required when the lingering pathogenic factor finally shows itself, although the nature of this support depends on how the pathogenic factor actually manifests: clearing phlegm if there is a lot of phlegm, clearing heat if there is a lot of heat, clearing stagnation of Liver qi. Each child must be considered individually and treated accordingly.

═══════

Before puberty, support the Kidney yang and Liver qi with such points as B-23 (shen shu) and B-18 (gan shu).

═══════

Emotional support

We saw earlier how a lingering pathogenic factor that persists through the seven-year transition may have a strong effect on the emotional level, leading the child to one-sided emotional development. During puberty, as the lingering pathogenic factor is expelled on the physical level, one finds similar turmoil on the emotional level, as the rather "stuck" emotions start to be freed. At this time it is common for children to show quite erratic behavior: obstinate, weepy, temperamental, excitable. If the child can be helped and supported with sympathy through these fluctuating moods, it will make an enormous difference to the transition. Likewise, if these moods are suppressed by anxious or rigid parents, it can be just as damaging as inappropriate medical treatment.

Physical support

Above all, during this time the child needs energy, and needs to conserve energy. This will usually be in direct opposition to its instincts, for the child feels the explosive Kidney yang energy rising up at the same time as it wants to rebel against its parents. Inevitably, there is a conflict between the child's desire to stay up late exploring the adult world, and its need to conserve energy so as to throw out any lingering pathogenic factor. If the parents have developed a good understanding with their child, this can be an opportunity for growth in both parents and child; in other circumstances, treatment and advice given to both parents and child can help facilitate the transition.

Health Problems that May Arise at Puberty

If the fouteen-year transition goes well, a child's health can take a turn for the better. Problems which had previously afflicted the child can be expelled once and for all. However, if the transition is not managed well—if, for example, the child is overworked, or the parents are over-rigid—a child who is comparatively healthy can take a turn for the worse and be left with a problem that can last for several decades, or even throughout life. These problems are related to:

- Kidney yang energy
- free flow of Liver qi
- penetration of a lingering pathogenic factor
- heat poison remaining in the system

Kidney yang energy

Briefly stated, if the child is overworked, either physically or mentally, at twelve to fourteen years of age, it can lay the foundation for a lifelong weakness of Kidney yang. When asked (but not before), the child will complain of being perpetually tired, of having a weak and aching back, and pain in the knees. This pattern may persist for many, many years.

Free flow of Liver qi

If the child is under emotional strain and has many late nights, it can injure the free flow of the Liver qi, and the child may suffer lifelong stagnation of Liver qi. In our description of the seven-year transition, we saw how a hot lingering pathogenic factor could lead to stagnation of Liver qi. At the fourteen-year transition this can become even more severe, leading to headaches, stiffness in the muscles, and asthma. In women the emotional stress caused by working for exams can lead to painful and irregular periods, a pattern which can last for many years.

Penetration of a lingering pathogenic factor

If the opportunity for expelling a lingering pathogenic factor is not taken, it may penetrate deeper, causing more severe problems. This will happen as a result of physical, emotional, or mental strain, or over-rigid parenting. If the child is not especially strong, and is encouraged to do lots of physical exercise, as well as working late into the night, it will not have the strength to expel any lingering pathogenic factor. Instead, it may simply remain in the body (see Case History 1 below) to cause trouble at a later date, or may actually penetrate deeper, causing a wide range of problems.

Heat poison remains

If the child does not have enough Kidney yang energy, and the heat poison remains in the system, this does not usually manifest straightaway as an illness. What does happen is that the child will have real problems in developing its own individuality, and in expressing itself. This is because heat poison is intimately connected with self-assertion and plain selfishness. This means that the child will have a difficult adolescence, with all sorts of trouble with relationships, a problem that may continue throughout adult life.

Case History 1

Jonathon was a healthy baby. He put on weight well and was very happy and a good sleeper. At the age of two this changed, after a whooping cough immunization booster. His sleep became disturbed and he often woke at night. During the daytime he was difficult to settle, having a short attention span, and found it difficult to be away from mother. This pattern continued throughout childhood, so that when he went to school, he had difficulty concentrating, and was always criticized for fidgeting and day dreaming. By the time he became fourteen, he had more or less conquered his fidgety behavior by taking large amounts of exercise. He played cricket in summer, rugby in autumn, and hockey in spring. All seemed to go well until he was seventeen. At this time he was working for his exams, played several matches a week, and had undertaken intense fitness training. The sleep problem that had given him trouble all through his life became worse. Finally, matters came to a head when he began to lose weight, at the same time as having very frequent urination. It did not take the school doctor long to establish that he was suffering from diabetes.

This is an example of a heat-type lingering pathogenic factor remaining in the system. If he had not been worked so hard in puberty, it is clear that he might have had the energy to expel the hot lingering pathogenic factor. As it was, the heat remained; combined with overwork, which depleted the Kidney energy, this led to the heat consuming the yin, which gave rise to diabetes.

Case History 2

Rachel was always a sunny child. Second in the family, she did not have the responsibility of her elder sister, and enjoyed being mothered by her. At this time it was normal for children to be given all the immunizations to protect them from disease. Consequently, she never had measles or whooping cough. She was rather active when young, always running around, and often had a red face. This desire for action was put to good use by the school, for they found that she enjoyed working off her energy doing gymnastics. In her they found a natural gymnast, and she was soon entered in one competition after another. Her parents were delighted to have such a star in the family, and spared no effort in taking her to all of the competitions, and paying for extra tuition in the evening.

At the age of fourteen, disaster struck. That winter she was competing in a very strenuous match, during which she got very hot and perspired a lot. Immediately afterwards she returned to the changing rooms, which were very cold, as the heating system had broken down. She got very chilled and was shivering all the time on the way home. The next day she had a high fever and spent the entire week in a fever. The fever eventually subsided, but left her very weak. At her doctors insistence, she was made to go back to school, and at her own insistence, was allowed to take up gymnastics again. That night she had a relapse with a mild fever that fortunately went down in the night. However, when she tried to get up the next day, she found that her legs would not support her, so that even two weeks later she was hardly able to stand. The conventional diagnosis of the disease later turned out to be fibromyalgia (ME), but at this time fibromyalgia was hardly known. Consequently, she had one test after another, each leaving her more tired and in more pain than the one before. Eventually, after six months, her condition was correctly diagnosed, but by this time she was bedridden and in great pain, a condition that lasted for the next five years.

This case illustrates that if the Kidney yang is insufficient, there will not be enough energy to expel the poison. If she had not pushed herself so hard before the age of fourteen, it is probable that she would not have depleted the Kidney energy so much, so that when she later became ill, she would have had the energy to throw off the pathogenic factor and expel the heat poison.

Case History 3

Duncan was always a sickly child. At birth he took a long time breathing, and during the first six months was not well. He was a poor eater, a poor sleeper, and did not put on as much weight as he should. Consequently, when he turned six months old—the standard time for immunization—he was given all the immunizations available. At about nine months he became seriously ill, vomiting continuously for several days. No clear diagnosis was given, but pancreatitis was suspected. He continued to be unhealthy throughout his childhood, with many days of absence from school due to sickness. Physically he was very thin, with thin bones, a great contrast to his younger brother, who was very sturdy. At the age of ten, Duncan grew stronger, and seemed to grow out of many of his childhood problems. He spent much less time off school and was more content there, although he was still physically rather thin, and easily became overtired. Although he had had many illnesses before the age of fourteen, they had been mostly cold-type illnesses; it was rare for him to have a fever. At fourteen he had not had measles or any sign of a rash. At thirteen he went to a new school and seemed to enjoy it. However, at fourteen he was put on the "fast track" at school, and given lots of homework. This was a great burden to him, and although he did not seem to get physically ill, he did seem to be depressed much of the time. Not surprisingly, he looked for different ways of relieving his depression. At fifteen he fell in love and had a passionate romance, which ended abruptly, leaving him much more depressed, and the girl deeply hurt. At sixteen he fell in love again, and after about half a year the affair again ended abruptly the same way.

Soon after this he came into contact with hard drug users and experimented with heroin. Fortunately, he had the good sense to see that drugs did not offer him the happiness that he was looking for, but it was close. At eighteen, once again, he fell in love, and again had the same shortlived relationship with the same turbulent ending.

This sort of pattern is very typical of someone who has has not yet managed to expel heat poison. They tend to be self-centered and look for satisfaction of their own desires, without much thought for the suffering they cause in others. It is tempting to think that the child's life could have been better if his energies had been better supported through puberty.

Life causes of illness	It is common in the United Kingdom to heap work upon work on a child at about the age of fourteen. A clever child will be encouraged to sit its national exams in nine, ten, or even more subjects, each one of which takes a lot of learning and a lot of course work. In addition, the child will be expected to play sports most days, and the child itself will also want to spend a lot of time socializing, often late into the night. The schools are keen for their pupils to collect prizes in as many subjects as possible, while the parents want their children to shine at an early age. All the attention is focused on present results, rather than seeing the educational process as a foundation for later life. This imbalance in priorities can mean that the child is under great stress—from physical exhaustion if the child is a champion at sports, from mental overwork if the child is brainy, and from lack of sleep and irregular lifestyle if the child socializes late into the night. Some children can cope with schedules like this, but for others it is the foundation for a lifetime of illness.
Growth spurts	We have mentioned this phenomenon before, but it is worth mentioning again. Growth spurts are controlled by the Kidneys—which govern the seven-year cycle—but the organ which supports growth is the Spleen. The reason for this is that there is a need to build bones and flesh, and to do this the child has to eat huge quantities of food. This requires considerable Spleen energy, and it is quite normal for children/teenagers to feel tired and listless while this is going on. If the child is healthy, it will consume huge quantities of food. If not quite so healthy, then the drain on the Spleen energy will mean that the child's appetite actually goes down, and then the child feels really very tired. The other organ to be affected is the Kidneys. This is only a secondary effect, and occurs if the child/teenager uses up too much energy during a growth spurt.
Knee problems	There is quite a common knee problem that occurs in teenagers, especially boys, known by the delightful name of osteochondritis dessicans. This involves growth of bone and inflammation at the insertion of the tendons, usually at the front of the knee. It has some similarities to arthritis.
	In my experience, this disorder appears in children who are simply overworked—physically and mentally—as well as going through a growth spurt. These children are usually very "results orientated" and "high achievers," being members of all sorts of sporting societies, and determined to win at all costs. I have found that it is useless to talk to them about reducing the amount of sports activi-

ties; it is like pouring water on a duck's back. However, acupuncture can be of great benefit in treating this disorder.

TREATMENT

The principle of treatment is to move the channels, using such points as:

G-34 *(yang ling quan)* and
S-36 *(zu san li)*

while tonifying the Kidney yin with points such as

K-3 *(tai xi)* or
B-23 *(shen shu)*

BCG immunization

In the United Kingdom it is common to give the BCG immunization (against tuberculosis) at about fourteen years of age. This can have quite a severe effect on the child, and at a very sensitive time in life. Of all the immunizations, this one is the most absurd. It is well known that an attack of tuberculosis does not confer immunity: if you have had it once, you may have it again. So the same is true about the immunity that the BCG immunization is purported to give. Recent studies by the orthodox medical profession (not just by dropouts!) have shown just that. The incidence and severity of tuberculosis is quite independent of whether immunization has been given.

In our opinion, the BCG immunization may possibly make matters worse. It can certainly make children much more emotional, and can make the teenage years even worse than they might otherwise be. What the BCG seems to do is to give the child the "TB miasm" that homeopaths are so fond of. This miasm does not seem to have a place in orthodox traditional Chinese medicine, but anyone with an eye for observing people knows that it is a reality.

What is the TB miasm?

The TB miasm is a state of being, an imbalance. In itself it is not a state of disease, and by no means is it the state of yin deficiency associated with the later stages of tuberculosis. It is more like an imbalance of the elements, in particular, one in which metal and water are both weak, while wood and fire are both strong. While this elemental imbalance describes a lot of what is happening, it is not the whole story. To get a clearer idea, here is a list of the more common signs and symptoms:

• restless
• always craves excitement, but is never satisfied, so craves even more stimulating activities
• if excitement is denied or obstructed, there is either anger or depression

- aversion to being confined or restricted
- loves open spaces; teenagers may think that the great plains of the USA are paradise on earth (until they get there)
- manic depressive: euphoria alternates with desperate gloom
- characteristic red spot on the cheek, like a boil; very occasionally it weeps, but more often it just stays there, growing slightly larger when the person is tired and run down, and smaller when the person is healthy

As can be seen from this description, it is a state of being rather than an illness. Moreover, it can easily develop into yin deficiency because these restless people tend to burn the candle at both ends.

TREATMENT

Just as this pattern does not seem to be recognized in traditional Chinese medicine, there also does not appear to be a treatment for it. To be sure, tuberculosis can be treated once it has developed, but I have not seen any descriptions of treatment of the miasm itself in the books.

In my experience, acupuncture can help the general health of the patient, and over a period of time can transform the pattern. However, it is slow to cure and can be stubborn, resisting both acupuncture and homeopathy. I think this is because the cause of this pattern is that the person has something deeply depressing that they don't want to look at. Consequently, they use stimulation or work, or anything that will take their mind off it. This is why if the homeopathic remedy Tuberculinum is given, it can lead to a very black depression. In itself this may not be dreadful, but it will only help if the individual can actually look at what is causing the depression and deal with it.

If there is a clear imbalance of qi, or any clear symptoms for that matter, these should be treated first. If there are no clear signs or symptoms, then points which calm the Liver and tonify the Kidneys and Lungs are often helpful. A typical prescription might include B-13 *(fei shu)*, B-23 *(shen shu)*, and Liv-3 *(tai chong)*.

Case History 4

Miss S was eighteen. She was full of enthusiasm and life, having been brought up by parents who took responsibility for their own child's health, and avoided giving medicine whenever possible. She had left school, and had just started as a trainee nurse, a vocation she had always wanted to follow since she was a child.

The first month was wonderful. The combination of living away from home, of being with other teenagers, and of studying nursing was exhilarating for her. This was to change abruptly.

On reviewing their records, the hospital authorities found that she had never been immunized against tuberculosis. Although only one case of tuberculosis had been seen in the town during the previous ten years (and that was treated at a different hospital), it was routine policy to give everyone the immunization.

When she was brought to me (JPS), I saw a sad, white-faced girl, with a large spot on her left cheek. She was drowsy and looked both frightened and as though she would burst into tears. This was some four months after she had started her nursing. The story was told to me once again: the first month to six weeks had been wonderful. She had enjoyed every minute. Then somehow everything changed. The nurses hostel, which at first had seemed a wonderful escape from home, became like a prison; her own room, which she had made beautiful with her own pictures and knick knacks, and which at first had seemed like her own favorite hidey-hole, now seemed like a cage. All she wanted to do was to go for long walks in the country.

At that time I was not very familiar with the ideas of homeopathy (and even had some prejudice against them), so it took a little time to find the reason for this sudden turnabout. It was only after some hours of study that the solution dawned on me: the TB immunization. On questioning, it turned out that this sudden flip in attitude came within a week of the immunization. So also did the large spot on her cheek, for which she was taking long-term antibiotic treatment.

Having unearthed this cause of illness, I decided to send her off for homeopathic treatment, which was dramatically successful. Within a few days she felt much better, and was back to her old bubbly self.

It has to be said that this was a very extreme and clear-cut case. Most do not have quite such an obvious cause or such a clear beginning. Indeed, it is true that even in this case there was an additional factor—getting overtired. Mummy was not there to make sure she got to bed early!

But if you look around, you will see many people who are healthy, but who have many of the features of the TB "miasm." Many of our patients may even have tuberculosis itself!

Since seeing this teenager, I have seen countless others like her. At first I would send them off for homeopathic treatment, but now I treat them with acupuncture, and only use homeopathy when I feel I have got stuck.

Special Problems Facing Girls at Puberty

The age we live in is very yang oriented. We are out of touch with the gentle rhythms of nature, insulated from the seasons. As a society we extol the virtues of speed, strength, movement, efficiency, leaving little time for stillness and contemplation. Straight lines rule, with towns, buildings, sculptures all constructed without a single curve. All of this emphasizes the yang at the expense of the yin. This has disastrous effects on men and women alike, but possibly more on women, many of whom feel that their yin nature is a weakness to be resisted and overcome.

This problem first comes to the surface at puberty when a girl starts her periods. She is likely to feel uneasy about them from the start, for in many circles there is the strange convention that nobody is supposed to know when a woman is having her period. Far from being proud of approaching womanhood, the girl finds she has to conceal even the slightest trace of it.

Worse still, no allowance is made for the natural changes in mood that come—the dreamy, otherworldly attitude that many women experience during a period. This is so at variance with the results-oriented, go-and-get-it attitude that is the norm, even in schools, that many girls (and women) fight against the feeling, and reject this valuable gift. Some women even call it "the curse."

To make matters worse, at this time it is common for schools to increase the load of school work, demanding that even more essays be delivered, thus imposing a level of stress that many would find intolerable at another time of life.

As individual practitioners, we cannot change society; we must work with what we are given. However, we can help our patients enormously. For many girls, even to have someone outside the family accepting that it is okay to be a woman can be immensely beneficial. Yet very often our work at this time is not based on any form of diagnosis, but should be educational in helping the child come to terms with being a woman.

Case History 5

Miss H was thirteen. She had to come to me with her mother, because she was suffering from painful periods. They had started six months ago, and from the outset were very regular, but extremely painful. She had to go to bed for a day, and even the next day she had to stay away from school.

I asked all the usual questions, and basically drew a blank. Yes, she was moody and emotional, but then show me the teenager who is not. Was she getting on alright at school? Yes, no problems, no bullying, popular in the class. Digestion, sleep, etc., all fine. Tongue, perfect. Pulse, great.

I was at a loss as to what to do, but remembered what one of my teachers in China had said: "If you are at a loss about what to do with painful periods, treat CV-3 *(ren zhong)* and Sp-6 *(san yin jiao)*"—which I duly did for several treatments.

Result: no change.

However, it was not such bad advice after all, for during those treatments it gave me something to do, somewhere to start. And during this time it gradually dawned on me that there was nothing wrong with this child, except that she hated the idea of periods. All her friends at school called it "the curse," and she thought that it was nasty and dirty.

Fortunately, her mother had quite a different view, and truly accepted the inconvenience as part of the process of being a woman, of which she was proud.

I was able to explain what I thought the problem was to her mother, and advised her to spend some time talking about the beneficial aspects of periods and of womanhood with her daughter. I also stopped treating her.

A few weeks later the mother said that she had managed to talk her daughter through a pain-free period.

Common Gynecological Problems

Once the periods start, all the related problems may occur. It is especially common to have painful or irregular or very heavy periods. These can be helped enormously by acupuncture. As far as the details of treatment are concerned, this is really outside the scope of this book, and is anyway not very different from the treatment of these problems in an adult.

Glandular fever (mononucleosis)

Glandular fever is normally viewed in orthodox medicine as invasion of a pathogenic factor: there is a "known" culprit, the Epstein-Barr Cocksackie virus. Chinese medicine also recognizes that an external pathogenic factor is involved, but the most important component is internal: stagnation of Liver qi.

The treatment approach to this problem, described in the next chapter, is the straightforward one set forth in Chinese medical texts. Of course, as in so many areas of medicine, matters have become much more complicated. A disease which used to be straightforward, and for which there was a simple treatment, now has new twists due to the complexities of life, not least of which is the interference in the body by orthodox medicine. For now glandular fever has taken on some of the functions of measles: ridding the body of toxins on the physical level, and making a big transition on the behavioral level. However, glandular fever appears during the teenage years or even later, while measles used to arrive before puberty. This makes understanding glandular fever much more difficult, for there is now a "good" attack of glandular fever, where the child makes an important transition, and consequently feels better after the illness; and there is a "bad" glandular fever, where the child just feels lousy, and goes on feeling lousy for perhaps years afterwards.

It is not easy to distinguish a "good" attack from a "bad" one. One important sign is a skin rash. If a rash comes with glandular fever (which was never the case in the past, when all attacks of glandular fever were "bad" ones), then the attack is likely to be a "good" one, and most beneficial to the system.

Case History 6

Harriet had always been a good girl, being teacher's pet at school, more through hard work than from actual aptitude. Her medical history was similar to many others at her school: the "normal" immunizations, the "normal" coughs thereafter, with occasional asthma attacks, all of which she "grew out of" at the age of seven years.

Her parents were teachers, so they assumed that Harriet would go to university and study an academic subject. Being a good girl, she had no trouble following this course, and decided to study history. The decision was based, perhaps, more on the fact that she liked the history teacher than on a real love for the subject. However, the combination worked well, and she duly got her grades and went off to university. When she arrived she had a big shock. She did not especially like the place, and worse, she did not like either history or the people who were teaching it. After one term, during which she became increasingly depressed, she gave up and went back home.

For six months she lived at home, and went out to work in a dress shop (she had always been very interested in clothes). While she was working there, with time to think, she gradually came to the conclusion that what she really wanted to do (and what she had really wanted to do for most of her life) was to be a dress designer.

One fateful night, she broached the subject with her parents. They were (predictably) furious and upset. No one in the family had ever worked in the "rag trade." The only suitable occupation for someone in that family was the academic life! But she held fast, for she knew what she wanted to do now. Next day she had scheduled interviews for herself, and within a month she had been accepted at a school for dressmaking, all despite the fierce opposition of her parents.

Then, one week after being accepted at the school, the glandular fever came. She was exhausted, and felt extremely ill. There was a fever, headache, and swollen, painful glands. The doctor quickly identified glandular fever, while making no comment about the rash which had appeared over most of her body. His prognosis was that she would have the fever on and off for a good month, and that she would not be really well again for two to three years.

The family was very discouraged by this, and so decided to try alternative medicine. To their surprise, they found that they could get an appointment within a week, which was just two weeks after the onset of the illness. Immediately after the first treatment (acupuncture) she felt better. After the second, the improvement continued. The acupuncture was supplemented by herbs, and at the end of three months she felt better than she had for a long time.

The parents noticed quite a change: she was much less fearful and more confident. The down side was that she had also become more independent and willful, often going her own way rather than obediently following the wishes of her parents.

This sort of transition is very similar to that experienced in measles, and it is clear that by at last doing what she wanted to do, and by going her own way, she had made an important transition in life.

The phenomenon of "acceleration"

Over the past seventy years there has been a trend toward earlier physical maturity such that the body's seven-year cycle has been accelerated. Physical maturity comes earlier, and some girls start to develop breasts as early as eight years of age, and have their first period before their tenth birthday. Likewise, boys start to grow facial hair at an earlier age, and their voices break earlier as well. However, the emotional development does not seem to be similarly accelerated. Consequently, one sees a split occurring between the physical and emotional aspects of the child. As far as disease is concerned, what seems to be important is the time when the deep emotional changes occur, which is usually at fourteen years. This means that the fourteen-year transition still occurs at fourteen years, even though physical maturity may come a bit sooner.

CONCLUSION

The seven-year transition is, as we have said, usually trouble-free. It is certainly not associated with the wild storms of puberty. By contrast, the fourteen-year transition at puberty is much more complex. In this chapter we have just scratched the surface. At times, I think there ought to be a medical/psychological speciality of puberty.

The main idea we want to get across is to allow the full expression of Kidney and Liver energies, so that the child can develop in the best possible way. Acupuncture can be of great help in making this transition relatively smooth.

❖

44 ❖ Glandular Fever
(Infectious Mononucleosis)

Glandular Fever

Infection ———┐
Immunization ———┘— Lingering pathogenic factor — Blocks channels, causes knots

Suppressed emotions, — Liver-yang rises — Heat condenses phlegm into knots
    especially anger

Exhaustion — Yin deficiency — Phlegm dries into knots

INTRODUCTION

Glandular fever is not a "new" disease, but the scale of its incidence is new. Like asthma and eczema, a few cases were known fifty years ago, but it was not as common a disease as it is now. It is very debilitating; it lays children low for a month or so during the active phase, and can impair their energy for up to two or three years. Little is offered by conventional medicine, while acupuncture can be of great help during the active phase of the disease, and can reduce the recuperation time to months instead of years.

The common age for glandular fever is the late teens, often at a time of stress, such as taking examinations. As such, it almost falls outside the scope of "children's diseases." However, it does affect especially those teenagers who are still completely dependent on their parents, so in that sense they could still be called "children." Glandular fever can also strike well before the teenage years, and recently there have been cases of children as young as three or four being diagnosed with this illness.

In this chapter we will only introduce the subject. It is perhaps not as full as it might be, in part because we are not particularly fond of treating the problems of steamy adolescence, and in part because the subject truly is vast, spreading as it does into the area of fibromyalgia (ME).

Conventional Approach

From the point of view of orthodox medicine, glandular fever is due to an invasion of a virus from the Epstein-Barr Cocksackie family. There is little more to be said. There is no treatment beyond rest and avoiding alcohol and stimulants. Occasionally, penicillin may be prescribed if there are swollen tonsils and sore throat.

TCM Approach

There is no exact counterpart of glandular fever in traditional Chinese medicine, but there is something very close. This is the pattern of *luǒ lì*. In the medical dictionaries this term is translated as scrofula, that is, tuberculosis of the lymph glands. However, a careful look at the symptoms and onset of *luǒ lì* shows that this is an inaccurate translation. To be sure, the term does include the biomedical pattern of scrofula, but it also includes other patterns, such as swollen glands in children, buboes, and also glandular fever. The common characteristic is swollen glands, perhaps boils or similar eruptions, and fever.

ETIOLOGY

There are three patterns of *luǒ lì* and glandular fever:

• stagnation of Liver qi
• lingering pathogenic factor
• yin deficiency

The common age of onset—the late teens—is a pointer to the main cause: stagnation of Liver qi. It is said that suppression of emotions causes stagnation of Liver qi. The stagnation of qi in the channels, especially the Liver channel, leads to stagnation of fluids, which then transform into phlegm. The phlegm "knots and ties up" the channels, causing them to swell and harden, giving rise to the symptom of swollen glands. In addition, the stagnation gives rise to heat, which is expressed as fever.

Other causes include our old friend lingering pathogenic factor, and yin deficiency. The etiology of lingering pathogenic factor should be familiar to you by now! The way that yin deficiency causes the glands to swell is as follows: the yin becomes exhausted, either by a long fever, overwork, or excessive sexual activity. Without yin, the body fluids dry up, stagnate, and transform into phlegm. The thick phlegm so formed cannot flow freely, thus the channels become hard and swollen. However, in teenage glandulaalr fever, these two patterns are not as common as stagnation of Liver qi.

As far as the Chinese texts are concerned, these patterns are discreet. In our experience, most teenagers have combinations of all three patterns, perhaps with one predominating.

Comment

As you can see, these explanations are quite different from that of conventional medicine. There is no mention at all of an external pathogenic factor. All the emphasis is on internal factors, in contrast to conventional medicine, which focuses exclusively on the external invasion.

A fulmination

It does seem extraordinary to us that there are so many intelligent people working in the field of medicine who are able to ignore a blindingly obvious fact concerning the incidence of disease in general, and of glandular fever in particular. The Cocksackie virus attacks every human being indiscriminately, but only those who are susceptible get a disease. Why is this all-important susceptibility so stubbornly ignored?

Emotional factors

So far, we have talked only about suppression of emotions. It is time to expand on this. The teenage years are a time of rebellion against authority, and of establishing independence. It is during the years from fourteen to twenty-one that the child's individuality develops, and splits away from that of its parents. The child becomes an adult, and gets in touch with it's own likes and dislikes, and it's own goals in life. Before this age only a few exceptional children really know what they want to do in life. After the age of twenty-one they should (in principle) know what they want to do—although more commonly they just know what they *don't* want to do—and they seek freedom to express themselves. It is during this age that people are especially sensitive to criticism about themselves, and especially crave freedom to do their own thing, or at the very least, to be "different." When this freedom is curtailed, or criticism of the new-found ego is perceived, huge emotions are generated. In the healthy and strong, these emotions find outlet in great arguments and slamming of doors. However, in the less healthy, the emotions remain inside and cause stagnation of qi.

Physical and emotional factors

In an earlier chapter we said that a lingering pathogenic factor could cause physical illness and emotional imbalance at a later age. Glandular fever is a prime example of this. On the physical level, the glands are already congested, and there is already thick phlegm in the system. On the qi level, the person is likely to be tired because the circulation of qi is impaired by the blocked channels. On the emotional level, frustration, depression, and feelings of worthlessness have become "built in" because the imbalance has persisted through the all important fourteen-year transition. Thus, we see that a child who has a lingering pathogenic factor is already half way to getting glandular fever. Just a little extra frustration is needed for the child to become ill.

Frustrations facing a teenager

It was bad enough in our time, but in many ways it is worse now! The pressures to do well in examinations seem to have increased enormously over the years. The schools seem to be able to think of nothing else apart from the number of children who achieve A-grade in their exams. There is less and less consideration of the child's welfare. By the time the child has completed its homework, there is no energy left for fun and amusement, and certainly none for self-expression and individuality. No wonder that the frustration and depression mount up inside.

There is also pressure on the home front. More often than not, both parents work, and it is simply inconvenient for a child to stay at home if it is unwell. Thus, children are packed off to school, even though they are pale-faced, with black pools around their eyes, drooping like a willow, and with aching back.

And then there is sexual frustration. In *Classic of the Simple Girl* it is noted that there is quite enough sexual energy at eighteen to make love regularly twice or three times a night. While a few teenagers do this, the good boys and girls who stay up late with their books certainly do not. Add to all this that the world is less safe, and children are less free to roam where they will in their spare time for fear of being raped, mugged, or simply run over!

Case History

Miss W was a delicate seventeen-year-old, and the daughter of a headmistress. The relationship was much as you might imagine between a busy, domineering mother and a shy, sensitive, and artistic daughter. The mother ensured that her daughter had an hour of "quality time" in the evening, but was mostly impatient with her daughter's inability to study subjects she found boring, and her tendency to day-dream.

Matters came to a head when the daughter went in for her public examinations a year early. Four months before the exams she came down with glandular fever. She was completely prostrated, spending three or four days a week in bed, and only two days in the week could she spend at her books (which her mother had thought-fully retrieved from school for her).

The mother brought her daughter to me (JPS) for treatment. I gave her acupuncture twice a week for ten weeks, and it did make a great difference to her energy, but I could not say that she was really cured. She never wanted to do the exams, and at this age was unable to break free of the mold in which her mother cast her. Her real love was painting and flowers, both of which subjects her mother considered worthless. The poor daughter did not at that age have the strength to follow her own way, and so could never be completely cured. In this case the acupuncture was only palliative.

SYMPTOMS

Glandular fever has two stages. The first is an initial attack lasting two to four weeks, resembling influenza. The second stage is the chronic lingering condition, and is the stage we commonly see. This stage can last for many years.

Stage One

The onset is sudden, like an attack of influenza. In fact, there is nothing to distinguish it from influenza at this stage, except that the glands are swollen and tender, and sometimes spontaneously painful. The glands most commonly affected are those in the neck and armpit, but the ones in the groin and abdomen may also be affected. This stage corresponds to an attack of wind-heat, and commonly lasts about two to four weeks; after this, the fever goes down.

Stage Two

This stage corresponds to *luǒ lì*. The fever goes down, but the glands remain swollen and tender, and the patient remains exhausted, for a long time. Even after a year the patient's energy may be limited, and he or she may find that when overtired, all the old symptoms will return. Tolerance to certain foods and drinks (especially alcohol) is much reduced.

In severe cases, the patient may have tuberculosis or cancer of the lymph glands, with associated signs of Lung and Kidney yin deficiency:

• night sweats, tidal fever, malar flush
• possible loss of voice
• body is weak and exhausted
• poor digestion

Within this stage there are two major categories—excess and deficiency. In both cases the child is exhausted, but in the case of excess there is at least some energy to work with.

TREATMENT

Stage One

Treatment principle: clear the heat and resolve the toxicity, transform the phlegm and disperse the knots

At this stage, the main treatment is to clear heat and expel wind. A useful prescription is:

GV-14 *(da zhui)*
LI-11 *(qu chi)*
LI-4 *(he gu)*

Method: treat every day or every other day, if you can, using a strong reducing technique

There is another prescription mentioned in practically all the acupuncture books, which is based on one found in the classic *Compendium of Acupuncture (Zhen jiu da cheng)*. The original prescription says to apply moxa at the following points:

bai lao (M-HN-30)
tip of the elbow
G-21 *(jian jing)*

In more recent texts, moxa is replaced with needles, and the prescription is often modified as follows:

bai lao (M-HN-30)
TB-10 *(tian jing)*
G-21 *(jian jing)*
TB-17 *(yi feng)*   Needle 1.5 to 2.5 units subcutaneously down the neck

We haven't actually used this prescription, so we can't say if it works.

Stage Two

Treatment principle (from Chinese text): clear the heat and transform the phlegm, soften the hardness and disperse the knots. If there are symptoms of yin deficiency, also enrich the Kidney and Lung yin.

The patterns described in the Chinese texts are not quite what we observe in England or the United States. By far the most common pattern is a mixture of a lingering pathogenic factor and stagnation of Liver qi. There is exhaustion as well, characteristic of a lingering pathogenic factor. In these circumstances, we find that the back *shū* points are effective, and recommend the following prescription:

bai lao (M-HN-30)

B-18 *(gan shu)*	Regulates the Liver qi and disperses the knots
B-20 *(pi shu)*	Tonifies the Spleen and transforms the phlegm
Sp-6 *(san yin jiao)*	

Additional points

Liv-2 *(xing jian)*	Clears the heat and brings down the Liver yang
LI-11 *(qu chi)*	Clears the heat
H-3 *(shao hai)*	Traditionally used for glandular congestion

If you are only treating once a week, this prescription is adequate. If you can treat twice a week, alternate this prescription with the following, to tonify the qi:

L-9 (tai yuan)
S-36 *(zu san li)*
Sp-6 *(san yin jiao)*

If the pulse is wiry rather than slippery, and the patient shows obvious signs of anger, alternate the above prescription with the following:

LI-4 *(he gu)*
Liv-3 *(tai chong)*

Excessive pattern

This pattern includes both acute attack and chronic inflammation or swelling in reasonably healthy patients. The main points listed above for stage two are usually sufficient. If there are especially painful or large and hard lymph glands, consider the following alternatives:

- needle the lymph gland with one to four needles
- pierce the lymph gland with a red-hot needle
- apply moxa on a ginger wafer
- use *tai yi* moxa. To get the smoke from the moxa (which includes many herbal additives) to condense on the skin without overheating, four or five layers of cotton wool are placed over the point or area to be treated, and the smouldering end of the moxa stick is pressed onto the cotton. If the stick is left in place too long, the cotton will begin to burn or the stick will go out. Therefore, when the patient complains of heat, the stick and cotton are removed. When the stick has become hot again the procedure is repeated, usually with new cotton.

Deficient pattern

This is chronic inflammation with more pronounced Lung and Kidney yin deficiency. All of the treatment regimens described above are applicable, but attention must be paid to tonifying the yin. Consider the following points:

B-18 *(gan shu)*	Tonifies the Liver yin
B-23 *(shen shu*	Tonifies the Kidney yin
B-17 *(ge shu)*	Tonifies the blood
B-13 *(fei shu)*	Tonifies the Lung yin
B-38 *(gao huang shu)*	Tonifies the yin of the entire body

Special techniques

There are a number of special techniques for treating glandular congestion. The reader is referred to *Acupuncture: A Comprehensive Text,* pages 589-90.

RESULTS

As you might expect, the results are quite variable. Sometimes you get stupendous results, with the teenager feeling much better in a short period of time, perhaps three or four treatments. More commonly, however, you can help the child get over the fever quite quickly, but it takes several months to restore their energy to full strength. It takes this long because they need to do two things: first, recover their energy, which is usually very depleted; and second, sort out their lives—perhaps it is the relationship with their parents, or how much work they do, or whether they can get the super-double-plus-starred-A-grade that they were hoping for on their exams.

Dietary advice

Pay attention to diet. Phlegm-producing foods such as cow's milk and cheese should be avoided as should red meat and greasy foods. For deficient patterns it is important to ensure that there is adequate nourishment.

Patterns of Luǒ Lì

For the sake of completeness, here are the common patterns of *luǒ lì* as viewed by the herbalist. These are somewhat different from those of the acupuncturist.

Lingering pathogenic factor

This is common under the age of fourteen. There isn't much more that I can tell you about it!

Liver yang rising

This is common in teenagers. In the Chinese books it is listed as Liver yang rising, but this refers to conditions in China. Somehow, Westerners—or at least the English—are much less yang, and it is more common to see stagnation of Liver qi. To be sure, there are terrific outbursts of anger, but it is rare to see red face, red eyes, red tongue, splitting headache, and so forth.

Kidney yin deficiency

This is more common in adults, who are more likely to overwork for years at a time. It may be one of the patterns of scrofula (tuberculosis) or of cancer of the lymph glands. Having said that, however, an individual in one of our case histories actually had phenomenal signs of yin deficiency with severe exhaustion, tidal fever, and night sweats. The Western diagnosis of her condition was fibromyalgia, a condition which does not appear in the Chinese texts.

Glandular Fever as a Transition

We have previously noted how children's diseases are often transitions, and are opportunities for the body to expel toxins while the child makes emotional and spiritual progress. We have also encountered this with chronic coughs. The same is sometimes true with glandular fever. Usually, the disease is due to the child succumbing to immense external pressures, but occasionally it is due to throwing off glandular disturbances that have been there since childhood. This is especially true if the child has not had measles, and the onset of glandular fever is accompanied by a measles-like rash. In this case, the illness serves exactly the same function as measles, and is a belated opportunity to expel 'womb poison'.

❖

Case History

Mr. C was the son of an ambitious mother. His father had been killed in the Second World War, and his mother was determined that all the glory that she imagined in her late husband should be distilled into her precious son. Her ambition for him was to become a famous musician, especially as he showed a natural aptitude for the violin at an early age. Accordingly, she employed the best teachers, and saw to it that from the age of seven he practiced his violin at least four hours a day after school. He came from physically strong stock, so that although he was a bit pale and nervous compared to his contemporaries (who spent a lot of time in the open air), he nevertheless grew up healthy and strong.

When he was eighteen he went for his auditions to the conservatory in the capital city. By this time he was an excellent musician, and knew many concertos by heart. But for some reason the examiner took against him, and awarded him very low marks. He made the infamous comment that far from making a world-class player, he "might hold down the post of back desk in the second violins in a provincial orchestra"!

Mr. C was furious. All the pent-up rage from having his life distorted and curtailed in the cause of music was let loose. All the frustration at having to stay indoors while his contemporaries were enjoying themselves came out. On top of this, there were almost certainly recriminations from his mother, behind closed doors.

The reaction on his body was devastating. He had a low grade fever for some months, with swollen glands and spontaneous sweating at odd times, and worst of all, two huge boils in his groin above the swollen glands. The boils swelled and swelled until they were a good two inches (5 cm) across, and poured pus.

This was a classic case of the stagnation of Liver qi type of glandular fever, with the buboes appearing at the groin on the Liver channel.

The story has a happy ending. Mr. C switched to the viola, and became a world class viola player!

45 ❖ Purpura

INTRODUCTION

Thrombocytopenic purpura is not especially common. In the acute form it affects young children between the ages of two and ten, and in its chronic form adolescents. In ninety percent of children in the West the disease is acute and self-limiting, and so is rarely a real threat to health. It is generally not a problem unless there is the complication of the purpura spreading to the mouth and intestines. Intracranial bleeding is rare, affecting less than half a percent of cases. In Western medicine there is no clear etiology (although it often develops after a viral infection), and there is little in the way of treatment. However, in our limited experience, acupuncture can be of help in curing an acute attack and in resolving a chronic condition.

In Chinese medicine, four distinct types are recognized. The first is due to attack by an external pathogenic factor, and is closest to the Western idea of a viral influence. The pathogenic factor especially attacks the Stomach and Intestines, thus points affecting these organs are used. The second type is due to heat in the blood and commonly occurs during febrile diseases. It is very uncommon for this type to appear in a chronic condition, but it sometimes does so in patients with lingering pathogenic heat as the result of a febrile disease or immunization. It then recurs from time to time, and is aggravated by warming foods. The third type is due to weakness and malnourishment, and is very uncommon among children in the West. When it does occur it may be from some hereditary cause. The fourth type, yin deficiency, is usually attributable to a long-term febrile disease weakening the body. This type is even more uncommon in the West, as febrile diseases are usually treated quickly with antibiotics.

ETIOLOGY

External attack of wind

Children's bodies are weak, their organs are soft, their qi and blood are lacking in strength, and the external protective qi is not fully formed. They are thus susceptible to attacks from external pathogenic factors, which battle with the protective qi and attack the channels and collaterals, causing the blood to extrude from the vessels and remain in the skin where it manifests as purpura.

The pathogenic factor may also enter the Intestines and Stomach where it causes abdominal pain and blood in the stools. If wind-heat combines with dampness, or if there is already dampness in the interior, damp-heat may ensue, with blood in the urine. Damp-heat is a very serious condition, and if not treated, may continue for an extended period of time.

Heat toxin accumulating inside

Heat toxin can accumulate inside and transform into fire, which affects the blood. It may then attack the blood vessels such that the blood moves recklessly and extravasates to the skin, giving rise to purpura. The fire may rise up to the sinuses, leading the blood, and causing nosebleeds. The accumulation of heat toxin can also injure the Stomach channel and cause vomiting of blood; entering the connecting channels of the Stomach which ascend to the teeth and gums, the pathogenic heat causes the gums to bleed. Or it may pour downward into the Large Intestine or Kidneys and Bladder, causing blood in the stools or urine. The disease is often one of sudden onset, and manifests in other heat symptoms such as red face, thirst, and irritability.

The continuation of pathogenic heat may also affect the Heart spirit, giving rise to restlessness, irritability, and even loss of consciousness. If it reaches the blood level, blood flows out of the channels and there is considerable loss of blood. The facial color then becomes bright white and there is profuse sweating, painful urination, low blood pressure, twitching, and cold limbs, all of which are characteristic of collapse from deficiency.

Injury to the organs, qi, and blood

This type of purpura is characterized by stomachache and occurs because the organs, qi, and blood are injured and the Spleen qi is deficient. When the Spleen is deficient it cannot create blood, and if the qi is deficient, it can neither move nor restrain the blood. Alternatively, this pattern can occur when Kidney yin is insufficient; the fire from deficiency burns upward, driving the blood from the channels.

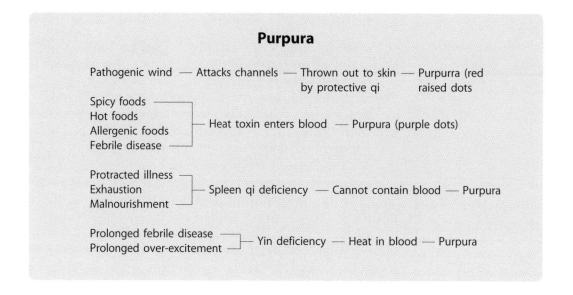

Purpura

Pathogenic wind —— Attacks channels —— Thrown out to skin —— Purpurra (red
by protective qi   raised dots

Spicy foods
Hot foods
Allergenic foods —— Heat toxin enters blood —— Purpura (purple dots)
Febrile disease

Protracted illness
Exhaustion —— Spleen qi deficiency —— Cannot contain blood —— Purpura
Malnourishment

Prolonged febrile disease
Prolonged over-excitement —— Yin deficiency —— Heat in blood —— Purpura

PATTERNS & SYMPTOMS

External attack of wind

- disease arises rather suddenly
- rash may cover the entire body (and oral cavity) and cause significant discomfort
- purpura, especially on the lower half of body and the lower limbs, but also on the shoulders; color is rather fresh red, in a rash with mounds, or as red spots, both big and small
- fever
- no desire for food or drink, indigestion
- possibly nausea and vomiting
- abdominal pain
- blood in stools
- blood in urine

Tongue body: red
Tongue coating: thick, greasy, possibly with red "thorns"
Pulse: floating, rapid

Treatment principle: expel the wind and clear the heat, cool the blood and stop the bleeding

Reckless movement of hot blood

- skin has purple dots or spots which may be raised and appear suddenly; in severe cases, the spots may be the size of coins
- facial color may be bright red or purple
- possibly nosebleeds
- possibly abdominal pain
- possibly blood in stools and constipation
- possibly blood in urine

- blood color is fresh red
- patient is agitated and restless

Tongue body: bright red
Tongue coating: thick, yellow
Pulse: slippery, rapid

Treatment principle: clear the heat, cool the blood, stop the bleeding

Spleen qi failing to restrain the blood

- spots are purple and flat, in the form of dots or larger spots, with a rather pale color
- facial color is dull
- spirit is tired, without strength
- dizziness
- palpitations
- dull abdominal pain, possibly poor appetite
- stools contain dark blood
- lips and tongue pale red
- possibly bleeding gums or nosebleeds
- possibly joint swelling

Pulse: fine

Treatment principle: reinforce the qi and contain the blood

Blazing fire from yin deficiency

- intermittent purpura, especially on the lower limbs
- intermittent dizziness, tinnitus, night sweats, malar flush, heat in the palms and soles

Tongue: red with little coating
Pulse: fine, rapid

Treatment principle: enrich the yin and reduce the heat, cool the blood and stop the bleeding

Note: when the bleeding stops (either naturally, or as a result of treatment) there may be a pattern of blood stasis, with symptoms of red petechiae, blood blisters, lumps in the abdomen, and blue dots on the tongue (see sequelae below)

TREATMENT

External attack of wind

CV-12 *(zhong wan)*	Clears the pathogenic factor from the Stomach and Intestines
S-25 *(tian shu)*	Clears the pathogenic factor from the Intestines
S-36 *(zu san li)*	Clears the pathogenic factor from the Stomach and Intestines
Sp-9 *(yin ling quan)*	Clears the damp-heat
Sp-10 *(xue hai)*	Clears the blood stagnation and benefits the skin

	Sp-6 *(san yin jiao)*	Clears the pathogenic wind from the Intestines

Method: dispersing method; treat once or twice a day
Prognosis: three to six treatments should be sufficient

Reckless movement of hot blood	Sp-10 *(xue hai)* Sp-6 *(san yin jiao)* Liv-3 *(tai chong)* B-40 *(wei zhong)*	Both points clear heat from the blood and benefit the skin Clears heat toxin Prick and bleed to clear the heat from the blood and cool the skin

Method: dispersing method; treat once or twice a day

Prognosis: depending on the cause of the heat in the blood, three to ten treatments

Spleen qi failing to restrain the blood	B-17 *(ge shu)* B-20 *(pi shu)* Sp-10 *(xue hai)* S-36 *(zu san li)* Sp-6 *(san yin jiao)*	Meeting point of blood Strengthens Spleen function of restraining the blood Regulates the blood and benefits the skin Tonifies the qi Tonifies the qi

Method: even method; treat daily or every other day; moxa may also be used

Prognosis: depends largely on the etiology and the strength of patient, and may vary from one treatment to very many

Blazing fire from yin deficiency	Sp-10 *(xue hai)* Liv-1 *(da dun)* K-3 *(tai xi)* H-6 *(yin xi)*	Both points clear heat from the blood Tonifies the yin Tonifies the yin and regulates the blood

Method: even method; treat once a day or every other day

Prognosis: depending on the etiology, from one treatment to many

Sequelae: blood stasis	Liv-3 *(tai chong)* Liv-2 *(xing jian)* LI-4 *(he gu)* B-17 *(ge shu)*	Resolves the blood stasis

If there is local stagnation or pain, points along the affected channel should be used.

Results of treatment	We have treated too few cases to generalize. Those which we did treat seemed to have very rapid relief from symptoms during acute attacks.

46 ❖ Anemia

INTRODUCTION

Anemia is not one of the mainstream children's diseases, and we have not treated many cases. However, it does occur, and the way it appears in babies is somewhat different from adults.

The Function of Blood

To start with, we thought it would be useful to provide a rather abstract discussion of the foundation of blood—as we understand it.

When you read through Chinese textbooks you will find very little on the function of blood, and what happens to a person when they don't have enough blood, and what cast of mind leads to blood insufficiency. The most that we have come across is sayings like, "The blood nourishes and cools" or "Blood deficiency is serious in men, but not in women" or "Women have more blood than men." But nowhere do you see anything about the manifestation of blood in daily life. For English speakers this is surprising, for we have many sayings relating to blood: "hot blooded," "full blooded," "thin blooded," "blue blood," and so forth, each of which has a strong association. We think it is likely that there are similar sayings in Chinese, but don't know.

So, in the absence of anything from the Chinese, one has to rely on the English language sayings, and on observation. Our personal opinion is that blood is the substance which allows a person to engage in life. It is the substance which transforms thought into deed. It is the connection between the Heart and the channels. In this, it has an intimate relation with qi, for without qi there is no movement or activity; but without blood, nothing gets done. Hence, when you meet anemia in an adult, you will very often find that the person cannot get anything done. It is a two-way thing: the person cannot concentrate, feels exhausted, is breathless upon going upstairs, cannot see anything through to the finish because of anemia. Likewise, if a woman feels unable to do anything, or to concentrate, or to finish anything (e.g., because she is surrounded by demanding children) then she can easily develop anemia. This is why anemic people sometimes have a very particular hopeless atmosphere about them.

The situation is quite different with babies and toddlers. At this young age there is not the same compulsive urge to do things, not the same tendency to frustration when you can't get anything done because of constant interruptions. Consequently, it is a much less common condition, and the presentation is somewhat different.

Causes of Anemia

So what are the causes of anemia in babies and toddlers? Why does it happen at all? We think the reason is that the babies do not want to engage in life. Something has happened to them which makes them feel that living in the world is just too much. It takes more effort than they have available to interact with the world.

When put this way, it becomes easy to appreciate the relation between qi deficiency and blood deficiency, and two well-known patterns which fit this category immediately spring to mind: Lung and Spleen qi deficiency, and lingering pathogenic factor. Lung and Spleen qi deficient children sometimes have a despairing, retreating look about them; likewise, children with lingering pathogenic factor often have a vague not-quite-all-there look. Both of these conditions are prime candidates for anemia, and we have seen both patterns in the clinic.

PATTERNS & SYMPTOMS

The patterns that we describe here are the ones that we have seen. They are based on the very limited number of children with these disorders who have come to the clinic, so they are far from complete. We welcome information from anyone who has experience with anemia in children.

As you can see from the appendix to this chapter below, the patterns we have seen are different from the Chinese ones. This is not surprising, for babies face quite different environmental problems here than in rural China.

We have seen two patterns:

- Spleen qi deficiency
- lingering pathogenic factor

Spleen qi deficiency

- pale (of course, because they are anemic)
- weak
- thin
- all the remaining symptoms of genuine Spleen qi deficiency

Lingering pathogenic factor

- pale, shiny
- not so thin; some are podgy
- ups and downs of health are more dramatic, for example, they may get a bit better and then have a massive fever from which they nearly die
- glands, of course

TREATMENT

Conventional treatment

Once straightforward anemia has been diagnosed, and other illnesses such as bone marrow disease, sickle cell, and so forth have been ruled out, the conventional treatment is simply to give iron supplements, or if this fails, a blood transfusion. This has the short-term effect of overcoming anemia. Additional treatment may be to include more iron in the diet.

We do not have enough experience to say whether this treatment is usually effective or not. Undoubtedly, it can be of use in treatment, and the few cases that we have seen have undergone this treatment, but experienced only a temporary response. In each of these cases the child relapsed within a month or two, which is why they were brought to us.

Acupuncture

Treatment is straightforward. A basic prescription would be:

- S-36 *(zu san li)*
- Sp-6 *(san yin jiao)*
- H-7 *(shen men)*

Method: needle all with the tonifying method

According to pattern

To begin with, the treatment is the same. As the child gets stronger, you must set about expelling the lingering pathogenic factor, and you may also have to be on hand to treat the sudden violent fevers which may arise as the lingering pathogenic factor is finally expelled.

Results of treatment

We have only seen a few cases, but they have responded well. It must, however, be said that these babies did have the combined Western and Chinese medical treatment. We have the feeling that a severely anemic child would not respond so well to acupuncture alone. A blood transfusion could be a terrific boost, which would enable the acupuncture to work. I have had this experience with an adult patient who suffered from severe rheumatoid arthritis. She had become very anemic as a result of the disease, so much so that the tendons in her arm had started to spontaneously snap. I gave her a lot of treatments, which did not seem to have much effect. Then after about three months of treatment she had a big blood transfusion. After this, the acupuncture treatments started to make a big difference.

Appendix

For the sake of completeness, we have provided a list of patterns as they appear in a typical book of traditional Chinese pediatrics. For those of you who are herbalists, this may be more important than for acupuncturists. Differentiation is not really that important for acupuncturists, because the treatment ends up as more or less the same. Identification of the pattern is more a help in understanding what is going on.

ETIOLOGY

The following causes of anemia are listed. They are the ones commonly seen in China, where life in the villages can be harsh. Lingering pathogenic factors are uncommon, because a child might not even survive a serious pathogenic factor!

Inherited

Blood is nourished during the period when the baby is in the womb. If the pregnancy is difficult, or the baby is nearly lost, or if the mother is undernourished or overworked, then this can result in anemia.

Spleen and Stomach deficiency

The *Inner Classic* notes that "The middle burner separates qi and fluids, transforms and digests, and is the foundation of blood." In children, the Spleen and Stomach are naturally weak, so it is difficult for the yang-supporting energy to recover. If the child has insufficient food, or becomes infected with intestinal parasites, or is weak after an illness (such as vomiting and diarrhea, accumulation disorder, or malnutrition disorder), the Spleen and Stomach are injured, the transportive and transformative functions are impaired, and the production of blood is insufficient, leading to anemia.

Heart and Spleen deficiency

The Heart rules the blood, and the Spleen contains the blood. Therefore, if the Heart is weak and the Spleen is insufficient, the blood will be weak and the qi will be wilted, leading to anemia.

Liver and Kidney yin deficiency

If a pathogenic factor persists for a long time, it obstructs the yin, and injures the five *zàng* (yin) organs, including the Liver and Kidneys. The Liver stores blood, the Kidneys store essence. The Kidneys create bone marrow, and marrow generates the Liver. Therefore, if the Liver and Kidney yin is deficient, bone marrow does not form, blood cannot be stored, and there is anemia.

Spleen and Kidney yang deficiency

The Spleen generates the post-natal body, and the Kidneys are the prenatal fountain. If the Spleen and Kidney yang are both deficienct, then the body is without nourishment and warmth, or support and growth. Essence and blood are not created, leading to anemia.

PATTERNS & SYMPTOMS

Qi and blood deficiency

The symptoms of this pattern are common to all the other patterns:

• lips, mouth, mucous membranes, and nails are white
• face is quite white, without a trace of pink
• small appetite

Tongue: body pale, coating thin and white
Pulse: fine

Treatment principle: support the qi and nourish the blood

Spleen and Stomach deficiency

Symptoms as above, plus:

• weak voice
• no strength
• stools greasy, sweet-smelling

Tongue: body pale, coating oily

Other possible symptoms include:

• abdomen cold and painful
• phlegm, tongue coating greasy
• constipation
• poor sleep, five centers hot, accumulation disorder

Treatment principle: nourish the Spleen, support the blood

Heart and Spleen deficiency	Symptoms as above, plus:

• palpitations
• shortness of breath
• insomnia

Other possible symptoms include:

• yang deficiency, edema
• skin has purple petechiae, or purple or red pimples
• blood in stools, nosebleeds
• swollen abdomen

In extreme cases:

• voice is deep
• dizziness
• loss of consciousness

Tongue: body pale, coating thin and white
Pulse: fine, weak

Treatment principle: reinforce and nourish the Heart and Spleen

Liver and Kidney yin deficiency

Symptoms as above, plus:

• dizziness
• tinnitus
• hard of hearing or even deaf
• eyes dry, tongue dry
• back and knees sore
• night 'robber' sweats
• nails concave

Other possible symptoms include:

• tidal fevers
• mouth ulcers due to fire from deficiency flaring up
• high fever

Tongue: body pale or red and dry
Pulse: fine, rapid, without force

Treatment principle: support and nourish the Liver and Kidneys

Spleen and Kidney yang deficiency

Symptoms as above, plus:

• aversion to food
• abdomen much enlarged
• accumulation from deficiency
• stools greasy, or with undigested food
• aversion to cold
• skin cold
• edema

Other possible symptoms:
- shortness of breath
- diarrhea
- limbs cold

Tongue: swollen, pale
Pulse: small, fine, weak

Treatment principle: warm and reinforce the Spleen and Kidneys

NOTE

- For a case history involving anemia, see Case 26 in Chapter 47.

❖

Part Three

Case Histories

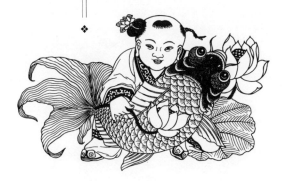

47 ❖ Case Histories

INTRODUCTION

In this chapter are a number of case histories from our own practice in treating children with acupuncture. Representative cases have been selected, rather than simply those which were most successful. As will be seen, some patients were not completely cured, or took an inordinate amount of time to recover.

In reporting the cases, we first discuss the appearance and behavior of the child, and then the main complaint as described by the parent, followed by answers to our questions. For the sake of brevity we have omitted unimportant facts. Therefore not all the records of histories and examinations are complete. This order of information reflects the sequence in which it is received in the clinic. With many babies and young children, one may only have a short time to observe when the child first enters the room, after which it may become distracted and wander off. Every opportunity to observe the child must therefore be taken when it arises.

RESPIRATORY DISEASES

Case 1: T. (boy) 18 months

Appearance

Sturdy. Hair is completely white, and abdomen is swollen. Face is a dull-red color, but he is not perspiring. Green nasal discharge.

Behavior

545

Rather inert and floppy, lying on bed. Very irritable, shouting from time to time, and pushing away helpers.

Main complaint	Influenza for one day. Otherwise is "healthy."
Questions:	
Chills and fevers	Has fever of 101°F (38°C).
Sweating	No sweating.
Head and body	Head smells a bit sour.
Thorax and abdomen	Abdomen is swollen, and gurgling noises can be heard. Has a slight croupy cough.
Food and taste	Appetite poor. Ate muesli yesterday morning and vomited it back at lunch time.
Stools and urine	Stools are green and smell dreadful, contain undigested raisins. No constipation. Diapers are wet several times during the day.
Sleep	Awakes two or three times during the night with a dreadful shout. Mother says his language "would be unprintable if he could speak."
Drink and thirst	Not thirsty. Occasionally sips hot honey and lemon.
Life	Parents are recently converted vegetarians and are most distressed that, despite their "good diet," their child has became ill. The whole family is vegetarian and eats a lot of whole foods.
Pulse	Cannot take.
Tongue	Cannot see.
Glands	Very swollen.
Immunizations	None.
Diagnosis	A clear case of wind complicated by accumulation disorder. The white hair is regarded as a sign of underlying Lung deficiency.
Treatment	Needled LI-4 *(he gu)* and *si feng* (M-UE-9). The fever was reduced, but not immediately cleared. It took several days for the fever to completely resolve, for it took that time to clear the stagnant food. The mother was advised to give the child more digestible food—advice which she did not take!

Case 2: S. (girl) 6 years

Appearance	Sturdy, well built. Face is rather pale, with dark rings under eyes. Coughing.
Behavior	Rather cross and irritated. A bit floppy and tired, always sitting down.
Main complaint	Cough. Has been coughing all through the night. She gets

a tickle in her throat and goes on coughing, unable to stop. A certain amount of wet phlegm comes up. She has had this cough for two days, and wants to perform (as a Christmas tree) in a school play in two days time. She does not feel especially hot or cold, but does not want to go outside. Pulse is rapid, slippery, and floating in the first position on the right hand. No visible finger vein, glands slightly swollen. Throat is a bit red. Her back is very sore in the thoracic area. Her mother wants to know whether she will be able to act in the play.

Diagnosis

About as straightforward as one is likely to get! This was a clear case of wind-cold, although there is the complication that she was exhausted, and had some signs of Kidney weakness (dark rings under the eyes). In fact, this was not genuine Kidney weakness, but lack of sleep.

Treatment

Cupping was given at the tender spots on the back. The soreness in the thoracic area is a strong indication that cupping will be effective. The mother wanted to know if she would be able to act in the play in two days' time. The answer I gave was that she could, provided she had treatment each day, that is, three treatments altogether. After the first treatment she was a bit better, and by the third (on the morning of the play) she was clearly well enough.

Case 3: M. (boy) 4½ years

Appearance

Forehead pale, cheeks red. Thick green nasal discharge. Dark skinned (Indian).

Behavior

Restless, irritable. Cannot sit still. Plays with one toy, but is soon bored and looks for another. Mother says that he is unlike her other children in that he hates to let her out of his sight. Moreover, he is often jealous if she shows love to his elder brothers and sisters.

Main complaint

Asthma. Starts with a cold, which quickly develops into a cough, and then asthma. Has had ten such coughs in previous eight months. The coughs are treated with antibiotics, but usually end up as asthma. Has had homeopathic treatment, which worked during treatment, but now that he has stopped, the symptoms have come back. When the cough comes, it is always hard and not productive. Much rattling in the throat, but no phlegm is brought up. Soon develops into wheezing with difficult breathing. The child takes Western medicine frequently when he has an attack. He has had this pattern since about the age of one.

Questions:
Chills and fevers

Often hot during attacks; when coughing, is very feverish and red.

Sweating	Much sweating during coughing attacks.
Head and body	Headaches during coughing and asthma attacks.
Food and taste	Appetite and digestion good. Eats anything. Family eats a lot of garlic, and a lot of curry. When first signs of a cold appear, mother gives him a lot of ginger and cayenne, believing these to be good for clearing colds.
Stools and urine	Tends to constipation. Bowel movements are rather smelly.
Sleep	Often coughs all through the night, with wheezing attacks that sometimes develop into full-blown asthma attacks. Otherwise sleep is good. Wakes perhaps twice a night. Mother often gives him chamomile tea.
Drink and thirst	Likes to drink a lot.
Life	Lives in house; good, loving parents. Older and younger brothers and sisters. Attends play school and enjoys it.
Immunizations	All the "normal" ones: DPT, BCG, measles.
Pulse	Rapid.
Tongue	Red.
Examination	Glands in neck swollen. Finger vein broad, almost black, reaches to qi gate.
Diagnosis	This is a clear case of hot lingering pathogenic factor type asthma. This pattern is in fact rather rare in Britain because of the cold and damp climate, and because of the liberal use of antibiotics, which themselves are rather cold and damp medicines.
	There are clear signs of lingering heat, with clinging to his mother, red tongue, a broad, dark vein, and swollen glands. With this imbalance the child would in any event be prone to further attacks, but the development into asthma was made certain by the mother giving him so many warming foods at the onset of a 'cold'.
Treatment	Needled L-5 *(chi ze)* and L-9 *(tai yuan)* weekly. There was gradual improvement. Overall, it took 18 treatments to cure the child. The first 10 were given weekly, then they were spaced out, first every two weeks, then every three weeks. Even at the end of treatment he was still a rather insecure child, although he did not suffer from chest problems and easily recovered from any coughs and colds.

ACUTE ATTACK—

After five treatments the child came to the clinic just at the onset of an attack, presenting with the following symptoms:

Appearance	Cheeks red. Thick green-yellow nasal discharge. Coughing intermittently—a hard cough, which rattles a bit. There is obviously phlegm in his throat, but he does not bring it up.
Behavior	Clinging to his mother, and a bit distressed. Every time he coughs, he cries a little and clings tightly to his mother.
Chills and fevers	Feels hot to touch on forehead.
Sweating	Sweating slightly.
Pulse	Rapid, slippery.
Tongue	Red with thin, yellow coating.
Glands	Very swollen and hard.
Finger vein	Dark, broad, reached qi gate.
Diagnosis	The child had an attack of wind-heat, which evolved into phlegm-heat, as could be deduced from the pain which he experienced every time he coughed, and the rapid, slippery pulse.
Treatment	Needled L-10 *(yu ji)* and L-5 *(chi ze)*, both with the dispersing method. About ten minutes later the child fell asleep. When he awoke in two hours he was clearly on the mend, with a looser cough and less fever and distress. This was somewhat better than expected, and the mother had been advised beforehand to obtain Western medicines in case the treatment was not effective. This was the turning point in the course of treatment. It is often found that a treatment administered during an acute attack is more effective and deeper in its action than treatment at other times. This is embodied in the Chinese saying, "A time of crisis is a time of opportunity."
	It is interesting to note that as his symptoms improved, the tongue became normal. The finger vein shortened and narrowed. He was treated for over a year (by myself [JPS] and other practitioners) to strengthen his constitution, after which the finger vein completely disappeared.

Case 4: W. (boy) 2 years, 4 months

Appearance	Face is white, especially forehead; cheeks are cherry red. Crusty-dried yellow nasal discharge. Carrot-colored hair.
Behavior	Restless, unable to settle on one thing or another. Irritable look in his eye. Tends to cling to mother.
Main complaint	Asthma for 12 months. Started with eczema at three months of age. At six months he got a severe chest infection. After that he suffered from repeated infections, each more severe than the last, until the year before, when the

chest infection became asthma. Since then each time he catches a cold it goes onto his chest, giving rise to an attack of asthma. During an asthma attack he has fever and a red face, with green nasal discharge.

Questions:	
Chills and fevers	Dislikes wearing much clothing.
Sweating	Sweats slightly on occasion at night, but gets very hot.
Head and body	Nasal discharge. Body well-formed. Rather large for his age.
Thorax and abdomen	Used to be very fat, with swollen abdomen. Becoming thinner during last six months.
Food and taste	Appetite used to be voracious. During last six months his appetite has diminished. Used to vomit a lot in the first 18 months.
Stools and urine	Used to be very constipated as a baby. Still only has one bowel movement every other day.
Drink and thirst	Thirsty.
Family	Brother vomits (see Case 12). Mother has asthma. Living conditions good.
Pulse	Weak.
Immunizations	First ones at three months. Eczema came immediately thereafter, and so did nasal discharge.
Glands	Neck glands swollen, very large.
Finger vein	Broad, dark blue.
Treatment	Needled L-5 *(chi ze)* and L-9 *(tai yuan),* or L-5 *(chi ze)* and L-7 *(lie que),* at times of infection. Treatment given once a week for eight weeks, supplemented with Blue Flag herbal tablets. Asthma was cleared, facial color good—white bits more pink, red bits less red. No nasal discharge. Behavior improved.
Follow-up	Came down with intermittent colds and needed treatment to strengthen the Spleen and Lung qi once a month for six months.
Comment	This is a very common situation (some deficiency, some excess), although here the pattern is clearly one of heat rather than cold. The red cheeks are an indication of accumulation disorder, and point to the underlying cause. The child had a voracious appetite, which led to accumulation disorder and the development of considerable heat. With the qi mechanism blocked, and his relatively rapid growth

(he is large for his age), there was not enough qi left to fight a pathogenic factor. The result was that the pathogenic factor remained lingering in his body.

The acupuncture treatment here was very simple, and did not take account of the accumulation disorder (except that L-5 *(chi ze)* does have an influence on the bowels). However, acupuncture was supplemented by the use of simple herbs. The Blue Flag tablets contain, among other things, *Iris versicolor* and *Phytolocca decandra,* both of which are indicated for a lingering pathogenic factor.

Case 5: H. (boy) 8 years

Appearance	Thin, smiling face. Green around the mouth and forehead, red cheeks. Obviously blocked nose.
Behavior	Very obedient, over-polite, restless. Can sit still, but plays with fingers all the time.
Main complaint	Asthma since age five. Child says that he constantly has a tight feeling in his chest. There is much coughing at night, bringing up phlegm with difficulty. Not much coughing in the daytime. He cannot do much physical exercise, although he spends a lot of time outdoors. Much sticky, yellow nasal discharge. Must use Ventolin bronchial dilator from time to time.
Questions:	
Head and body	Body is very thin. Occasionally gets eczema which used to be worse, but has been considerably helped by homeopathy.
Thorax and abdomen	No problems, except constant wheezing.
Food and taste	When young, much vomiting. Appetite all right now, but rather small.
Stools and urine	Used to have chronic diarrhea (four times a day, very loose). This was cured by homeopathy.
Sleep	Often awakened by wheezing during sleep. Difficult to fall asleep.
Drink and thirst	Often thirsty. Used to drink a lot of milk, now drinks fruit juice. Does not seem to make much difference what he drinks.
Family	Educated at home. Father away most of the time. Has dominating elder sister, and three younger sisters. Mother has forceful personality.
Life	Pertussis at age three. Treated with acupuncture.

Pulse	Both middle pulses forceful and wiry-slippery, rapid.
Tongue	Red, especially at tip. Yellowish coating at root.
Immunizations	DPT and polio at age two, polio again at age five.
Treatment	Has had homeopathic treatment, which did not affect asthma. Had one course of acupuncture plus herbal treatment lasting about a year. Acupuncture was mainly given at L-5 *(chi ze)*, L-9 *(tai yuan)*, S-36 *(zu san li)*, and Liv-3 *(tai chong)*. Provided only slight improvement. Treatment was then abandoned for a year, as the mother had another baby. After this his elder sister went to the local school instead of being educated at home, and the mother had the time to continue treatment. Second course of treatment was much more successful, and he had months at a time when there were no symptoms. Gradually, as he grew older, his character became more forceful, and his asthma disappeared.
Comment	This boy's problem started with accumulation disorder, which was never cured. This opened the way for asthma, which became serious when he was expected to restrain his emotions and conform to an essentially feminine behavior pattern, which did not accord with his true nature.

Case 6: W. (boy) 3 years, 1 month

Appearance	White face with red cheeks. Very strong. Has penetrating look in eyes. No blue between eyes.
Behavior	Wilful and a bit restless. Won't do anything he is told to do, but continues doing what he likes.
Main complaint	Asthma since he was "scratched by a cat" when he was one. Prior to this he had a few colds, but nothing serious. Occasionally must take nebuliser outside the asthma attacks, and has on occasion been hospitalized because attacks are so severe. Attacks are bought on by "colds," and also by dusty environment.
Questions:	
Chills and fevers	Dislikes wearing any clothes.
Sweating	Sometimes sweats at night.
Food and taste	Appetite good, but irregular—may refuse food at lunch time, then be hungry two hours later. Total quantity of food consumed is not excessive.

Sleep	Good. Sometimes awakened by cough, which is productive.
Life	Was well until age one. Parents are wealthy, the father having made a large fortune. When his son was about six months old, father gambled heavily and was obliged to move into a smaller house when his son was about one.
Pulse	Cannot take (too restless).
Tongue	A bit red.
Finger vein	Broad, dark.
Glands	Slightly swollen below ears.
Immunization	Had booster at age one, shortly before asthma attack.
Treatment	Needled L-5 *(chi ze)* and L-9 *(tai yuan)* weekly, with some mild herbal treatment to assist (Hydrastis, Inula, Hyssopus, Tussilago). After the first three treatments he had diarrhea for two days, but not much improvement in his asthma. However, the mother was noticeably more relaxed and calm and commented how much better she felt. At the fourth treatment needled L-9 *(tai yuan)* and S-40 *(feng long)*. Diarrhea again followed treatment. No asthma, even though he had a cold shortly after treatment. Behavior is more calm, much more placid and less wilful. Still some nighttime coughing. At the fifth and sixth treatments needled L-9 *(tai yuan)* and S-40 *(feng long)*. Continued to improve. By the sixth treatment the finger vein had become very faint. During the week he had a severe fever, but no wheezing. His behavior returned to very calm as soon as the fever had subsided.
Comment	The main problem here was phlegm caused by a lingering pathogenic factor. The absence of blue between the eyes meant that this child was not suffering from shock; it is therefore unlikely that the cause of his problem was being scratched by a cat. The child had a strong constitution, but the way was opened for a pathogenic factor because of the two stresses occurring at once—the immunization and the emotional trauma in his family. After the first treatments the phlegm was released, coming out in the stools in the form of mild diarrhea. It was interesting that it was the mother rather than the child who felt better after the first few treatments. This is because the mother was providing the extra qi that the child needed. Because the child required less support, the mother was less drained.

Case 7: D. (boy) 6 years

Appearance	Huge for his age. Very pale face, almost white hair. Red lips, slightly blue around the mouth. Bright eyes, cheerful.
Behavior	Rather restless. A bit obstinate—tends to do the opposite of what is asked.
Main complaint	'Bronchitic asthma' since age two-and-a-half. Has frequent attacks (about once a month) which start with the symptoms of a cold in the head (i.e., runny nose) which becomes catarrhal. The catarrh rapidly clogs up his air passages and causes an asthma attack. He also vomits catarrh. Attacks occur primarily during the winter months. Wind can start him coughing, which sometimes precipitates an attack. Attacks are treated with antibiotics, which usually do not work, then steroids. Takes Becotide as a preventive measure. Cannot run around without coughing.
Questions:	
Head and body	Often has nosebleeds, and eczema which comes and goes.
Food and taste	Appetite good. Eats anything, except during an attack.
Stools and urine	Stools are very large.
Sleep	Good except at time of attack.
Life	Father unemployed, 62-years old. Sees no reason to take up further employment and is very happy.
Pulse	Slow, forceful, and slippery.
Tongue	Red.
Glands	Very large glands in neck and under ears.
Finger vein	Quite large and dark.
Treatment	In some ways this boy is typical of long-term patients: there are some signs of heat (red lips, red tongue) and some of cold (pale face); some of deficiency (upset by wind, easily catches cold) and some of excess (phlegm, strong pulse, bright eyes). This means that whatever treatment is given, some symptoms are bound to be aggravated. If tonification is used, then a lot of phlegm may be released and he may get a severe cough; if dispersion is used, he may be exhausted and suffer from diarrhea. When deciding how to proceed, it is helpful to go right back to first principles and ask whether he is more deficient or more excessive. Does he in fact need a bit of extra energy to help expel the phlegm, or can he withstand a dispersing treatment without becoming exhausted? In this case I decided on dispersion, needling S-40 *(feng long)* with

dispersion and L-9 *(tai yuan)* with tonification. He did get diarrhea, but was not exhausted by it.

After six treatments he was markedly better, rarely needed to use his inhaler, and never suffered serious attacks. However, he was still "chesty" and obviously not well. Treatment continued once a week for some six more months, with no noticeable effect. The treatments were varied, and each time a new prescription was chosen (whether acupuncture or herbal) there was some improvement, but he soon relapsed.

The clue to this mystery was provided at last when the mother, instead of the father, brought the boy to the clinic. Upon questioning her it turned out that she had a severe, chronic cough. I offered her treatment, which at first she was unwilling to accept, as she did not think that her own problem had anything to do with her son's. She did eventually accept treatment, however, and as she improved, so did her son, who was eventually cured completely. This again illustrates the strong influence that parents (especially mothers) have on their children's qi.

Case 8: J. (boy) 4 years

This boy had a violent nighttime cough for three weeks which had failed to respond to antibiotics, and had been confirmed as pertussis. The cough was paroxysmal and nearly always ended in his vomiting some sticky, ropy phlegm. The boy's appetite (not surprisingly) was very poor.

He was treated with acupuncture using the points *si feng* (M-UE-9) and L-9 *(tai yuan)* once a week for three consecutive weeks. After the first treatment he slept well for three days without coughing at night, and his appetite was much improved. However, the effect of the treatment gradually wore off, and by the time of the second treatment he was again coughing all night. After this treatment he had two very good nights, then three which were not so good. His condition picked up after that and he did not experience any further nighttime coughing.

A third treatment was given to consolidate the result, and herbs were prescribed to strengthen his Lungs, to be taken over the following two months. These included *Prunus serotina*, *Gentiana lutea*, and *Leptandra virginica* for the lingering effects of the pertussis, and then *Hydrastis canadensis*, *Inula helenium*, *Hysoppus officinalis,* and *Tussilago farfara*. Ideally, acupuncture treatment should have been given twice or three times a week to prevent relapse.

Comment	The boy's mother was delighted with the results of the treatment. She knew that pertussis could last for months and weaken her son's constitution. The effect of the acupuncture (i.e., relapses in between treatment, but gradually improving) was typical for a strong child who is treated soon after the onset of pertussis. If no herbs had been given, he would have needed more acupuncture treatments.
	It is more common to see weaker children, later on in the illness. Then treatment has to be given several times a week. Moreover, once the main symptoms have been cured, consolidation treatments once a week may be needed for up to six months.

Case 9: G. (girl) 7 years

Appearance	White face, dull eyes. Sits in a chair, blankly looking into the distance. The child appears to have a robust constitution.
Behavior	Inert. Does not seem to understand what is said. Only moves with great difficulty.
Main complaint	Tonsillitis. Has had a high fever, during which she complained of pain in the throat, for two days. The fever has come down after sweating through the night, but she still has great pain in the tonsils, which are red with some yellow spots.
Questions:	
Chills and fevers	Obviously feels cold.
Sweating	Not sweating now.
Food and taste	No appetite. Refuses all food that is offered, or just looks blankly upon it. When food is put on spoon and held to her mouth, she takes no interest.
Stools and urine	Urinated twice today. No stools.
Sleep	Sleeps at night.
Drink and thirst	No thirst.
Pain	Difficult to determine the nature of the pain, but when she speaks at all, it is to complain about the pain in her throat.
Life	Her mother has been away for two months visiting a sick grandmother in Germany, during which time the child has been staying with a friend.
Pulse	Very weak.

Tongue	Pale body, white coating.
Glands	Swollen.
Diagnosis	As described on paper, this case sounds as though it might be very serious. However, there was no feeling of alarm when observing the patient. This was because her skin looked fairly normal, her weight was good, she was not sweating, and she sat in the chair without totally collapsing. These were all signs that she was not suffering from collapse of yang.

It is not unusual for the whole qi mechanism to stop working during a febrile disease. As long as there are reserves of energy, this condition is not dangerous. This type of case is common in China: very strong, clear symptoms of qi deficiency with a lingering pathogenic factor. Although temporarily qi deficient, this girl was basically robust (a farmer's daughter, by the way) and had great reserves of physical energy.

Treatment	Needled S-36 *(zu san li)* to tonify the qi and LI-4 *(he gu)* to invigorate the circulation of qi, especially to the throat. The result was that the pain was reduced in a few minutes, and she started to take an interest in life. Only one treatment was necessary because the problem was due to disruption of the qi mechanism; this was not a case of exhaustion of qi.

Acute tonsillitis and its immediate sequelae respond well to acupuncture, especially if there is a lot of energy left.

DIGESTIVE DISEASES

Case 10: T. (girl) 7 months

Appearance	Dull, white face with a hint of unhealthy pink on cheeks. A bit green between the eyes. Dull, lifeless eyes which are wet and puffy. Her whole face is a bit puffy.
Behavior	Lies inert, showing little interest.
Main complaint	Restless at night. Cannot sleep for more than an hour. Sometimes just wakes, and sometimes wants to feed all through the night, settling down at 5 A.M.
Questions:	
Chills and fevers	Often looks cold, and feels cold and moist to the touch.
Sweating	Sometimes sweats when trying to pass stool.
Head and body	Legs are cold and clammy at night.

Thorax and abdomen	Abdomen a little swollen and flabby.
Food and taste	Prefers to take only breast milk. Despite repeated attempts to interest her in other foods, the most she ever takes is one teaspoon of millet porridge.
Stools and urine	Constipated since birth. Passes stool only once a week, and even then with great difficulty and struggle.
Drink and thirst	Not especially thirsty.
Immunizations	Polio, tetanus, and diphtheria given at three months, but not pertussis. No unusual reaction.
Life	Parents are loving, but are now very exhausted and worried.
Tongue	Pale with slightly milky coating.
Vein	None visible.
Diagnosis	The diagnosis was deficient-type accumulation disorder. The deficiency came from the mother's anemia in pregnancy (she was a strict vegetarian). When babies have no reaction to immunization, this is sometimes regarded as a good sign, but in fact is usually a bad sign, for it shows that the pathogenic factor introduced is not being fought and is therefore almost certainly lingering in the body. This pattern is becoming more common as children with weak qi, who would normally have died soon after birth in earlier generations, are kept alive by modern medicine.
Treatment	S-36 *(zu san li)* and *si feng* (M-UE-9) were needled weekly. There was slow-but-sure improvement. Although *si feng* (M-UE-9) was used, great care was taken to ensure that S-36 *(zu san li)* was tonified. This means basically that the practitioner should avoid causing any pain (which induces dispersion) when inserting the needle. This may be difficult owing to the toughness of the skin and the wriggling of the child.

After the third treatment the child was having a bowel movement every day, although it obviously caused a lot of pain and discomfort. She could then sleep for two hours at a time, but awoke with a scream or shout. She exhibited more energy and was more lively. Her face was less puffy. The problem had thus shifted from deficiency to excess. At this juncture an even needle technique was chosen for treating S-36 *(zu san li)*.

After the sixth treatment she passed stool every day, and with less trouble. Stools were hard to begin with, but then became soft. She showed a lot of nasal catarrh, and some spots on the chin and around the mouth, as she threw out the pathogenic factors introduced in the immunization. These had been there all the time, but were not the most important problem when she first came to the clinic; one could even not have realized that they were there. Her cheeks were bright red and her appetite was much better. Sleep was still bad, and she still awoke with a terrible shout.

After the seventh treatment her bowel movements were regular and normal. I then needled H-7 *(shen men)* and S-36 *(zu san li)* for two treatments. After this she slept well.

Case 11: J. (boy) 7 months

Appearance	Forehead a little pale. Most of face red. Cheeks especially red. Green around the mouth.
Behavior	Sleeping at time of appointment.
Main complaint	Colic, that is, crying and writhing for two hours after eating. Appears to be in pain at this time. Condition has worsened during past three months.
Questions:	
Chills and fevers	Appears to be hot, especially at night.
Sweating	Often sweating on head, especially after eating. Often covered in sweat at night.
Head and body	Occasional thick, yellow wax in ears. Recently experienced some ear pain (i.e., rubbing ears).
Thorax and abdomen	No chest infection. Occasional nasal discharge. Abdomen is swollen, with blue veins.
Food and taste	Started weaning at four months. Huge appetite—eats large helpings of everything that family eats, including cereals, meat, vegetables, a lot of bananas, yoghurt, quite a lot of milk.
Stools and urine	Stools often loose, foul-smelling, green.
Sleep	Awakes at night every two hours. Does not scream if light is on, but gradually starts to complain if no attention is given, working himself up into a great rage.
Immunizations	None as yet.
Tongue	Milky coating, red body.
Finger vein	Broad, purple.
Glands	Not swollen.

Diagnosis	This is a typical case of excess-type accumulation disorder caused mainly by eating unsuitable foods. This generates internal heat, which in turn leads to insomnia and overeating. The most important aspect of treatment was advising the mother to give simple foods: just milk and baby rice.
Treatment	Needled *si feng* (M-UE-9) once a week. After the first treatment he passed huge, foul-smelling stools four times that day. His sleep was very bad the following three nights, and he was thoroughly bad-tempered. After that, he started behaving better and was happier. The same pattern was repeated after the next treatment, but not as severe. In all, six treatments were required to cure him. The mother was advised to be careful with new foods and to limit the child's diet for a year. Normally this will not be difficult for a young child, as it should be content with a bland diet. Those who are not are either greedy or have Stomach heat.

Case 12: W. (boy) 6 months

Appearance	Face white and puffy. Lower eyelids puffy and swollen. Eyes red.
Behavior	Rather listless and inert, but eyes are bright.
Main complaint	Vomiting since birth. Vomits perhaps 30 minutes to two hours after feeding. Vomit is curdled milk, mixed with "water."
Family illnesses	Elder brother has asthma (see Case 4), and his health was very similar when he was young, with constipation, vomiting, and gurgling in his chest. As time passed, the chest problem turned to asthma. Mother also had asthma when young. She is very worried that this child might also develop asthma.
Questions:	
Sweating	Occasional sweating on forehead after feeding.
Thorax and abdomen	Abdomen distended. Chest is congested, with gurgling noises on breathing.
Food and taste	Appetite good, but not too large.
Stools and urine	Constipated. Only passes stools every three or four days. Becomes lethargic, irritable, and sleepy after two or three days without passing stools.
Pain	May have abdominal pain before passing stools.
Finger vein	Not visible.

Glands	Not swollen.
Immunizations	DPT.
Diagnosis	The diagnosis was clearly qi deficiency with accumulation of dampness. The deficient qi led to a deficient type of accumulation disorder. There were some slight traces of heat (red eyes), but this was not relevant to his main problem.
Treatment	Weekly acupuncture was performed, with the following results:

1. *si feng* (M-UE-9) (left hand). The next day he passed huge stools several times, then nothing for five days, followed by small stools each day.
2. *si feng* (M-UE-9) (right hand). Stools more or less regular: always something each day, but some days more than others. Vomited afternoons only.
3. *si feng* (M-UE-9) (left hand). Stools regular. No vomiting. Phlegm in chest disappeared. No puffiness in face.
4. One month later, stools had become irregular during preceding week. Treated *si feng* (M-UE-9) (right hand). Regularity returned. Advised mother to bring the child for treatment every six weeks.

Comment	*si feng* (M-UE-9) should generally only be used for conditions of excess. The reaction to this treatment, namely, that huge stools were passed followed by constipation for five days, is typical of what one should expect from using a dispersing treatment for a deficient type of accumulation disorder. A better method would have been to include S-36 (*zu san li*) as well. If this had been done, the boy would probably not have experienced the five days of constipation. Note that it is our standard practice to alternate left and right hands when using *si feng* (M-UE-9).

Case 13: H. (boy) 22 months

Appearance	Face and lips are red. Skin around mouth is a bit dry, with beginnings of a red rash. Looks remarkably healthy, but mother looks worn out. Her face is also red.
Behavior	Very active. Normally independent spirit, but now clings to mother, Very restless, moving from one position to another, never finding a comfortable place. Mother says behavior at home is terrible: rushing around, never still, unable to settle on anything.
Main complaint	Vomiting. Since age one the child has had recurrent attacks of vomiting, which last three or four days. The general pattern is that he vomits through the night until

all the food has come up; then he is hungry and asks for food, which is vomited five minutes later. Throughout the day he calls for food every hour or two, which again is vomited five minutes after eating. Sometimes he can hold down liquid; on this day he held down a small amount of dry toast. The day before he vomited phlegm for the first time.

These attacks occur about once a month. Their family doctor says that nothing is wrong, but the mother is on the verge of a nervous breakdown. She does not feel that this pattern of vomiting and sleeplessness is normal.

Questions:	
Chills and fevers	Never feels cold.
Sweating	Face and forehead sweat a lot, especially at night. Feet often sweat, and are smelly.
Food and taste	Normally has a good appetite (in between attacks).
Stools and urine	Stools always loose, three to four times a day, neither watery nor green. Smell is sometimes bad. Undigested food is often found in stools.
Sleep	Generally good, except during attacks.
Drink and thirst	Always thirsty.
Life	History of chest problems for first six months, but he is all right now.
Pulse	Rapid.
Family	Mother has a red face and full color in cheeks.
Immunizations	Pertussis at age one.
Diagnosis	This is an example of obstructed heat in the Stomach and cold in the Spleen. In children it is common for the Spleen and Stomach to be a bit disconnected, with one being hot and the other cold. This is one reason why children often eat too much.

The main source of the heat is 'womb heat', that is, passed to the child from the mother during pregnancy. It has been aggravated by the pertussis immunization. In cases of obstructed heat, children are often more irritable and restless after treatment, with insomnia, for up to a week.

Treatment	Acupuncture was performed every week, but ideally should have been given two to three times a week.

1. Needled P-6 *(nei guan)* and S-44 *(nei ting)*. Two to three hours after treatment the child had a very runny nose. For the rest of the week his behavior was terrible, even

worse than before. His sleep was bad, waking for two to three hours each night. The stools were slightly better formed. Not so thirsty.

2. Needled S-44 *(nei ting)* and *an mian* (N-HN-54). His behavior and sleep were better, although the stools were loose again (six times a day), and he was again thirsty. The rash around the mouth was reduced.

3. Needled S-44 *(nei ting)* and Sp-6 *(san yin jiao)*. His appetite was much reduced after treatment, his bowels were much better, and his sleep and behavior were normal. His color was also improved (not as red).

4-6. Same treatment as in third week. His appetite, feeding, and bowels showed occasional relapse, but by the sixth treatment all of the problems were resolved. Thereafter the red color disappeared, and he has continued to be in good health.

Case 14: J. (girl) 7 years

Appearance	White face, black rings under eyes. Sometimes shows three-white-eye (also known as *sanpaku* in macrobiotics).
Behavior	Listless, very shy. Very floppy: must sit down, and cannot stand up.
Main complaint	Vomiting. Recurring attacks with fever. Mother says it is always due to a virus. She had four attacks this year, which is typical. Has always had difficulty digesting food, and was a very colicky baby. No recent attacks, but mother would like to strengthen her. Mother herself looks pale, and is resentful. She is entering the hospital shortly to have surgery for a prolapsed uterus.
Questions:	
Chills and fevers	Often feels chilly. Hates going outside.
Sweating	No sweating.
Thorax and abdomen	Chest is quite clear. Occasionally gets coughs, but not troubled by catarrh.
Food and taste	Appetite very poor. Very choosy about food and will only eat white bread and honey, peas, fish sticks, and very little else.
Stools and urine	Not incontinent, but sometimes gets diarrhea with vomiting. It seems as though stools are always loose, but it is difficult to be sure because the family prefers not to talk about them.
Sleep	Difficulty falling asleep. Often gets wound up over television programs, and although she is put to bed at 9.30 P.M., is often up again and again until 11:30 P.M.

Drink and thirst	Not especially thirsty. Will only drink milk and nothing else.
Life	Lives indoors most of the time and takes very little exercise, although there are green fields nearby. Spends a lot of time watching television. Never walks anywhere; is taken to school by car.
Pulse	Weak.
Tongue	Pale, with pronounced crack down the middle.
Glands	Not swollen.
Diagnosis	The diagnosis is deficient Spleen and Kidney yang. In the last century this pattern was quite common, and was due to child labor. It had become very uncommon 20 years ago, but is reviving due to ignorance of the need to look after children's health while they are growing, in particular to ensure that they get enough sleep and fresh air.
Treatment	After much thought, it was decided not to give any treatment. The mother was only half-hearted in her commitment to treatment. Moreover, it was felt that treatment without a change in lifestyle would be ineffective. In any event, the mother was not prepared to make any changes.

Case 15: L. (boy) 2½ years

Appearance	Face is white, a little grey around the eyes, and green in between. Eyes are bright.
Behavior	Quite active, easily irritated, impatient.
Main complaint	Diarrhea. He caught a "germ" which was going around the family three weeks previously. Most of the family recovered within three days, but his diarrhea persists, some days with, some days without. Stools are always green, unformed, and have a sour, acidic smell. There is sometimes undigested food in the stools.
Questions:	
Chills and fevers	Hands feel damp and cold.
Sweating	Sometimes sweating on the head, especially before an attack of diarrhea.
Thorax and abdomen	No cough. Abdomen is swollen.
Food and taste	In spite of diarrhea, appetite is now good. Appetite was poor for first three days of attack, but soon recovered. Eats a lot of bananas and yoghurt, and drinks milk from the refrigerator. Is given cucumber and a lot of fresh brown bread.

Sleep	Very poor since diarrhea attacks. Awakes several times at night, screaming. Grinds teeth while asleep.
Immunizations	DPT at six months, polio at nine months. Only slight reactions.
Life	Plenty of money. Father is away much of the time, and mother has career in television.
Pulse	Cannot take.
Tongue	Greasy coating.
Glands	Not swollen.
Diagnosis	It might be thought from the history that the condition was one of a lingering pathogenic factor. In fact, however, the problem was due to heat in the Stomach, which led the child to overeat. This in turn gave rise to injury from food. The heat was not at all obvious (he had a pale face) but could be deduced from the amount of food that he ate and the cold nature of the food that he liked. The key to the diagnosis was the nature of the stools—which had a sour smell—and this can only come from accumulation disorder. It was this symptom which led me to ask about the child's diet.
Treatment	The aim of treatment was to clear the heat from the Stomach. Without doing this, the child would continue to eat excessively, and any treatment would be in vain. Points used were S-36 *(zu san li)* and S-44 *(nei ting),* bilaterally. The parents were advised to give the boy only a small amount of food, and to avoid very cold foods, such as cucumbers. After three weekly treatments his appetite was much reduced, and although he still had diarrhea, it was much less severe. This gradual effect in easing of the symptoms is common in accumulation disorders. Three additional treatments were then given using S-36 *(zu san li)* and Sp-6 *(san yin jiao).* These last treatments were probably unnecessary to effect a cure, but certainly accelerated it.

Case 16: M. (boy) 17 months

Appearance	Pale, a little gray around the mouth, watery nasal discharge, and a slightly sore upper lip.
Behavior	Listless and shy, clinging to mother.
Main complaint	"Not well." Had an attack of gastroenteritis two months before which was so severe that he had to be hospitalized to prevent dehydration. Since then he has never recovered, and his behavior has been very clinging. Is prone to occasional attacks of mild diarrhea lasting one day. Occasionally vomits undigested food.

Questions:	
Chills and fevers	Tends to feel the cold.
Sweating	No sweating, although his skin is often damp.
Thorax and abdomen	Abdomen is sometimes swollen.
Food and taste	Appetite is poor. He is very choosy about food, and never eats more than half of what he is given.
Stools and urine	Stools are pale and always contain undigested food. They have always been loose since the gastroenteritis.
Sleep	Sometimes wakes to vomit. The vomit is watery, does not have much smell, and contains undigested food. Has periods when he wakes every two hours, needing comfort. These periods last about a week.
Drink and thirst	Not thirsty. Mother does not understand where all the moisture in stools and skin could be coming from.
Immunizations	All the usual, at three and six months. No measles.
Life	Mother and father are professionals. Both go out to work and are reluctant to reduce their standard of living.
Pulse	Very weak.
Tongue	Normal.
Finger vein	Very slight thin, red on left hand.
Glands	Not swollen.
Diagnosis	This is a typical case of Spleen qi deficiency with dampness, due to an attack of diarrhea. These cases used to dominate pediatrics in the past, but with improved hygiene in modern times they are now not so common.
	A contributory factor to the child failing to get better is the lack of attention he gets from his parents. When both parents have demanding jobs, there may not be enough energy to spare when a child gets ill.
	The diarrhea can take a surprisingly long time to cure. This is because after a bad attack of diarrhea, the villi in the intestines are actually destroyed and take time to regrow.
Treatment	Needled S-36 (*zu san li*) and Sp-6 (*san yin jiao*) with the tonifying method. Used both needle and indirect moxa at CV-12 (*zhong wan*). Treatment was given weekly for twelve weeks, with gradual improvement. After the sixth treatment the parents started thinking about how they could spend more time with their child. It is one of the marvels of acupuncture that by treating the child, the parents start to see things in a new light!

Case 17: G. (girl) 5 ½ years

Appearance	Broad face and big head, but rather slender body. Eyes seem too large and a bit odd, and lips are full. Otherwise looks basically healthy. Color quite good, with red cheeks.
Behavior	Rather shy, quiet, unadventurous.
Main complaint	Poor appetite for a year. Used to be quite pudgy, but over the past year has become skinny.
Questions: *Head and body*	Was born with a very severe squint. Had two operations at age one, but recovered quickly.
Thorax and abdomen	Abdominal skin is rough. Easily catches cold, which quickly becomes a cough. Has rarely taken antibiotics.
Food and taste	Appetite very poor. Never finishes food on plate. Very choosy about food.
Stools and urine	Normal.
Sleep	Good.
Drink and thirst	Not thirsty.
Life	Was very upset at arrival of younger sister just over a year ago. Behavior was very odd, and was obviously jealous. Always clinging to mother. She is now just getting over it and coming to terms with having a younger sister.
Pulse	Very forceful in middle positions, both sides.
Tongue	Greasy coating at root.
Glands	Not swollen.
Treatment	The diagnosis was obstruction of qi in the middle burner, a problem which usually affects adults rather than children. The cause was jealousy of her younger sister. I treated her with acupuncture at S-36 *(zu san li),* Sp-6 *(san yin jiao),* and G-34 *(yang ling quan),* along with such Western herbs as *Gentiana lutea* and *Leptandra virginica.* This treatment had only a very temporary effect, as it did nothing to change her jealousy. However, she was helped (although not completely cured) by using the Bach Flower Remedies. Holly (for revenge, suspicion, and jealousy) seemed to make the most difference.

MISCELLANEOUS DISEASES

Case 18: P. (girl) 5 years, 3 months

Appearance	White, puffy face. Blank look in the eyes, eyelids a little red. Eyes tremble and turn sideways from time to time. Dribbling at the mouth. Lips a little red.

Behavior	Stands completely still most of the time, except occasionally has trembling attacks when her hands and head seem to shiver for about 10 seconds.
Main complaint	"Epilepsy." When she was four-years old she had a series of high fevers with a urinary tract infection, and during one particularly high fever she had a "fit" which lasted 40 minutes. Since then she has had 10 major fits, but is now "controlled" by using strong drugs: Epilim and Triludan. In spite of this, she has continued to have "abnormal brain activity" on EEG.
	Her current condition is that she suffers from very frequent minor fits, perhaps 10 to 15 a day. Her mother describes these as "absences," as they are characterized by momentary blankness, after which she cannot remember where she is or what has happened for about half an hour before the blankness. She considers the fits "controlled" because she does not have any major convulsive spasms.
Questions: *Chills and fevers*	Is worse in cold weather. Feels cold and damp to the touch.
Food and taste	Appetite is poor most of the time, but occasionally has a voracious appetite. She avoids cold foods, and cold energy foods.
Stools and urine	Occasionally constipated. Still gets mild cystitis, but not so severe that it requires antibiotics. Very occasionally wets bed at night.
Sleep	Sleeps well at night, and also two hours during the day.
Drink and thirst	No thirst.
Pulse	Left side is weak and soft. Right side is so weak that it is imperceptible.
Diagnosis	Her current condition is that of chronic convulsions, or chronic Spleen wind. One of the causes attributed to this pattern in Chinese texts is "taking too much cold medicine for acute convulsions," and that is what has happened here. In this case the "cold medicines" are the anticonvulsant drugs. A straightforward case of chronic convulsions does not involve epilepsy, and can be cured in about 10 to 20 treatments.
Treatment	Simple treatments were given on a weekly basis. The points included S-36 *(zu san li),* Sp-6 *(san yin jiao),* and L-9 *(tai yuan),* all needled with a tonifying method, and CV-12 *(zhong wan),* with needling followed by indirect moxibustion. These points were used at every treatment, occasionally omitting L-9 *(tai yuan),* and occasionally adding CV-4 *(guan yuan).*

There was gradual improvement throughout the course of treatment. After 12 treatments she was much brighter, and suffered only one or two absences a day. Her mother then felt able to start reducing the drugs. At this time, she started a continuous nasal discharge.

Three weeks after the first reduction in drugs she had a high fever and a slight convulsive fit. This was the first fever she had experienced since taking the drugs, and in fact was a good sign, as it was an indication that the body was expelling the pathogenic factor. However, the mother was quite rattled by this, and it took some persuasion to encourage her to continue treatment.

After 20 treatments she started talking for the first time since the fits began. The expulsion of catarrh was by now quite severe, and could even keep her awake at night. After 30 treatments she had stopped taking all medication. Thirty additional treatments were needed to bring about a complete cure. At this time the EEG was improved, she was not experiencing any more fits, her pulse was normal, and her behavior was as normal as that of any other child.

Case 19: M. (girl) 9½ years

Appearance	Very overweight. Red face. At times three-white-eye.
Behavior	Shy. Walks in a heavy, lethargic way.
Main complaint	Fits, convulsions. 'Petit mal'. At first the fits were brought on by fevers, but now they can be brought on by excitement as well. Before a fit she becomes intense and agitated. They first appeared during a severe attack of tonsillitis at the age of three, when she had a high fever. Since then she has been taking large doses of drugs: Epinutin and Tegritol on a regular basis, and Valium when she has an attack (which prevents the attacks from getting out of control). In addition to convulsions, she is tired all the time.
Questions:	
Chills and fevers	Always hot. Must use deodorant three times a day.
Sweating	Often sweating, especially at night. Awakes in the night covered in sweat and very hot. Her bedroom is hot in the morning due to the heat she has given off.
Head and body	Left side of body is weak. Some brain damage leading to reduction of use in left hand. Limited range of motion, and can only lift very light objects.
Thorax and abdomen	Abdomen is swollen and distended.
Food and taste	Appetite is very good. Likes a lot of sweet foods, and easily puts on weight.

Stools and urine	Normal.
Sleep	Good. Rather too heavy on account of medication.
Drink and thirst	Thirsty. Drinks a lot of fluids all the time.
Life	Family is well-off, very supportive and happy.
Pulse	Weak, deep. Especially weak at the proximal positions.
Tongue	Body is pale blue. Greasy coating at root.
Glands	Slightly swollen.
Finger vein	Long and blue, reaches to qi gate bilaterally.
Immunizations	All the "usual" ones when very young. Some boosters at three years of age.
Birth	Difficult birth with fetal distress and forceps delivery, which led to the slight brain damage. It is thought that the epilepsy is due to this difficult birth.
Treatment	For first five treatments used LI-11 *(qu chi)*, S-40 *(feng long)*, and Liv-8 *(qu quan)*. She was taken off all dairy products and sweet foods. The result was that she became more spirited, had more energy, and there was a reduction in the heat signs: face was less red, skin was less hot, she no longer had night sweats, and her feet were not smelly.
	After eight treatments she became rather emotional and aggressive. The pulse turned more slippery, but was still weak at the third position. The points for later treatments included those above, plus LI-4 *(he gu)* and Liv-3 *(tai chong)* to encourage the free flow of Liver qi, and B-23 *(shen shu)* to tonify the Kidneys. No other points were used. The finger vein disappeared completely after about 20 treatments. While her left hand became stronger, she never gained full use of it.
	She recently came back for treatment after suffering her first attack in two years. This occurred just before her first period. The treatments have focused on B-23 *(shen shu)*, as her back caves in when she becomes tired.
Comment	The combination of heat (red face, sweating, feels hot), phlegm from a lingering pathogenic factor (overweight, heavy movement), and slight brain damage at birth are the three factors contributing to epilepsy. To these three factors a fourth has recently been added: fright, since she gets attacks when startled. The heat was the easiest to eliminate with acupuncture, taking only five treatments. After this she had no more attacks of epilepsy, except when the drugs were first reduced. Each time the drugs were reduced, even by a small amount, she was tired and irritable for about five days after the treatment. To prevent

an attack during this time, she was given two or even three treatments a week, instead of the usual one. The drugs were reduced gradually and in small steps—once every three weeks—taking nine months altogether. After she was completely off drugs, she still had monthly booster treatments for the next year.

The smooth course of this treatment is not really typical of epilepsy. There are usually crises and relapses. The steady progress is attributable to her strong constitution and the unwavering support of her family, especially her mother, who did everything she could to ensure that the treatment was a success.

Case 20: B. (boy) 10 years

Appearance	Healthy looking. A bit pale, but suntanned. Huge ears, well set. Eyes good. Voice is a bit nasal, and has a strangely cavernous quality and is too deep—more like a man's voice.
Behavior	Good. Polite, but not too polite.
Main complaint	Bedwetting all of his life. Has tried all conventional methods, but nothing has worked. Bed is unbelievably wet in the morning on most days. According to him, it is even wetter when he is at his boarding school! Although he urinates before going to bed, he wets very soon after going to sleep. Otherwise his health is good and he has no other problems, just occasional coughs or influenza when epidemic goes around the school.
Questions:	
Sweating	Only when hot. Especially sweats after running 800-yard race.
Head and body	No nasal discharge.
Thorax and abdomen	Has always had a hard, dry cough, which comes and goes.
Food and taste	Appetite is very good. Especially fond of milk and cheese. Has a pint of milk for breakfast, and more throughout the day. Likes "spotted dick" (a very stodgy steamed pudding made with flour, suet, and raisins) which is served at school every Thursday.
Stools and urine	Urine is copious, even through the day. Can go 15 times during the day, each with large amount. Also has "accidents" during the day, when he wets his pants slightly. Bowels are all right; goes in the evening.
Sleep	Very heavy. Can sleep through anything. Is like a drugged person in the mornings.

Drink and thirst	Not especially thirsty.
Family	Grandfather used to wet bed until age 16.
Life	Prosperous family. He is away at boarding school during term. At three months of age he had a very severe attack of bronchitis and nearly died. It was many months after that before he was "fully recovered."
Pulse	Strong and slippery. On both sides there is a pronounced Special Lung pulse.*
Tongue	Large, pale. Greasy, white coating.
Glands	Quite swollen in throat.
Comment	About half the cases of bedwetting seen in the clinic are straightforward, and are more or less cured within 10 treatments or so. The other half are complicated. This is a rather extreme case of a commonly-seen "complicated" pattern. At first sight it looks straightforward: there is clearly Kidney weakness (frequent urination, urinary incontinence, deep voice) and a lingering pathogenic factor in the Lung (chronic dry cough, special Lung pulse, history of severe Lung infection). But the other signs and symptoms would seem to contradict this diagnosis: no one with Kidney and Lung weakness can run 800 yards; the pulse is strong and slippery; his spirit is good, and so is his appetite.

There is a saying in Chinese medicine to the effect that when the symptoms and pulse do not match, the condition is serious. In acute disease this is certainly true. For example, if a person has a high fever but a slow and weak pulse, something is badly wrong. But in my (JPS) experience, in cases of chronic disease this means something different: that the cause of the illness is not on the physical level. If an imbalance is attributable to a problem like overwork, the symptoms are straightforward and fit into a clear pattern. However, the more that the cause is found on an emotional or subconscious level, the more that paradoxes will be found in the symptoms.

In this case, acupuncture treatment was given. It was partially successful in that his sleep became less heavy, and the urinary frequency and "accidents" during the day

---

*This is a pulse described by Dr. J. F. Shen that is found on both sides, about half a unit distal and medial to the first-position pulse. According to Dr. Shen, it means either that the person has had pulmonary tuberculosis, or that the Lung has been injured. Often this injury is due to an illness such as pertussis attacking the Lungs, or chronic asthma. While the pulse quality is often slippery, this pulse is "special" because it is found in a place where a pulse cannot normally be palpated.

were reduced; but the main problem of urinary incontinence at night did not change.

After some discussion with his parents, and meditation on the child, it became clear that the problem was not just on the emotional level, but was really karmic in origin. It related to a very violent and savage streak in his character, which had to be suppressed.

Case 21: A. (boy) 18 months

Appearance	Sturdy-looking child. Cheeks a little red. Blue between and under eyes.
Behavior	More or less normal. Tends to cling to mother a bit.
Main complaint	Insomnia for 11 months. Difficult to fall asleep, light sleep, wakes up repeatedly through the night. Not helped by night light. Sleep was perfect until he reached seven months.
Questions:	
Chills and fevers	Sometimes a little hot after meals. Hands get cold in cold weather.
Sweating	Only when very hot.
Thorax and abdomen	Occasionally catches cough from elder sister. Abdomen not swollen, nor tender on palpation.
Food and taste	Appetite good. Cereal with milk for breakfast, fish, meat, and vegetables for lunch, toast and jam for tea.
Stools and urine	Bowels normal: once a day.
Pregnancy and Birth	Mother had high blood pressure during pregnancy. Birth normal.
Life	House with garden. At seven months he could walk. Mother fitted gate to stairs to stop him from falling down. However, he got through and fell downstairs and broke a leg, but did not cry. Since then he has had insomnia.
Immunizations	Pertussis, polio at eight months.
Tongue	A little red.
Pulse	A little rapid, variable in speed.
Glands	Not swollen.
Diagnosis	This is a typical case of fright-type insomnia. All of the physical signs are normal, but the child is in fear. The fright became "locked in" because he did not cry when he should have.

The point chosen for treatment was H-7 *(shen men),* needled bilaterally. In this case one treatment was enough, although one would normally expect three to five treatments. After the treatment there was a violent discharge of accumulated heat, giving him a sore anus and very bad sleep for four or five days. This is a characteristic reaction when treating fright in young children. After these discharges he no longer had insomnia, although he remained a light sleeper.

Case 22: R. (boy) 4½ years

Appearance	Looks healthy. Cheeks a little red, face slightly red. Slightly green between the eyes. Nasal discharge (thick).
Behavior	Very wild. Rushes up and down the whole time throwing toys around. Cannot sit still at all. Always talking. Has been this way since birth.
Main complaint	Hyperactivity and insomnia. Is active from about 3 A.M. through to 11 P.M. Often quite violent and destructive, for example, throwing plates on the floor at 4 A.M. Never sleeps more than four hours at night, often only two hours. Does not sleep during the day.
Questions:	
Chills and fevers	Never cold. Can run around in freezing weather with hardly any clothes on, but feels no cold.
Sweating	Not much, sometimes sweats in very hot weather.
Head and body	Development is normal.
Thorax and abdomen	No chest problems. Blue veins on abdomen. Abdomen is not swollen.
Food and taste	Obsessive desire for oranges: can eat ten a day if allowed. Drinks orange juice. Also drinks about three pints of milk a day. Appetite good. For breakfast, packaged cereal with milk (the milk often has artificial color and flavor). Mid-morning, packet of flavored crisps. For lunch, packaged or tinned food. No fresh vegetables. For afternoon snack, biscuits (packaged) with color and flour, and much milk. For dinner, packaged or canned food, with orange juice to drink.
Deafness and tinnitus	Some hearing difficulty (it is believed), although it is hard to get him to sit still long enough to do a test. There is some speech difficulty.
Pregnancy	Mother ate 12 oranges a day during pregnancy.
Life	Three-room flat. Elder brother goes to school. A bit short of money.

Immunizations	All the usual: DPT, polio.
Pulse	Will not keep still long enough for pulse to be taken.
Tongue	Will not show tongue.
Glands	Huge glands under ears; more glands stretching in chains down his neck.
Diagnosis	This is a rather bad case of hyperactivity from eating oranges in pregnancy . . . and ever since.
Treatment	First, the child had to stop eating oranges and foods containing artificial colors and flavoring. Without this there was no point in giving treatment. The points used were H-7 *(shen men)* with an even method, and Liv-2 *(xing jian)* and Liv-3 *(tai chong),* both with a strong dispersing method. Even though a strong dispersing method was used, he did not particularly mind.

After 10 treatments his behavior was much better, and he became a much more loving child. He started to complain about having his treatment. This I usually regard as a sign of progress. After 20 treatments he slept about six hours at night, and could usually be trusted to remain on his own without wrecking things. His parents stopped bringing him for treatment at this point, although he would still be classified as hyperactive, and would have benefitted from further treatment.

Without treatment, mild cases of womb toxin do eventually improve over a period of about five to seven years—provided the child does not take any more oranges!

Case 23: S. (boy) 4 years, 8 months

Appearance	White face with red cheeks. Red lips. Tall for his age.
Behavior	Rather shy and sensitive.
Main complaint	Recurrent, almost continuous ear infections for six months since he transferred from play school to full school. Repeated treatment with antibiotics. Ten months before coming to the clinic, because of poor hearing, he underwent surgery in which his adenoids were removed and tubes placed in his ears. This was done because his speech, coordination, and walking were all backward.
Questions:	
Chills and fevers	Frequent fevers with ear infections.
Sweating	Sweating with fevers.
Head and body	No nasal discharge.
Thorax and abdomen	Some dull abdominal pain from time to time.

Food and taste	Appetite is all right most of the time, but there are periods of a week or so when he has a poor appetite and is very choosy about his food. Dislikes meat.
Sleep	Was very bad until 3 1/2 years of age. Still has difficulty falling asleep, and wakes several times during the night.
Deafness and tinnitus	Hearing is still poor. Ears are full of yellow, sticky matter.
Drink and thirst	Not especially thirsty, but often asks for lemon juice and then does not finish it.
Immunization	All given: DPT, polio, measles.
Life	Supportive family with enough money.
Pulse	Liver-Gallbladder pulse is full and slippery. Others are small and deep.
Tongue	Body red, gray coating at root.
Glands	Very pronounced in neck and groin.
Diagnosis	This is a typical example of ear infection due to a lingering pathogenic factor which has left behind some heat (red tongue, insomnia) and phlegm obstructing the channels (irregular appetite, abdominal aches, swollen glands). The fullness of the Liver-Gallbladder pulse is related to obstruction in the Gallbladder channel, while the weakness in the other positions is due to the failure of qi to flow into the other channels, and also from genuine weakness attributable to his growing too fast.
	Using acupuncture alone, a complete cure is possible, but difficult—it would take 20 to 40 treatments. Likewise, herbs alone are not especially effective, as they do not work too specifically on the channels, and do not have the effect of bringing qi to a local area (the ears, in this case). The combination of herbs and acupuncture is thus more effective than either therapy by itself.
Treatment	Acupuncture was given weekly at TB-5 *(wai guan)* and TB-17 *(yi feng)* to move the qi in the channels, and at G-34 *(yang ling quan)* to clear the phlegm. Blue Flag herbal tablets were also prescribed. After six treatments the boy was noticeably better, with no matter coming out of the ears. He also had more energy, and was more cheerful. Treatment was then reduced to every two weeks for another five treatments.

Case 24: G. (boy) 2½ years

Appearance	Red cheeks, tear-stained. Yellow discharge from ear. Hair is dishevelled and appears as though he has been sweating.

	Very thin and a little undersized for his age.
Behavior	Crying intermittently. Very fearful, afraid of people, places, toys, children. When frightened he clings to his mother and buries his head in her bosom, weeping and crying with fear.
Main complaint	Otitis media in both ears almost continuously for nearly one-and-a-half years. Has been regularly taking antibiotics during this time. When he does so, the inflammation and fever come down, but a week or so later the inflammation returns. During the last two to three months the effect of the antibiotics has diminished; they do not seem to work anymore.

Questions:

Chills and fevers	Almost continuous fever, generally not high, but always higher in the afternoon. Does not feel hot.
Sweating	Sweats from time to time. Occasionally drenched in sweat at night.
Head and body	Severe pain in ears most of the time. Head looks too large, arms and legs too thin.
Thorax and abdomen	Abdomen is thin.
Food and taste	Hardly eats anything, just picks irregularly at food.
Stools and urine	Not much urine, and sometimes smells bad. Occasional diarrhea as reaction to antibiotics.
Sleep	Awake through the night almost continuously. Sleeps from about 7 A.M. to 11 A.M.
Deafness and tinnitus	Becoming rather deaf.
Drink and thirst	Always crying out for something to drink, but after a sip or two pushes it away and starts crying.
Pain	Continuous.
Life	Mother is very distraught and does not know what to do. She is close to a breakdown. Family is close-knit, and apart from this disaster is happy and contented.
Pulse	Cannot take.
Tongue	Will not stick out.
Glands	In neck are enormous.
Immunizations	The "usual" at three and six months. Mother not very coherent about them.
Diagnosis	This is a case of chronic otitis due to yin deficiency, and as such is uncommon in the West. Acupuncture is not really indicated because it is not quite soothing and calming enough, and can easily aggravate the panic. The only way acupuncture can help is by treating the mother—which

was not done in this case. The child eventually got better when the mother finally gave in and took her child to someone else to look after for a week, during which time she could recuperate herself. This broke the circle of mother and child infecting each other with feelings of panic and despair.

Case 25: A. (boy) 9 months

This was a strong baby, but rather catarrhal. He did not get chest infections, but had a lot of minor irritations such as colds and diaper rash. At nine months he developed acute conjunctivitis with a fever. His eyes were red and oozing a yellow discharge, and they were obviously causing him some pain, as he rubbed them frequently and cried. His face was a bit red and his forehead was hot. His mother, who was a nurse, had never given him antibiotics, and did not want to do so now. He was therefore brought to me.

The acupuncture treatment took about a minute, with the brief insertion of needles at G-20 *(feng chi)* and LI-4 *(he gu)*. The boy became much calmer over the next few minutes, and by the time they reached home was fast asleep. He perspired freely in his sleep, and three hours later awoke with his temperature down, feeling much more cheerful. His eyes were still red, but he did not rub them. By the next day, all of the redness and discharge had disappeared.

Comment   This was a clear case of wind-heat affecting the eyes. Such quick response is typical when there is a clear diagnosis and the child is reasonably strong. By way of contrast, chronic conjunctivitis is much more complex, and although it can be cured more quickly in children than in adults, it can still take months.

It is sometimes said that acupuncture works more slowly than Western medicine. This is not true when treating infectious diseases in children. In the time that it would have taken to prepare and obtain a prescription, the fever was down and the cure was on its way. Moreover, acupuncture has the effect of strengthening the child's resistance to disease.

Case 26: C. (boy) 12 months

Appearance   Pale face, chubby. Eyes are bright, lips a bit pale.

Behavior   Rather quiet for a boy, but looks around with great interest.

Main complaint   Anemia. Three months previously the whole family came down with a severe cold, with runny noses and catarrhal cough. This boy got worse than the others in his family, and became more and more listless and exhausted. The doctor was called out four times within a month, and finally took a blood test. The hemoglobin was found to be 4.2g per deciliter, instead of the normal 10 to 12g per deciliter. He was hospitalized and had injections of iron and folic acid, which brought his hemoglobin up to 10g per deciliter. Since leaving the hospital he had frequent fevers, and, what is worse, his hemoglobin had been gradually falling. At the time he came to the clinic it was 7.4g per deciliter.

Questions:	
Chills and fevers	Frequent fevers. Has had three courses of antibiotics in two months. The antibiotics give him diarrhea.
Thorax and abdomen	Abdomen is a little swollen.
Food and taste	Poor appetite most of the time. Had colic for the first six months of life, which was cured by homeopathy, and by taking him off cow's milk. He is still slightly allergic to cow's milk.
Stools and urine	Diarrhea with antibiotics. Constipation with iron pills.
Sleep	Was bad when he had colic, but his sleep is better now. However, still wakes up twice a night.
Tongue	Pale, with a red tip.
Finger vein	Very faint, thin, red.
Immunizations	Had usual immunizations at seven months.
Treatment	Needled S-36 *(zu san li)*, Sp-6 *(san yin jiao)*, and CV-12 *(zhong wan)*, all with the tonifying method. After the first treatment his appetite improved noticeably, and after four treatments he had a large appetite. His blood count then started to increase. Two months after the fourth treatment he caught another cold and did not recover fully, so came for further treatment. After that his health was good, and he easily recovered from infections. At the end of treatment the hemoglobin was 12g per deciliter.
Comment	This baby was essentially healthy, but had two attacks in quick succession: first the immunizations, and then an attack of wind-cold. These so lowered his qi that the whole qi mechanism stopped working, giving rise to anemia.

The combination of acupuncture and conventional medicine is more effective in treating anemia than is either alone. Progress is slow in treating children (or adults for that matter) who have iron deficiency anemia. They improve much more quickly if they receive an injection of iron or a blood transfusion.

Appendix 1 ❖ What Acupuncture Can Cure

INTRODUCTION

This appendix is a bit of a mixed bag, and touches on many diseases. It includes brief summaries of most of the illnesses that are covered in this book, and many other illnesses that have not been included. It is not a complete list, but it does give some idea of what can be done in a wide variety of situations. It should also be helpful in determining when an illness should be referred out. If a pattern is specifically covered elsewhere in this book, it is called out.

Abdominal pain

Cold, accumulation, or deficiency

See Chapter 10. Responds well to acupuncture. Other common patterns include blood stagnation (after injury or surgery) and worms.

Abscess, boil

Heat poison

Responds reasonably well to acupuncture. If a baby has an abscess, then something very odd is happening, but it is common in teenagers. May be a further development of glandular disturbance (see Chapter 44). In older children a prescription such as B-18 *(gan shu)*, GV-12 *(shen zhu)*, and Liv-3 *(tai chong)* is often helpful.

Acne (teenage)

Damp-heat rises up

In theory this should be easy to cure, but in practice it is not. The cause is the child's frustration and pent-up anger. If the child is going to school, and just does not want to be going to school, there may not be much that can be done.

Adenoids swollen	Accumulation of phlegm

The basic cause is accumulation of phlegm, sometimes with a lingering pathogenic factor. The adenoids often become so swollen that the child becomes a "mouth breather," because the nasal cavity has become so reduced that it is easily blocked by phlegm. There are times when it is advisable to remove the adenoids surgically. Often the adenoids can be reduced in size enough by acupuncture for the child to have no further trouble; but there are also cases when the lack of air flow in the nasal cavity allows one infection after another to develop. The child's qi can then become severely depleted. Generally, we don't advise surgery until at least twelve treatments have been given. These will go some way toward building up the child's health. (See also *Surgery* below.)

Allergy	Lingering pathogenic factor

Covered under asthma, Chapter 18. Acupuncture is said to be very useful for anaphylactic shock from allergy. The treatments for collapse of yang and restoring the spirit are helpful: GV-26 *(ren zhong)*, CV-1 *(hui yin)*, P-6 *(nei guan)*.

Anemia	Qi deficiency, Blood deficiency, lingering pathogenic factor

Covered in Chapter 46. Responds well to acupuncture.

Anorexia nervosa	This would be classified as *yì bìng*, a "thinking" or "emotional" type disorder, in TCM. It does not respond well to acupuncture.

Anus itching	Thread worms

See Chapter 10 on abdominal pain.

Anus sore	Damp-heat pouring down

In babies, usually due to accumulation disorder. In older children (even as young as four) there is usually an emotional component (or else they spend time sitting on radiators!)

Anxiety	See also *Exam nerves* below. Anxiety is very common in children. As adults we don't really see the problem, but children can be frightened by quite simple things, such as a picture of a dog eating meat. I (JPS) remember myself being quite scared by the picture on the Tate & Lyle Golden Syrup tin of bees making their nest in a dead lion! Usually the anxiety passes, but sometimes it builds up and gets worse and worse so that the mother is really anxious about her child. In the early stages, the Bach remedies are particularly to be recommended. Moxibustion can also be

of help. Very gently moxa (with indirect moxa) CV-4 *(guan yuan)* and B-23 *(shen shu)* to assist the parents and child in sorting the problem out.

Arrythmia (heart)	Stagnation of qi

It is quite common to find the pulse lurching around, without a good rhythm. In children it nearly always means stagnation of qi in the diaphragm or abdomen, often combined with qi deficiency.

Arthritis	Wind-cold-dampness

Something is badly wrong if a child gets arthritis. I have seen one case of rheumatoid arthritis in a five-year-old, but it was an orphan refugee from a war zone. I am convinced that acupuncture can be helpful.

Ascariasis

See Chapter 10. Acupuncture is not the treatment of choice, but can help if the child continues to get worms.

Athlete's foot	Dampness

The fungus that causes athlete's foot can only survive if there is dampness in the system. To cure, it is normally necessary for the child to have a completely sugar-free diet, as sugar easily creates dampness.

Autism	*Shén* disturbance

See Chapter 33. In so far as autism is a disturbance of the spirit, it does not respond directly to acupuncture. However, in the few cases I (JPS) have seen, the spirit disturbance was accompanied by severe stagnation of qi and heat, both of which would affect the spirit. Acupuncture is certainly of help in the cure, and sometimes is the key to unlocking the problem.

AIDS

Reliable information is hard to come by. I (JPS) have only treated one child who is HIV positive (who went from strength to strength); but the consensus is that if a child is looked after well, fed well, and given low key supportive treatment, then HIV need not develop into AIDS.

Backache	Kidney deficiency

In our generation, backache was a problem of adults only. Now children are getting weak and aching backs as young as nine or ten due to a combination of stress at school and a crazy lifestyles. Acupuncture can be of great benefit in supporting these children if there is no possibility of changing their lives or reducing their workloads.

Alopecia	Phlegm-dampness
	Not especially common now, but does seem to affect children more in their teens. Due to phlegm accumulating in the scalp, and is thus similar in cause to eczema. Like eczema, there is an emotional component, so the results of treatment are quite variable: some miracle cures, some complete failures!
Boils	See *Abscess.*
Bone pains	See *Growing pains.*
Brain damage	See *Mental retardation* in Chapter 30. Acupuncture can sometimes be helpful.
Bronchitis	Phlegm-heat in Lungs
	Acupuncture is wonderful at curing this, far quicker than antibiotics. See Chapter 16.
Cancer	As with adults, acupuncture has three uses: 1. To reduce the side effects of chemotherapy. Treatment may be required every day. 2. To support the qi, to enable other therapies to be more effective. 3. To relieve pain. It does seem that acupuncture is very effective in this role, although it can hasten death.
Candida	Damp (heat)
	Acupuncture can be of help, although dietary changes are usually necessary.
Cavities (dental)	Kidney weakness
	See *Teeth.*
Cerebral palsy	See Chapter 35.
Chicken pox	Acupuncture can be of help, but is not really the treatment of choice. Homeopathy is especially effective both in treatment and in prophylaxis when an epidemic is going round.
Cholera	Invasion of cold-dampness
	Not much seen in United Kingdom or developed countries. However, acupuncture has a very good reputation in curing it. In extreme cases, scarring moxibustion on the abdominal points S-25 *(tian shu)*, CV-4 *(guan yuan)*, and CV-12 *(zhong wan)* may be needled (according to text).

Cholesterol	Some children have a hereditary tendency to high cholesterol. This does not cause immediate danger, but left without treatment or diet change can lead to death from heart attack from about thirty years of age. Acupuncture is largely ineffective.
Chorea	See Chapter 39.
Colic	Cold See *Abdominal pain* above, and Chapter 10.
Conjunctivitis	Very quick results with acupuncture. See Chapter 24.
Convulsions	Acupuncture is the number one therapy for acute convulsions, with almost instant results. See Chapter 38.
Coeliac disease	Allergy to gluten is extremely common in a mild form, especially in the very young. Acupuncture can be of help in strengthening the digestion so that at least small amounts of wheat can be digested, but once this point has been reached, it makes sense to avoid wheat as much as possible.
Croup	A harsh cough. If it comes during an acute attack, it is relatively more severe than an ordinary cough, because it means that the phlegm has become very hard and difficult to bring up. In the past, before the days of antibiotics, it was seen as a good sign when the cough "broke" and became softer and more productive. In a chronic cough, croup is a sign of a lingering pathogenic factor, often from whooping cough or whooping cough immunization.
Cystic fibrosis	May respond to acupuncture; little is known at present. We would be glad to hear from anyone who has experience in treating it.
Dandruff	Dampness Basically a mild form of eczema, appearing in the scalp. As such it is due to dampness, and can be treated by acupuncture.
Deafness	Phlegm, nerve injury This is covered in Chapter 25 on otitis. By far the most common cause is phlegm blocking the cavities in the ear. Responds well to acupuncture. Occasionally, deafness is due to damage to the nerves of the ear, either from disease, an immunization, or dampness. In principle this can be helped a great deal with acupuncture, but it takes lots

of treatments (50~150), and is painful. Most parents, on behalf of their children, have a fear of the likely pain, and will not submit them to a long and painful treatment, even though it is the only hope of saving their hearing.

Delirium

The delirium of high fevers responds very well to acupuncture. The principle of treatment is to bring back the spirit and clear heat. Besides the classic prescription of GV-14 *(da zhui)*, LI-11 *(qu chi)*, and LI-4 *(he gu)* to clear heat, one can use GV-26 *(ren zhong)*.

Dermatitis

See Chapter 28. Results are often good, but are basically unpredictable.

Diabetes mellitus

Arises from the combination of long-lasting internal heat and being overtired for a long time. The continuing presence of heat consumes the yin of the three *zàng* organs relating to water metabolism: Kidneys, Lungs, and Spleen.

If diabetes arises in children, and there are clear signs of heat (such as red face, red tongue, rapid pulse), then it will respond to acupuncture. Frequent and many treatments are required, but there is a very good chance of curing the condition for life. If, on the other hand, there are no signs of heat, the prognosis is poor. Also, once the child has been put on insulin, it is very difficult to break the habit. It is a truly addictive drug.

Diarrhea

See Chapter 8.

Diphtheria

Almost unknown in the United Kingdom now, it used to be a very dangerous disease in children. It is not dangerous in developed countries for three reasons: first, the level of nutrition is such that the toxins do not build up in the body; second, children are now encouraged to speak out (in contrast to previous generations when children should be "seen and not heard") so the qi does not get stuck in the throat in the same way; and third, because antitoxins now exist.

Down's syndrome

See Chapter 32. A lot of help can be given to these children.

Dwarfism

There are two sorts: the first is due to dysfunction of the pituitary gland, in which the proportions of the body are retained, but the child simply does not grow. It is hard to be sure, but our belief is that this type responds to acupuncture. Certainly we have seen small children growing very rapidly after treatment. This is discussed further in Chapter 29. The other type is known as achondroplasia, where only the growth of the long bones is affected. We have limited experience with this type, which seems to suggest that the condition itself cannot be helped, but the bowing of the legs due to shortening of the muscles can be avoided by regular treatment while the child is growing. We would be glad to hear from anyone who has experience with either type of dwarfism.

Dysentery	See *Diarrhea*.
Dysmenorrhea	The treatment of gynecological disorders is outside the scope of this course on pediatrics, but the transition through puberty is discussed in Chapter 43. Often the first few periods are painful. If they do not quickly settle down into a regular and pain-free pattern, then treatment should be given, otherwise the pain may recur for many years. It is above all important to avoid stress and overwork during these years. The treatment is basically the same as for adults, with one important difference: the pain may be due to anxiety and fear of the periods themselves, and of becoming a woman and leaving childhood behind. See also *Premenstrual tension*.
Eczema	See Chapter 28.
Encephalitis	The main form of this is myalgic encephalitis. See also *Meningitis*.
Energy	Low energy can, of course, be helped by acupuncture. Collapses of energy which happen again and again may be due to food allergies; when they occur without obvious cause, it may be due to a lingering pathogenic factor.
Epilepsy	See Chapter 40. Acupuncture is one of the prime methods for curing epilepsy.
Exam nerves	Some children become almost paralyzed by nervousness when exam time comes. They seem to be rather thin, jumpy children from success-oriented families; but sometimes even children from "well-balanced" acupuncturist's families get nerves! I have not found acupuncture to be especially helpful in treating this condition. The Bach remedy Mimulus is helpful, and so is the homeopathic remedy Gelsemium.
Eye strain	Often a cause of headaches. Children's eyes very rarely get strained from bad use or overuse, and eye strain is usually a symptom of more general strain. Can be helped enormously. See Chapter 36.

Fat	See *Obesity.*
Fissure (anal)	Sometimes occurs after a period of constipation. Passing stools then becomes very painful, so the child becomes more constipated, thus aggravating the condition. There is often an emotional component, but it usually responds well to acupuncture. In addition to other points to move the bowels, such as TB-6 *(zhi gou)* and GV-1 *(chang jiang)*, B-57 *(cheng shan)* is helpful in bringing qi to the anus.
Fits	See Chapter 38. Acupuncture is the number one therapy for fits.
German measles (Rubella)	In itself, German measles rarely leads to anything other than mild discomfort, and it is not worth giving acupuncture (itself a mild discomfort). The real danger is to the unborn baby in the first three months of pregnancy, and it is unlikely that acupuncture will have the slightest effect.
Glandular fever	Stagnation of Liver qi with dampness Acupuncture can be of great help, both during the attack, and in preventing the long drawn out recuperation period when the child never feels really well. This is discussed in Chapter 44.
Growing pains	Dampness in channels These are due to dampness and phlegm. Often the pains are felt along the Gallbladder channel.
Hemorrhoids	Damp-heat It is unusual to have really swollen veins in the anus in children, but inflammation and pain is quite common. See *Anus* and *Fissure.*
Hay fever	Lingering pathogenic factor, Liver yang rising See Chapter 26. As in adults, hay fever in children responds well to acupuncture. There is a significant emotional component, which is why it is much more common after seven years of age. There is also a lingering pathogenic factor component.
Headache	Really, children should not get headaches at all, because the root cause is overthinking, and they should not be forced into this. However, the truth is that in the United Kingdom, lots of children are forced into doing much too much mental work, too early on, and this gives rise to headaches. Other causes are eye strain, and poison in the system from lingering pathogenic factors, especially the measles immunization.

Heart problems	The main heart problems that children have are congenital defects. Acupuncture can be of some help, surprisingly, for hole-in-the-heart babies, when the hole is not too big. By bringing qi to the chest, the heart can heal itself, often surprisingly quickly. The situations where it cannot help include when the hole is too large, and when the child is very angry, even after a lot of treatment. It seems that there is a particular sort of anger, which is quite unremitting (different from Liver anger) which injures the heart. It is my (JPS) opinion that if this anger remains, then even with surgery, the child is unlikely to have a long life. If parents decide to have surgery for their child—which is certainly indicated for some children—then acupuncture can be of help both before and after the operation, to assist in recovery. See also *Surgery*.
Heatstroke	Acupuncture has a good reputation for curing heatstroke, although, living in England, we have little experience. Spooning *(guā shā)* the inside of the elbows and backs of the knees (common places for eczema) is also supposed to be helpful.
Hemiplegia	This is described under cerebral palsy in Chapter 35. See also *Stroke*.
Hepatitis	Damp-heat invades the Spleen and Liver; also Spleen qi deficiency The diagnosis and treatment of hepatitis in children is the same as in adults. We have no direct experience, but it should respond well to acupuncture.
Hepatitis (neonatal)	Damp-heat, Spleen qi deficiency Neonatal hepatitis has two forms: excessive type related to damp-heat, and deficient type related to Spleen qi deficiency. Both are "womb diseases," the excessive type arising from dampness in the mother, and the deficient type usually from blood deficiency in the mother. The conventional treatment is 1. to wait; 2. to expose children to ultraviolet light. In some cases the hepatitis persists, and rather drastic surgery is performed. This is usually quite unnecessary if the baby avoids damp-producing foods, such as cow's milk. Acupuncture can be of great help in serious cases.
Hernia	The two common hernias are inguinal and umbilical. Both are due to weakness of the abdomen, but they can occur in babies who are otherwise quite strong. One of the most common causes is roaring with rage for too long! This

only happens in strong babies. The traditional treatment for umbilical hernia of bandaging a copper coin over the umbilicus has some foundation in science. Copper has a strong effect in benefiting the muscles, hence the use of copper bracelets for rheumatism.

Herpes simplex	Damp-heat See *Thrush*.
Hiccough	Rebellious qi The immediate cause of hiccough is stagnation of qi in the diaphragm. The traditional method of curing it is to drink water from the wrong side of a mug. If it continues for a long time, it can be cured by needling P-6 *(nei guan)* and S-40 *(feng long)*. If hiccoughs keep recurring, it may be due to stagnation of qi in the middle burner, or to deficient Stomach energy.
Hip deformity	Congenital hip deformity (Perthes disease, "clicking hips") is usually associated with qi deficiency and a lingering pathogenic factor. Mild cases can be completely cured by acupuncture alone. Intermediate cases respond to acupuncture with herbs. When there is serious bone deformity, orthopaedic splints or even surgery are needed to prevent repeated dislocations.
Histamine reaction	See *Hay fever*.
Hydrocephalus	Can be quickly spotted by the unusual enlargement of the head. Prompt action must be taken to prevent brain damage. Acupuncture can certainly be of help, and can obviate the need for surgery, but frequent treatment must be given (every day, or every other day) to strengthen the Kidneys, and to relieve the pressure in the head. Use such points as GV-16 *(feng fu)*, GV-20 *(bai hui)*, and B-23 *(shen shu)*.
Hypoglycemia	Yin deficiency with heat This is much more common in children than is realized. In the early years the sugar level in the blood is not really stable. After about the age of four or five it should settle down. Factors which interfere with the sugar balance are (obviously) eating refined sugar, and (less obviously) computer games and lingering pathogenic factors. This is the reason why immunizations can lead to diabetes. In some families, hypoglycemia is hereditary. This seems to come when all members of the family are rather vague and "in the clouds." If this is a real problem, the Bach remedy Clematis can sometimes be of help, so also can treatment to strengthen the Kidney qi, such as B-23 *(shen shu)*.

Impetigo	Damp-heat
	Would be classified under the heading of eczema in Chinese medicine (see Chapter 28). Although it is believed to be due to bacteria, and responds to antibiotics, it nevertheless responds even more quickly to acupuncture. In the cases that we have seen, the damp-heat has been due to accumulation disorder.
Incontinence of urine	In some senses, bedwetting at night is "normal," and children do eventually grow out of it, while incontinence of urine during the daytime can never be considered normal. It is invariably due to local weakness of qi, and is often associated with Kidney deficiency, sometimes due to damp-heat. It responds well to acupuncture.
Infectious diseases	Acupuncture is really one of the quickest and best treatments for all infectious diseases in babies and children. The times when it is ineffective are when the child is very weak, or has had a life-threatening infection so many times that it gives in. Normally, one can say that there is no need for children ever to take antibiotics.
Inflammation	Acupuncture is especially good at taking down bad inflammations. In acute disorders like tonsillitis and acute otitis media, the pain caused by the inflammation can disappear within minutes, and the inflammation itself within a few hours. In chronic cases such as inflammation of the anus or foreskin, the inflammation usually comes down within a few days.
Iritis	In the textbooks, iritis is attributed to Liver yang rising or Liver yin deficiency. Predictably, the only case we have seen was one of yang deficiency! It appeared that the child was suffering from well-disguised fear. We were unable to identify the cause of the fear, and did not have any long-term success, although there were good short-term results.
Jaundice	See *Hepatitis.*
Lactation	Acupuncture is very helpful in promoting milk production.
Lordosis	See *Postural defects.*
Measles	See Chapter 20.
ME (Myalgic encephalomyelitis) and fibromyalgia	Fibromyalgia in children? Surely it does not happen! Well, it does. The youngest case we have heard of was in a five-year-old, although it is very uncommon at this age. Much

more common is at puberty. As with asthma, there are a multitude of causes, all of which play a part. From the point of view of TCM, there are a number of different patterns, and different writers have put their emphasis on different aspects: dampnes, yin deficiency, Liver stagnation, depression. One thing that they all seem to have in common is a lingering pathogenic factor, and deficiency of the body. The deficiency allows the pathogenic factor to penetrate deeply. Whatever the cause, it is certain that children's energy should not be overtaxed in puberty. Acupuncture can be of help (with other remedies) on the long road to recovery.

Meconium

This is the green mixture of bile and phlegm in the neonate's guts that is passed soon after birth. In old China, it was said that a baby should pass this before being given any food, otherwise there was a chance that eczema would develop. A teaspoonful of Three Yellow Decoction *(sān huáng tāng)* was routinely given at birth to clean out the guts. This practice is at variance with the modern practice of putting the newborn babe straight to the breast.

Meningitis

Much feared in England at present, due to recent "outbreaks." This has formed the basis of a nationwide campaign to immunize against Haemophylus Influenza B (HIB), a particularly vicious immunization, with very doubtful benefits. From the point of view of TCM, meningitis comes from three causes: 1. great external heat, that is, hot weather; 2. internal heat, for example, from accumulation disorder, or more commonly a lingering pathogenic factor; and 3. deficiency of protective qi. Thus, a healthy child has little to fear, unless it gets very distressed in hot weather, or becomes overtired. A weak child is much more at risk—but then it is also more at risk from the immunization.

Nosebleed

Full heat, rebellious qi, Lung weakness

Nosebleeds are really quite common in children. Usually, besides internal heat, there is some hereditary Lung weakness. There also may be Kidney weakness, such that rebellious qi can readily rise up. In most children, severe nosebleeds are an indication that they are overtired.

Obesity

Dampness

It is normal for babies and toddlers to look obese. If the obesity persists after five or six years, however, it should be taken seriously. From the point of view of TCM, obesity is accumulation of dampness. This may come from damp-producing foods (especially sweets), poor quality food (e.g., supermarket food), or simply eating too much. It may also be attributed to a lingering pathogenic factor, usually of a damp nature, especially when the original pathogenic factor was treated with antibiotics. If the obesity remains beyond the seven-year transition, it is difficult to cure. If it remains beyond the fourteen-year transition as well, it is extremely difficult to cure, and usually takes some major life event. This can be helped by acupuncture, but herbal medicine with dietary changes appears to be more effective. However, the obese children that we have treated seem to be reluctant to continue treatment for any length of time.

Osteochondritis dessicans

Also known as Schlatter's disease, a growth of bone below the knee. It occurs in teenage years when a child suffers from Kidney deficiency due to a combination of overwork and rapid growth. It responds well to acupuncture, although repeated treatments are necessary if the child cannot avoid the pressure of overwork (as is usually the case). Treatment consists of strengthening the Kidneys and moving qi in the channels of the legs, especially the Stomach and Gallbladder channels.

Rett's syndrome

Another rare pattern, of which acupuncturists see an abnormal number. This one is characterized by severe scoliosis, which worsens as the child grows. At about twelve years, it usually gets so bad that the child needs "Harrington rods" in the spine in order to stand upright at all. Other signs are very poor development. Although the child starts out normal, they gradually become more ill, so that by the age of three they cannot speak or stand. Although allegedly due to a defective gene, a colleague reports that it responds very well to acupuncture. She began treating a child at age eleven, and far from getting worse and more bent over at this age, the scoliosis actually improved, as did her general health and development.

Paralysis (infantile)

The sequelae of polio (see Chapter 35). Acupuncture is the main therapy for curing this, but results are variable, with some complete cures and others receiving only little benefit. For best results, treatment should start as soon as possible, within three months. After two years, it is unusual to see any improvement.

Perthes disease

See *Hips*.

Petit mal

See *Epilepsy*.

Pharyngitis	Although usually treated with antibiotics, pharyngitis is much better treated with acupuncture. Often represents a symptom of general heat in the body trying to come out.
Piles	See *Hemorrhoids.*
Platelets	Heat in blood, Spleen qi deficiency
	Thrombocytopenic purpura, a disease of the blood where there are insufficient platelets for good clotting action, responds to acupuncture. It is commonly due to heat in the blood (perhaps from an immunization), or less commonly, inability of the Spleen to restrain the blood. Further details of treatment are provided in Chapter 45.
Pleurisy	It does respond to acupuncture, but only rather slowly.
Pneumonia	Pathogenic factor
	Pneumonia responds well to acupuncture. It is our belief that the recovery is much quicker than if conventional medicine is used. However, treatment must be given quickly and frequently. For further detail, see Chapter 17. One of us (JPS) had pneumonia while in China during the winter. The effects of acupuncture were instantaneous: when CV-17 *(shan zhong)* was needled, it felt like delicious cool water being poured in to soothe the fierce pain in the chest. The fever subsided within twelve hours, and the next day I was up and about.
Polio	In principle, polio can be treated with acupuncture. In practice, the onset is so rapid that any damage that occurs is likely to happen well before reaching any therapist. The best approach is to strengthen the child so that when he or she is infected by the polio virus, it never goes beyond the superficial level. See Chapter 35.
Postural defects	Although acupuncture is not the therapy that one would think of first for postural defects, so many of these problems now come from real imbalances of the channels and organs (rather than simply from the acquisition of bad habits) that acupuncture is often very beneficial. For example, bent upper back may come from Lung weakness, lordosis from Kidney weakness, kyphosis from Lung and Spleen weakness, scoliosis from left-right imbalance.

Premenstrual tension (PMS)	It seems somewhat dotty to talk about gynecological problems in a children's textbook, but it is increasingly in our province. Both of us have treated girls of just nine years of age for premenstrual tension! The treatment principles for gynecological problems in children are the same as for adults, although the treatment can be much gentler. This is discussed a little bit more in Chapter 43 on the stages of growth and development.
Projectile vomiting	Heat in blood
	In conventional medicine attributed to malformation of the stomach, which may be treated by surgery. Usually responds well to acupuncture, and is a characteristic sign of the heat pattern of vomiting.
Psoriasis	In adults, psoriasis is very difficult to cure completely, even with herbs, but in children it seems to be easier. We have treated several cases in children between the ages of seven and fourteen, all with good results. In each case there was a significant anxiety component in their life (such as not getting along with their teacher) which became apparent as a result of treatment.
Purpura	See *Platelets.*
Pus	Heat poison
	In conventional medicine pus is seen as a by-product of inflammation. In traditional Chinese medicine it is viewed as a manifestation of "poison" (toxin). If a child has signs of poison, such as repeated attacks of boils, or of prevalent conjunctivitis, then he or she should avoid eggs, chicken, and peanuts.
Pyloric stenosis	See *Projectile vomiting.*
Ringworm	Dampness in skin
	This skin disease looks as though it is caused by a worm, but is in fact caused by a fungus or mold. As such, it is due to dampness collecting in the skin layer. In conventional medicine it is considered to be highly contagious. It responds well to acupuncture. The principle of treatment is to clear the dampness under the skin.
Roundworm	See *Abdominal pain.* The best way to treat is with herbs which stun the worms. However, if a child keeps on getting worms, it means that food is not passing through quickly enough, and is a sign of accumulation disorder or of Spleen qi deficiency.

Salmonella	The common type of salmonella poisoning (in England usually from infected egg yolks) corresponds to the cold-damp type of diarrhea, and responds well to acupuncture and especially to moxibustion.
Scarlet fever	We have no experience in treating scarlet fever, but it seems likely that it would respond to acupuncture. We would like to hear from anyone who has such experience.
Scoliosis	See *Postural defects*.
Seborrhoea	Usually a sign of phlegm-dampness.
Sinusitis	The patterns for sinusitis in children are the same as for chronic cough. The treatment of the underlying pattern is the same, with additional points to move the qi in the nose, such as GV-23 *(shang xing)*.
Strabismus squint (cross-eyed)	Some types of strabismus squint respond well to acupuncture. See Chapter 37.
Stroke	Stroke is an old-age disease. However, I (JPS) have seen one case of stroke in a child, which has been recorded on video! Quite unbelievably, this child of about ten years of age suffered from sudden paralysis on one side of the body, due to a buildup of tension. The pulse was wiry, and the tongue red and coated, as one would expect in a stroke patient.
Surgery	Much of our work is to keep children out of the hands of surgeons! However, there are times when surgery really is the best treatment. Acupuncture can be of help in assisting the cure. Treat both before surgery and (if possible) afterwards. The treatment principle is to treat any underlying imbalance—in much the same way as one would prepare a child for an immunization—and to bring qi to the affected area. For example, in surgery for hole-in-the-heart one might tonify the qi with a point such as S-36 *(zu san li)* and bring qi to the chest with such points as P-6 *(nei guan)*, B-15 *(xin shu)*, and CV-17 *(shan zhong)*.
Sweating	The causes of sweating are the same in children as in adults: heat, or severe qi deficiency. Night sweats may be due to yin deficiency, but are more commonly due to damp-heat from accumulation disorder.
Teeth	Poor development, and late appearance of teeth, are mainly due to Kidney deficiency. This can also be the result of a lingering pathogenic factor. If the first teeth are badly

formed (e.g., crumbling or blackening) there is not a great deal that can be done. However, with treatment, one can make sure that the second set of teeth are well formed.

Undescended testicle

I (JPS) have treated quite a number of cases, all of them successfully. They all had weakness in the lower burner. Some of them showed overall weakness, and the main treatment was to tonify the entire body with such points as S-36 *(zu san li)*, Sp-6 *(san yin jiao)*, and CV-12 *(zhong wan)*; while others were just weak in the lower burner, with emphasis on such points as B-23 *(shen shu)* and B-32 *(ci liao)*. In a number of cases it was obvious that the mother wanted the boy to be girlish, dressing him up and cutting his hair in what she regarded as a girlish way. In others, the desire for the boy to be a girl was more subtle and muted. However, these parental feelings did not seem to affect the treatment.

Tetanus

There is much fear of tetanus, which appears unfounded. This accounts for the over-protection in the form of "tetanus jabs," even though there is evidence that repeated tetanus immunizations may be behind neurological diseases such as multiple sclerosis. Acupuncture may be of great help in treating tetanus, although of course you have to be there to give the treatment!

Thrush

Dampness

Both oral and vaginal thrush respond very well to acupuncture. See Chapter 13.

Thyroid (hypo)

Underactive thyroid is sometimes diagnosed in babies and toddlers, and is then treated with thyroxine. This seems a big mistake to us, for the babies are usually just deficient and damp, and a few treatments will cure the condition. The alternative may be to take drugs for life.

Tinea

See *Ringworm.*

Tonsillitis

Acute tonsillitis responds exceptionally well to acupuncture. See Chapter 23.

Travel sickness

See Chapter 11.

Tuberculosis

It was thought that tuberculosis would disappear as prosperity increased, but in England, where both wage differentials and relative poverty have increased, tuberculosis is on the rise, in spite of mass immunization. At present there are drugs which control it, but in time it seems likely that drug resistant strains will become common. When this happens, other natural therapies will really be needed.

Typhoid fever	See *Salmonella.*
Ulcer (mouth)	Responds well to acupuncture. See Chapter 13.
Umbilical hernia	See *Hernia.*
Urethritis	See Chapter 42.
Urinary reflux	Urethritis often has urinary reflux as its root. Conventional treatment is long-term low–dose antibiotics, a treatment which has devastating side effects in a minority. Our experience indicates that reflux is due to weakness in the lower burner, and that many children can be cured by tonifying the Kidney energy in 10 to 20 treatments. To get some idea of the progress of treatment, feeling the energy in the back is helpful, but the only reliable guide is conventional medical tests.
Verruca	Verruca means wart, but the term is usually used in common language for warts on the feet. See *Warts.*
Vomiting	See Chapter 11. Responds very well to acupuncture.
Warts	Warts can only grow if there is dampness in the system. Warts on the hand are more likely to be from the Spleen and Lungs, while warts on the feet from the Spleen and Kidneys. Very often, when the dampness is cleared, the warts go away. They are much easier to cure in children than in adults.
Whooping cough	See Chapter 22. Acupuncture is the treatment of choice.
Worms	See Chapter 10.

❖

Appendix 2 ❖ Table of Hot and Cold Foods

This table shows the heating and cooling effects of some common foods. Patients who suffer from a cold condition should eat predominantly warm foods and vice versa. The heating and cooling effects of foods can be balanced within one meal, to a certain extent. For example, melon (cold) can be combined with ginger (hot) to provide a neutral effect. Milk (cool) can be simmered (warmed) with onion (warm) to provide a neutral drink that reduces the amount of phlegm produced. The table is provided only as a guide, and some people will react differently. For example, Chinese people find that lamb is extremely hot and brings out rashes in many, while for most Western people, lamb is between warm and hot.

Cold		Cool	
	Apple		Aubergine
	Banana		Barley
	Celery		Calf's liver
	Cottage cheese		Cow's milk
	Cucumber		Crab
	Grapefruit		Cress
	Lettuce		Green lentils
	Marrow		Lamb's liver
	Melon		Lemon
	Mussels		Mung beans
	Pear		Pork
	Yoghurt		Soft cheeses
			Soused herring
			Spinach
			Steamed foods
			Tea (green)
			Tofu (bean curd)
			Tomatoes (raw)
			White wine

Neutral

Broad beans
Brown rice
Coconut
Corn on the cob
Dates
Eggs
Grapes
Herring
Mushrooms
Peas
Potatoes
Plums
Runner beans
Strawberries
Veal
Wheat
White cabbage

Hot

Almonds
Beets
Brown lentils
Brussel sprouts
Cayenne pepper
Cinnamon
Cloves
Eels
Garlic
Ginger
Goat's meat
Lamb
Peach
Pepper

Warm

Blackberry (cooked)
Carrots
Chocolate
Chicken
Cocoa
Coffee
Figs
Goat's milk
Greens (brassica)
Mint tea
Oats
Onion
Orange
Parsnips
Peanuts
Pig's liver
Pumpkin
Radish
Red beans
Red wine
Roasted foods
Sesame seeds
Smoked foods
Tea (Indian)
Tomatoes (cooked)
Turnips
Venison

❖

❖ Bibliography

The material for the etiology, pathogenesis, and differentiation of traditional patterns was largely based on the two books of pediatrics noted below by the Shanghai College of Traditional Chinese Medicine. *Pediatrics in Traditional Chinese Medicine (Zhong yi er ke xue),* although a modern book, was written by experts in the field from all over mainland China. The youngest contributor was 64 years old, and the oldest 78 years old. It was written at a time of comparative freedom of expression, and can therefore be taken to represent the mainstream of traditional Chinese medical thought.

The only classical works we consulted were *Explaining the Puzzles of Pediatrics (You ke shi mi)* and the *Great Compendium of Acupuncture and Moxibustion (Zhen jiu da cheng).* The first is a handbook for the treatment of children, based on herbal medicine, but its etiology, pathogenesis, and differentiation of patterns are similar to those presented here, though not so complete or detailed. The *Great Compendium of Acupuncture and Moxibustion* has a large section on the treatment of children. On reading this work, with whole sections devoted to jumbles of symptomatic treatments, one is struck by the advances that have been made in acupuncture over the past four hundred years.

The material for prescription of points was taken from the books noted below by the Tianjin College of Traditional Chinese Medicine Number One Affiliated Hospital, Li Wen-Rui and He Bao-Yi, the Academy of Traditional Chinese Medicine, Yan Hong-Chen and Cheng Shao-En, the Cheng-du College of Traditional Chinese Medicine, the Shanghai College of Traditional Chinese Medicine, and my (JPS) notes from the Nanjing College of Traditional Chinese Medicine. Some material for prognosis was obtained from the collections of case histories edited by Jiao Guo-Rui and Sun Xue-Quan, but for the most part the prognoses are based on our own experience with English and American children.

The material for Chapter 1, "Differences Between Children and Adults," and Chapter 4, "Diagnosis," was drawn from *Pediatrics in Traditional Chinese Medicine (Zhong yi er ke xue)* by the Shanghai College of Traditional Chinese Medicine, supplemented by our own experience. The material for the causes of disease was based on our own experience.

Academy of Traditional Chinese Medicine. *Simplified Edition of Acupuncture (Zhen jiu xue jian bian).* 针灸学简编 Beijing: People's Health Publishing Company, 1978.

Chengdu College of Traditional Chinese Medicine. *Acupuncture (Zhen jiu xue).* 针灸学 Chengdu: Sichuan People's Press, 1981.

Dong Hao-Kui and Li En-Fu. *Therapeutic Massage for Organs and Channels (Zang fu jing luo an mo).* 脏腑经络按摩 Shijiazhuang: Hebei People's Publishing Company, 1981.

Jiao Guo-Rui, ed. *Abstracts of Clinical Experience with Acupuncture (Zhen jiu lin chuang jing yan ji yao).* 针灸临床经验积要 Beijing: People's Health Publishing Company, 1981.

Jin Yi-Cheng. *Pediatric Tuina (Xiao er tui na).* 小儿推拿 Shanghai: Shanghai Science & Technology Press, 1980.

Li Wen-Rui and He Bao-Yi, eds. *Practical Acupuncture (Shi yong zhen jiu xue).* 实用针灸学 Beijing: People's Health Publishing Company, 1982.

Li-Xue-Geng. *Flying Needle Therapy for Children (Xiao er fei zhen liao fa).* 小儿飞针疗法 Fuzhou: Fujian Science & Technology Press, 1981.

Nanjing College of Traditional Chinese Medicine (Notes from lectures and clinics) 1981-82.

Shanghai College of Traditional Chinese Medicine Shuguang Affiliated Hospital. *Clinical Handbook of Pediatrics in Traditional Chinese Medicine (Zhong yi er ke lin chuang shou ce).* 中医儿科临床手册 Shanghai: Shanghai Science & Technology Press, 1980.

Shanghai College of Traditional Chinese Medicine. *Pediatrics in Traditional Chinese Medicine (Zhong yi er ke xue)*. 中医儿科学 Shanghai: Shanghai Science & Technology Press, 1979.

Shanghai College of Traditional Chinese Medicine (O'Connor, John and Bensky, Dan translators). *Acupuncture: A Comprehensive Text (Zhen jiu xue)*. 针灸学 Chicago: Eastland Press, 1981. [Chinese edition published in 1974.]

Sun Xue-Quan, ed. *Collection of Clinical Experiences with Acupuncture (Zhen jiu lin zheng ji yan)*. 针灸临症积验 Jinan: Shandong Technical Press, 1982.

Tianjin College of Traditional Chinese Medicine Number One Affiliated Hospital. *Practical Acupuncture (Shi yong zhen jiu xue)*. 实用针灸学 Tianjin: Tianjin Science & Technology Press, 1980.

Wang Quan. *Explaining the Puzzles of Pediatrics (You ke shi mi)*. 幼科释秘 Beijing: People's Health Publishing Company, 1980. [Originally published in 1774.]

Yan Hong-Chen and Cheng Shao-En, eds. *Anthology of Acupuncture Prescriptions (Zhen jiu chu fang ji)*. 针灸处方集 Guilin: Guilin People's Publishing Company, 1983.

Yang Ji-Zhou. *Great Compendium of Acupuncture and Moxibustion (Zhen jiu da cheng)*. 针灸大成 Beijing: People's Health Publishing Company, 1978. [Originally published in 1602.]

❖

❖ Glossary

Accumulation disorder
积滞 *(jí zhì)*

Occurs when food moves too slowly through the intestinal tract. Intestinal blockage from accumulation (or accumulation and obstruction) is very common among babies and children. It corresponds roughly to the retention of food disorder *(shǐ zhì)* seen in adults. It is very common in Western children. In fact, when treating young children this disorder is so common that one should routinely check to see if it is present (see Chapter 7).

Basal yang
元阳 *(yuán yáng)*

The essence of the body which fills up the brain and spinal column and is the precursor of bone marrow. It is related to constitutional strength. When *yuán* appears on its own it usually refers to *yuán qì,* that is, basal qi (also known as ancestral, original, or source qi), which is the constitutional qi given to the child by its parents. It is sometimes thought to reside in the lower abdomen, at the 'dantian', but in clinical practice refers to the constitutional reserves of strength.

Blood stasis
血瘀 *(xuè yū)*

Refers to inadequate blood circulation associated with blood clots, bruises, varicose veins, or even blood getting 'stuck' in the channels.

Collection or knot
结 *(jié)*

This is our imperfect solution to translating the Chinese character which literally means knot, but in traditional Chinese medicine suggests the idea of something collecting, clotting, clumping, or congealing. It sometimes refers specifically to the phenomenon of the intestines going into spasm.

Heat in the five centers
五心热 *(wǔ xīn rè)*

A sensation of heat in the chest, the palms of the hands, and the soles of the feet. Traditionally, these are signs of yin deficiency, although in practice they are rarely seen now in the West.

Lingering pathogenic factor 邪余 *(xié yú)*	When an illness is left untreated, or if it is checked by inappropriate treatment which prevents it from running its natural course, or if it is only partially treated, it may leave behind some trace of the original disease. These conditions are regarded in Chinese medicine as ones in which the pathogenic factor lingers or is not completely cleared from the body (see Chapter 3).
Qi mechanism 气机 *(qì jī)*	Refers to the dynamic, functional aspects (especially those with directional qualities) of the internal organs which are responsible for generating qi: the Stomach, Spleen, Intestines, and Lungs. In children it is common that when any one part of the qi mechanism is dysfunctional, the entire mechanism will be affected.
Release the exterior 解表 *(jiě biǎo)*	Exterior diseases (those in the superficial layers) such as colds, rashes, or mild coughs are treated by 'releasing' or relieving the exterior. This almost always involves activating the protective qi to open the pores and allow for a therapeutic sweat. Cupping is often effective.
Rebellious qi 逆气 *(nì qì)*	Qi which rises up instead of descending; sometimes referred to as counterflow. Usually refers to a cough, where the Lung qi rises instead of descending; or to vomiting, where the Stomach qi rises instead of descending.
Sensory orifices 心窍 *(xīn qiào)*	Literally, these are the 'holes of the heart'. They are in the head and are the sensory orifices through which the spirit should pass on waking and going to sleep. If the holes are blocked there will be some disturbance of consciousness. In recent times the term has been adopted to mean the functioning of the brain. These are also known as the clear or pure orifices *(qīng qiào)* or the upper orifices *(shàng qiào)* to distinguish them from the orifices in the lower part of the body (urethra and anus) which are turbid.
Stifling sensation 闷 *(mèn)*	This character shows the heart being squeezed between the two sides of a door, which accurately portrays this sensation. It can range anywhere from difficulty in taking a deep breath, to an ache, to a crushing sensation in the chest.
Stomach passage 脘 *(wǎn)*	This character means the passage leading from the Stomach to the Intestines (including the pyloric sphincter). It is one of the characters in the point CV-12 *(zhong wan)*.
Toxin 毒 *(dú)*	In the past, communicable diseases were thought to be transmitted by poison or toxin spreading from one person to another. The term *bìng dú* (disease toxin) now means bacteria or virus, but in traditional Chinese medicine it can mean internally generated toxin which gives symptoms such as boils, or the rash in measles.

Unit 寸 *(cùn)*	The unit of body measurement used in acupuncture also known as *cùn*. On babies the unit is approximately one quarter of an inch.
Womb heat 胎热 *(tāi rè)*	Refers to a condition passed from the mother to the child. It occurs when the pregnant mother consumes too much hot or spicy foods, or the weather is uncomfortably hot during pregnancy, or when the mother herself has a hot disposition. Common symptoms include tantrums, insomnia, and vomiting (hot type).
Womb toxin 胎毒 *(tāi dú)*	This is said to occur because during the time the fetus is in the womb, toxins build up due to the lack of any excretory function. The mother's behavior (eating unsuitable foods such as oranges, taking drugs) can increase the severity of this condition.
Yang brightness fever 阳明热 *(yáng míng rè)*	A fever which has progressed to the yang brightness stage in the system of disease differentiation according to the six stages. It is characterized by bright red face and very high fever, and either profuse heat, sweating, intense thirst, high fever, and a big, overflowing pulse (yang brightness channel stage), or a fever that worsens in the afternoon, fullness and pain in the abdomen, restlessness, constipation, and a deep, forceful pulse (yang brightness organ stage).

❖

❖ Point Index

❖ General Index